Cancer Prevention:
The Causes and Prevention of Cancer
Volume 1

Cancer Prevention – Cancer Causes

Volume 1

Cancer Prevention:
The Causes and Prevention of Cancer – Volume 1

Edited by

Dr. P.H. Graham A. Colditz, M.D.,
Harvard University, Boston, MA, U.S.A.

and

David Hunter, M.B., B.S., Sc.D.
The Harvard Center for Cancer Prevention, Boston, MA, U.S.A.

Springer-Science+Business Media, B.V.

A C.I.P. Catalogue record for this book is available from the Library of Congress.

ISBN 978-94-017-3860-6   ISBN 978-0-306-47523-8 (eBook)
DOI 10.1007/978-0-306-47523-8

Printed on acid-free paper

© 2000 Springer Science+Business Media Dordrecht
Originally published by Kluwer Academic Publishers in 2000.

Contents

Contributors

We are grateful to our colleagues who contributed to this volume. It is their participation that makes this volume a unique contribution to the field of cancer causes and prevention.

Joaquin Barnoya, M.D.
John D. Boice, Jr., Sc.D.
Willard Cates, Jr., M.D., M.P.H.
David C. Christiani, M.D., M.P.H.
Susan J. Curry, Ph.D.
William DeJong, Ph.D.
Karen M. Emmons, Ph.D.
Alison E. Field, Sc.D.
A. Lindsay Frazier, M.D.
Karen Glanz, M.P.H., Ph.D.
Laura Gomberg, M.S.
Susan E. Hankinson, Sc.D.
Lydia M. E. Jones, M.D.
Ichiro Kawachi, M.D., Ph.D.
Francine Laden, Sc.D.
Anthony D. LaMontagne, Sc.D., M.A., M.Ed.
I-Min Lee, M.B.B.S., Sc.D.
Frederick P. Li, M.D.
John B. Little, M.D.
Kimberly Lochner, Sc.D.
Jennifer B. McClure, Ph.D.
Stacey A. Missmer, M.Sc.

Richard R. Monson, M.D.
Charles S. Morrison, Ph.D.
Nancy Mueller, Sc.D.
Kavita Nanda, M.D., M.H.S.
Lucas M. Neas, Sc.D.
Elyse Park, Ph.D.
Nancy A. Rigotti, M.D.
Beverly Rockhill, Ph.D.
Pamela J. Schwingl, Ph.D.
Howard D. Sesso, Sc.D.
Glorian Sorensen, Ph.D.
Alexander M. Walker, M.D., Dr.P.H.
Martin A.Weinstock, M.D., Ph.D.
David W. Wetter, Ph.D.
Walter C. Willett, M.D., M.P.H.

Editors:
Graham A. Colditz, M.D., Dr.P.H.
David Hunter, M.B., B.S., Sc.D.

Acknowledgements

We are grateful to our colleagues who contributed to the peer review of materials included in the earlier reports from the Harvard Center for Cancer Prevention, which served as the starting point for this volume. Jennifer Hamilton provided outstanding support to make this volume move from the idea to reality. Her tireless efforts are truly appreciated.

Preface

This Cancer Prevention book series aims to complement the research reported in the journal *Cancer Causes and Control*. Volumes in this series will summarize the state of the science from causes to prevention of cancer. The scope will be international.

The past 20 years has seen an explosion of epidemiologic material on the causes of cancer. Examples include the growing number of studies of physical activity and colon cancer which have emerged and the numerous studies of components of diet such as alcohol and the risk of specific cancers. Major shifts in resource allocation now focus on translation of this new knowledge to actual cancer prevention programs. Researchers, practicing clinicians, and those who write and implement public health policy need this information summarized in an easily accessible format.

The abundance of knowledge, increasing understanding of how to communicate risk of cancer to the public, and greater public awareness of cancer, make the coming years ones in which we will see many new attempts at widespread cancer prevention programs. For example, the U.S. Centers for Disease Control and Prevention launched a national colon cancer awareness campaign in early 1999.

Activities such as this call for an academic series that summarizes the scope of cancer causes, the potential for prevention, and strategies to achieve realistic goals. This series will include volumes that address the prevention of individual cancers, in addition to separate books on the magnitude of the relation between lifestyle and cancer risk. In essence, some books in the series should be disease focused, others should address behavior or lifestyle factors, and yet others will focus on general issues such as risk communication or methods for evaluation of prevention strategies.

The Harvard Center for Cancer Prevention has prepared the first volume in this series. The Harvard Center for Cancer Prevention was established on the premise that prevention offers the best hope for significantly reducing the suffering and death caused by cancer. As the burden of cardiovascular disease continues its substantial fall [1] and cancer mortality suggests a small decline, the relative importance of cancer continues to rise. To bring the growing knowledge about cancer and options for prevention to the public we have worked to meet educational goals bringing together in the first report from the Harvard Center for Cancer Prevention general information on the causes of cancer [2] and on strategies for prevention [3].

In this volume we expand on materials to summarize the evidence on causes of cancer and to set forth a series of strategies to promote the prevention of cancer. *Cancer Causes - Cancer Prevention* is designed to provide a comprehensive overview of what we know about cancer risk in the United States (and other established market economies) and the preventive measures we can take to reduce the burden of cancer. In the first half of this volume, we review the causes of human cancer considering a wide range of potential sources of risk such as smoking, diet sedentary lifestyle, occupational factors, viruses and alcohol. We concluded that cancer is indeed preventable. Over 50 percent of cancer could be prevented if we could implement what we already know about the causes of cancer.

In the second half of this volume, we summarize research on prevention programs, public education campaigns, and social policy measures for preventing cancer. Working in schools, health clinics, and workplaces as well as through the mass media and in the political arena, social scientists and health educators are designing innovative and effective health promotion programs to help people quit smoking, eat healthier, and exercise more.

We conclude with a series of recommendations for achieving a reduction in cancer risk through diet, activity, weight control, and safe sex practices.

We do not include a detailed discussion of the efficacy of screening tests for cancer. In large part, these have been thoroughly reviewed by the U.S. Preventive Services Task Force [4]. Recommendations for breast, cervix and colon screening are now widespread in the U.S. Barriers to access and utilization of screening services are being addressed through efforts of the Centers for Disease Control and Prevention (breast and cervix) and through the availability of funding for colon screening among the Medicare population. The continuing review of these options for screening by the U.S. Preventive Services Task Force assures us that the evidence for screening will be comprehensively reviewed and kept current.

Many of the messages in the text of this book are incorporated into the Harvard Center for Cancer Prevention web site which provides tailored feed back to individuals identifying strategies to reduce risk for the leading causes of cancer death. This material can be accessed at www.yourcancerrisk.harvard.edu.

Graham A. Colditz, M.D., Dr.P.H.

Editor-in-Chief, Cancer Causes and Control

REFERENCES

1. McGovern P, Pankow J, Sharar E, *et al.* (1996) Recent trends in acute coronary heart disease. Mortality, morbidity, medical care, and risk factors. *N Engl J Med* **334:** 884-90.
2. Colditz GA, DeJong D, Hunter DJ, *et al.* (1996) Harvard Report on Cancer Prevention. Volume 1. Causes of Human Cancer. *Cancer Causes Control* **7**(Suppl 1)1-59.
3. Colditz GA, DeJong D, Emmons K, *et al.* (1997) Harvard Report on Cancer Prevention. Volume 1. Prevention of Human Cancer. *Cancer Causes Control* **8**(Suppl 1).
4. U.S. Preventive Task Force (1996) *Guide to Clinical Preventive Services.* (2nd ed.) Baltimore, MD (USA): Williams and Wilkins.

1

CAUSES OF HUMAN CANCER

Chapter 1

Smoking

Beverly Rockhill, Ph.D. and Graham A. Colditz, M.D., Dr.P.H.
Channing Laboratory, Department of Medicine, Brigham and Women's Hospital and Harvard Medical School, Boston, MA

INTRODUCTION

Decades of epidemiologic research have demonstrated that tobacco is a uniquely hazardous substance. It is known to cause over two dozen chronic diseases (many of which are major contributors to overall mortality), acute respiratory diseases such as pneumonia and influenza, and various persistent respiratory symptoms such as cough and wheezing which, while not deadly by themselves, may greatly reduce quality of life. The overall effect of tobacco use on public health is thus enormous. Scientific consensus on the causal relationships between smoking and various diseases was first reached in the 1960s, and was documented in the first *Surgeon General's Report on Smoking and Health*, released in 1964 [1].

The cigarette has been such an important image in American culture that it is difficult to believe it is primarily a twentieth-century phenomenon [2]. As a result of developments in agriculture and industrialization, cigarette smoking became increasingly popular in the U.S. in the early decades of this century. Figure 1.1 shows the trend in total and *per capita* tobacco consumption in the U.S. in this century [3]. A decline in *per capita* consumption began in this country in the 1960s, following the release of the *Surgeon General's Report* and the sustained, organized effort on the part of the public health community to educate citizens about the health hazards of smoking.

3

G.A. Colditz et al. (eds.), Cancer Prevention: The Causes and Prevention of Cancer - Volume I, 3–16.
© 2000 *Kluwer Academic Publishers.*

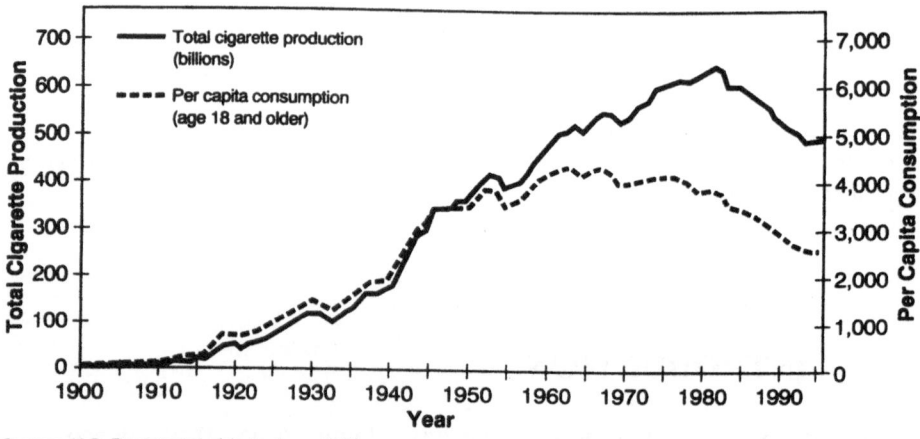

Source: U.S. Department of Agriculture, 1996.

Figure 1.1 Total and per capita cigarette consumption in the United States, 1900-1995

Trends in tobacco consumption in Britain, as well as other industrialized nations, paralleled for the most part the pattern in the United States, perhaps with a slight time lag [4]. At the same time, lung cancer was assuming prominence as a new epidemic. Figure 1.2, which appeared as a figure in one of the first epidemiologic reports on smoking and lung cancer [4], shows data on trends in tobacco consumption and lung cancer mortality in Britain. Meanwhile, in the United States, lung cancer went from being an extremely rare occurrence (there were 400 reported deaths from lung cancer in this country in 1900) to being a leading cause of cancer mortality (in the 1980s, lung cancer became the leading cause of cancer mortality in the U.S., a position it still occupies). Richard Doll one of the first epidemiologists to analyze the association between smoking and lung cancer, reported in one of his early papers on the subject [4 (p. 739)] that ...

"In England and Wales the phenomenal increase in the number of deaths attributed to cancer of the lung provides one of the most striking changes in the pattern of mortality....this remarkable increase is, of course, out of all proportion to the increase of population--both in total, and, particularly, in its older age groups."

In his Discussion, Doll carefully stated that

"it must be concluded that there is a real association between carcinoma of the lung and smoking. The habit of smoking was...invariably formed before the onset of the disease (as revealed by the production of symptoms), so that the disease cannot be held to have caused the habit; nor can we ourselves envisage any common cause likely to lead both to the development of the habit and to the development of the disease 20 to 50 years later. We therefore conclude that smoking is a factor, and an important factor, in the production of carcinoma of the lung" [4] (pp. 744-745).

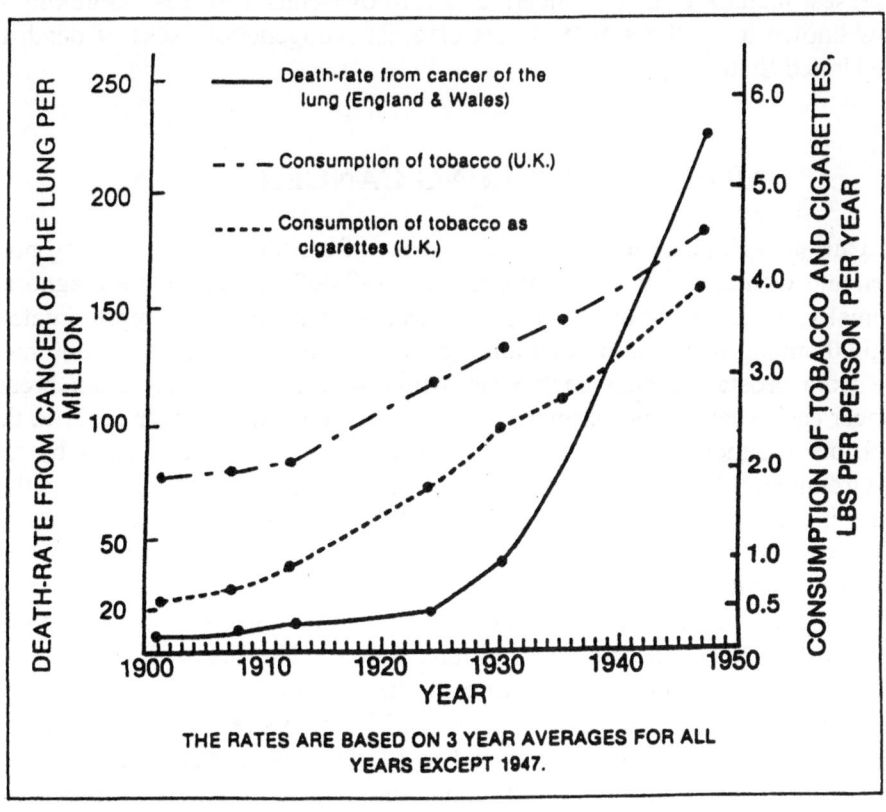

Figure1.2 Death rate from cancer of the lung and rate of consumption of tobacco and cigarettes

Epidemiologic analyses such as Doll's helped provide the motivation for the *1964 U.S. Surgeon General's Report.* The authors of this *Report* reviewed existing epidemiologic data and concluded that among men who smoked cigarettes, the death rate from lung cancer was ten times higher than among nonsmokers. The authors of the report wrote "Cigarette smoking is causally related to lung cancer in men; the magnitude of the effect far outweighs all other factors." Although at the time there were fewer studies of women, available data indicated the same association.

The epidemiologic evidence available to the writers of the *1964 Report* was already extensive: 29 retrospective and seven prospective studies of smoking and lung cancer [2]. In the years since the initial Report, voluminous evidence has continued to accumulate. This evidence has shown that smoking causes lung cancer in women as well as men, and it has also shown strong dose-response relationships between smoking and a variety of diseases, including many cancers and cardiovascular diseases. Smoking is now known to be the single largest external (nongenetic) cause of death in the United States [5].

1.   SMOKING AND LUNG CANCER

Currently, lung cancer the leading cause of cancer mortality among both men and women in the U.S.; an estimated 172,000 new cases are diagnosed annually, with an estimated 153,000 deaths each year [6], approximately 88,000 among men and 65,000 among women. (In comparison, 40,000 men die from prostate cancer each year, while 46,000 women die from breast cancer each year.) Approximately 98 percent of all lung cancer cases in the U.S. are diagnosed in smokers, and based on estimates compiled by the Environmental Protection Agency, a sizeable proportion of lung cancers that arise in nonsmokers may be attributable to passive smoke exposure [7]. Lung cancer has one of the poorest prognoses of all cancers, with a 5-year survival probability of less than 13 percent [6].

Abundant   epidemiologic   evidence   shows   strong   dose-response relationships between smoking and lung cancer. The risk of lung cancer is highly dependent on the number of cigarettes smoked per day. For instance, a prospective study conducted among British doctors [8] found that, among current smokers, those who smoked 1 to 14 cigarettes per day had a relative risk of lung cancer of around 8.0 (compared to never smokers); this relative risk increased to 13.0 for those currently smoking 15 to 24 cigarettes per day, and to 25.0 for those currently smoking 25 or more cigarettes per day. Risk is also highly dependent on degree of inhalation and duration of smoking. Those smokers who inhale deeply are at greater risk of lung cancer than smokers who do not inhale. Similarly, those who begin smoking at an early age (in the teen years or before) have a much higher risk of lung cancer than those who begin smoking later in life, because of the longer cumulative exposure.

2.   SMOKING AND OTHER CANCERS

Over the past half-century, there have been numerous studies of the role played by cigarette smoking in the pathogenesis, pathophysiology, and natural history of a variety of diseases in addition to lung cancer. Smoking is now known to be a cause of many types of cancers, including cancers of the mouth, lip, oro- and hypopharynx, larynx, esophagus, pancreas, bladder, kidney, and stomach. In addition, recent evidence indicates that smoking may increase the risk of colon cancer. Cohort studies with long duration of follow-up, such as the British doctors study mentioned above, the American Veterans Cohort Study, the Nurses' Health Study, and the Health Professionals' Follow-up Study, show that having smoked 30 or more years ago increases the risk of colon cancer [9]. Such data are suggestive of a long latency period between smoking and colon cancer. Smoking also increases the risk of colon polyps, which are precursors to colon cancer.

That smoking should be a cause of so many different types of cancer should not be surprising: inhalation is a very effective way of distributing chemicals throughout the body, and tobacco smoke contains at least 50 chemicals that are known to be carcinogenic in animal experiments, including radioactive polonium, benzene, 2-naphthylamine, 4-amino-biphenyl, and various polycyclic aromatic hydrocarbons and nitrosamines [10]. As is the case with lung cancer, risks of virtually all other smoking–related cancers rise with average number of cigarettes smoked per day, degree of inhalation, and years of smoking.

In their oft-cited book *The Causes of Cancer*, Doll and Peto [11] state that "No single measure is known that would have as great an impact on the number of (cancer) deaths as a reduction in the use of tobacco". Estimates have placed the contribution of smoking in the range of 11 percent to 30 percent for all cancer deaths in the U.S. [5]. Table 1.1 [12] shows, for men and women separately, the proportions of various cancers attributable to smoking. These attributable fractions pertain to the United States in 1990. The attributable fraction is a measure that takes into account both the prevalence of smoking as well as the relative risk associated with smoking; it will increase as either of these quantities rise. The attributable fraction indicates the proportion of disease incidence in the population that could be prevented if the exposure (smoking, in this situation) were to be eliminated from the population. The attributable fractions from smoking for cancers of the lip, oral cavity, and pharynx, cancer of the larynx, cancer of the esophagus, and lung cancer are all very high; 80 to 90 percent of the incidence of these various cancers in the U.S. could be eliminated if smoking prevalence dropped to zero.

Table 1.1 Estimated attributable risks for 10 selected causes of death from cigarette smoking, males and females, United States, 1965 [12].

Cause of Death	Males (%)	Females (%)
CHD, age 35-64	42 (40-45)[a]	26 (23-30)
CHD, age ≥65	11 (9-14)	3.3 (2.1-5.1)
COPD	84 (79-88)	67 (57-76)
Cancer of lip, oral cavity, and pharynx	74 (59-85)	27 (12-51)
Cancer of pharynx	84 (61-94)	47 (8-90)
Cancer of esophagus	57 (36-76)	14 (6-29)
Cancer of lung	86 (82-88)	40 (31-50)
Cancer of pancreas	41 (30-53)	14 (6-30)
Cancer of bladder	53 (39-66)	36 (20-56)
Cancer of kidney	36 (19-56)	17 (5-42)
Cardiovascular disease, age 35-64	28 (21-36)	28 (22-33)
Cerebrovascular disease, age >65	2.0 (0.6-6.6)	1.3 (0.2-6.5)

[a]Numbers in parentheses are 95 percent confidence intervals.

3.   AGE AT STARTING SMOKING

Both epidemiologic and experimental evidence suggest that the risk for lung cancer varies more strongly with duration of smoking than with the average number of cigarettes smoked [13, 14]. This dependence of risk on duration of smoking implies that starting smoking at an earlier age, which increases the potential number of life-years of smoking, will increase lung cancer risk relative to starting smoking at a later age. Based on mathematical models of lung carcinogenesis, which assume that lung cancer risk rises exponentially as a function of duration of smoking, the risk at age

50 years for a person who began smoking regularly at age 13 years will be 3.5 times as great as the risk for a 50-year old who began smoking at age 23 years [15]. Although this type of analysis has not been done for other smoking-related cancers, one can infer from the epidemiologic data that, for a given adult age, risk for a smoking-related cancer increases in inverse proportion to the age at which smoking began [15]. Further, recent studies indicate that earlier onset of cigarette smoking is associated with heavier smoking [16, 17]. Heavier smokers are more likely to experience smoking-related health problems and are least likely to quit [12]. Early age at initiation of smoking therefore influences intensity as well as duration of smoking, and thus strongly increases the likelihood of long-term health consequences.

Almost all first use of tobacco occurs before the time of high-school graduation [15]; if adolescents can remain "tobacco-free", the great majority will never begin smoking. Cigarette manufacturers recognize this, and continue to target young people to insure that there will be adults who are addicted to smoking. Smoking prevalence among adolescents declined sharply in the 1970s [15], but the decline has slowed, and recent evidence indicates that there may be a rise in the proportion of adolescents who smoke [18]. Both male and female adolescents are now equally likely to smoke.

4.   BENEFITS OF SMOKING CESSATION

Scientific data on the benefits of smoking cessation were reviewed in detail in the *1990 Surgeon General's Report* [19]. In the last quarter-century, half of all living Americans who have ever smoked have now quit. The 1990 Report concluded that smoking cessation has major and immediate health benefits for men and women of all ages. Former smokers live longer than continuing smokers; for instance, people who quit smoking before age 50 years have, on average, half the mortality risk of dying in the next 15 years compared with continuing smokers. This reduction in mortality comes from a reduction in risk of nearly all smoking-related diseases. Among former smokers, the decline in risk of death compared with continuing smoking begins shortly after quitting, and continues for at least 10 to 15 years.

Smoking cessation reduces the risk of many cancers compared with continuing smoking. This is likely due to cigarette smoking acting both as an early initiator of carcinogenesis, as well as a late-stage promoter of existing genetic damage. Quitting smoking thus lowers the probability of late-stage propagation of such damage. For example, after ten years of abstinence, the risk of lung cancer is about 30 percent to 50 percent to that of continuing smokers. With a longer period of abstinence, there is a further decline in risk [19]. (It is very likely, however, that the lung cancer risk of a former smoker never declines to that of a never-smoker.) Smoking cessation also reduces the risk of laryngeal cancer, and halves the risk, after five years of cessation, for cancers of the oral cavity, esophagus, bladder, and pancreas, compared to continued smoking [19, 20].

The specific magnitude of benefit derived from smoking cessation depends on factors such as the number of years spent smoking, the number of cigarettes smoked per day, and the presence or absence of disease at the time of quitting. There is also evidence to suggest that smokers who have already developed cancer may benefit from smoking cessation. Several studies indicate that persons who stopped smoking after cancer diagnosis have a reduced risk of acquiring a second primary cancer, compared to those who continue smoking [19].

Because of the addictive nature of tobacco (specifically, nicotine) and because of the cumulative nature of health damage due to smoking, strategies to reduce tobacco use should focus on primary prevention rather than smoking cessation, though the latter should not be ignored, particularly when smoking is widely prevalent in the population.

5.   SMOKING AND CONFOUNDING

Litigation by states and individuals against the tobacco industry has rekindled debates about whether observed smoking-cancer associations are confounded by other factors not considered in analyses. For instance, the tobacco industry maintains that a good deal of the increased disease and mortality risk observed among smokers is due to other factors that tend to be more prevalent in smokers, including lower socioeconomic status (and the behaviors and health care variables that are associated with such lower status), greater alcohol consumption, and so forth. Although some of the early epidemiologic studies of smoking and lung cancer did not collect data on other health-related variables and thus were unable to adjust for any covariates besides age, studies in recent decades have become increasingly sophisticated in their ability to collect data on, and statistically control for, potential confounding variables. These recent studies have shown negative health effects of smoking as strong, or even stronger, than the earlier studies, after controlling for potential confounders. It is highly unlikely that there exists a risk factor still unknown and unmeasured by epidemiologists that could account for the high relative risks observed for smoking and a variety of diseases. Such a factor would have to be highly unequally distributed in the population (being almost universally present among smokers and almost nonexistent among nonsmokers), and would have to be very strongly associated with disease risk (*e.g.*, relative risk of at least 10.0 or more).

CONCLUSION

Smoking is linked to a multitude of major chronic diseases, and as a result, it is the single most important non-genetic cause of premature morbidity and mortality in most industrialized societies today. Figure 1.3, based on data from the British Doctors' Cohort Study, shows the large differences in survival curves according to smoking behavior [21]. By age 70 years, only 50 percent of those who smoked 25 or more cigarettes a day remained alive, while the corresponding percentage for never smokers was 80 percent. Those who smoked fewer than 25 cigarettes a day had intermediate mortality risk. This figure starkly illustrates the role of smoking in causing premature death.

In 1964, when the first *Surgeon General's Report* was released, 42 percent of American adults smoked; in 1995, this percentage had declined to 24.7 percent (47 million) of American adults [22]. Given such progress over the past quarter-century, it is possible to envision a smoke-free society, but maintaining the current rate of progress will be challenging. The prevalence of smoking remains disproportionately high among blacks, blue-collar workers, and persons with lower educational attainment.

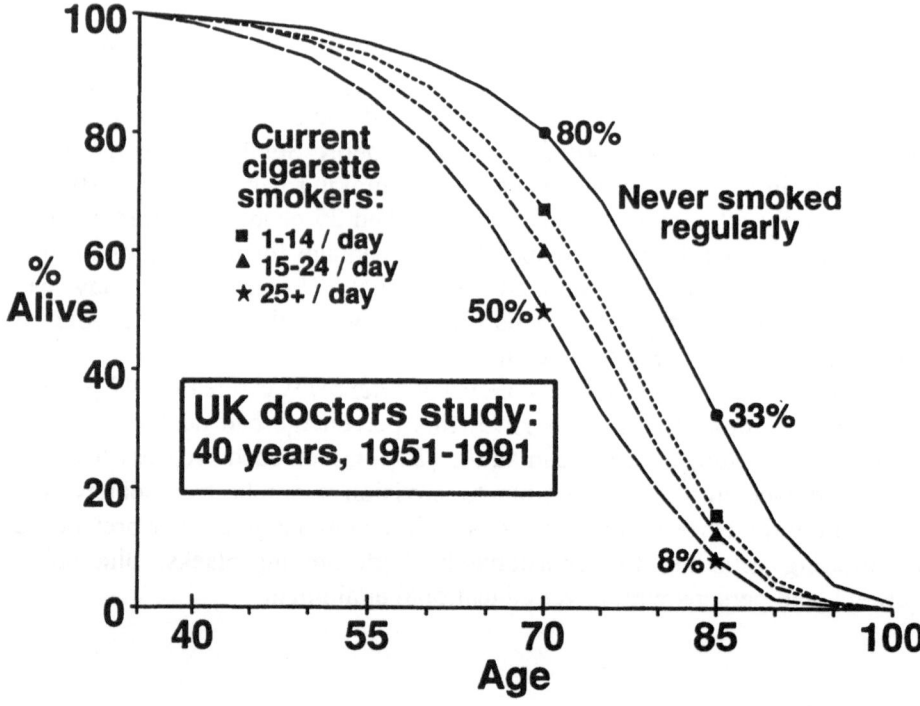

Figure 1.3 Effects of cigarette smoking on survival to age 70 and to age 85, in 40-year prospective study of male British doctors. Source Doll, Peto, *et al.*, 1994

Epidemiologists are increasingly conducting research into genetic markers of disease risk, and the field of smoking-related diseases is no exception to this trend. In the past several years, many reports on genetic markers of susceptibility to the harmful effects of cigarette smoking have been published. On the whole, this body of research has failed to uncover genetic markers that are highly effective in discriminating between those persons not at increased health risk from smoking and a pool of persons who are at increased health risk from this behavior. This failure should not be surprising. Cigarette smoke is a highly toxic substance, linked to a large variety of disease outcomes. There are undoubtedly many complex pathways, containing both genetic and nongenetic elements, which act to determine the health consequences of smoking for any given individual. It is likely that no individual is immune to all of the negative effects of cigarette smoking, and the large research attempt to identify markers of cigarette smoke susceptibility seems misguided from a public health standpoint. The evidence is overwhelming that the population pattern of tobacco consumption is the single most important determinant of the future population burdens of lung cancer, chronic obstructive pulmonary disease, chronic bronchitis, and emphysema; it is also an important determinant of future cardiovascular disease trends. From a public health perspective, the most efficient and ethical means of reducing premature morbidity and mortality due to smoking is to lower the prevalence of smoking to as close to zero as possible, rather than to seek to segregate the population into those susceptible and not susceptible to the effect of this carcinogenic behavior.

Finally, a decline in tobacco use in the United States, while obviously beneficial from the standpoint of our nation's public health, may have the unintended consequence of contributing to the dramatic increase in tobacco-related epidemics worldwide, as the multinational U.S.-based tobacco firms desperately seek new markets for their product. Such a consequence shows the importance of extending the conventional epidemiologic focus on the individual-level association between smoking and disease to one that encompasses the macro-level forces that influence tobacco consumption, and thus influence the burden of premature morbidity and mortality within populations.

SUMMARY POINTS

* The overall effect of tobacco use on public health is enormous. Smoking causes over two dozen chronic diseases, many of which are major contributors to mortality in industrialized populations. Cigarette smoking is the single biggest contributor to premature mortality in the United States.
* Cigarette smoking is the most important risk factor for lung cancer, which, since the 1980s, has been the leading cause of cancer mortality in the United States among both men and women. Approximately 98 percent of lung cancer cases in the United States occur in smokers. Lung cancer has one of the poorest prognoses of all cancers, making primary prevention critical. Smoking is also a cause of cancers of the mouth, lip, oro- and hypopharynx, esophagus, pancreas, bladder, kidney, and stomach, and appears to be a cause of colon cancer as well. It is estimated that 80 to 90 percent of the incidence of these various cancers could be eliminated if smoking prevalence were to drop to zero.
* The risk for lung cancer, as well as many other smoking-related diseases, varies strongly with duration of smoking. Starting smoking at an early age thus greatly increases the risk of future adverse outcomes.

- Almost all first-use of tobacco occurs before the time of high school graduation; if adolescents can remain "tobacco-free", the great majority will never begin smoking.
- Smoking cessation has major and immediate health benefits for men and women of all ages. Cessation leads to a reduction in mortality risks from nearly all smoking-related diseases, compared to mortality risks in continuing smokers.

RECOMMENDATIONS

- Recommendations to the individual are clear and simple: Do not start smoking, and if one has already started, quit.
- Preventing smoking initiation among young persons is the most important component of a strategy to reduce smoking prevalence to zero.
- Epidemiologists and other public health researchers must extend the conventional individual-level focus on smoking and disease to one that encompasses macro-level forces that influence tobacco consumption in populations. These forces include aggressive and deceptive marketing by the tobacco industry, and government policies that support or even require the marketing of U.S. tobacco products to industrializing nations anxious to create economic ties to this country.

SUGGESTED FURTHER READING

1. U. S. Department of Health and Human Services (1989*). Reducing the Health Consequences of Smoking: 25 Years of Progress. A Report of the Surgeon General.* Rockville, Maryland: U.S. Department of Health and Human Services, Public Health Service, Centers for Disease Control, Center for Chronic Disease Prevention and Health Promotion, Office on Smoking and Health.
2. U. S. Department of Health and Human Services (1994). *Preventing Tobacco Use among Young People. A Report of the Surgeon General.* Atlanta, Georgia: U.S. Department of Health and Human Services, Public Health Service, Centers for Disease Control, National Center for Chronic Disease Prevention and Health Promotion, Office on Smoking and Health.
3. U. S. Department of Health and Human Services (1990). *The Health Benefits of Smoking Cessation. A Report of the Surgeon General.* Rockville, Maryland: U.S. Department of Health and Human Services, Public Health Service, Centers for Disease Control, Center for Chronic

Disease Prevention and Health Promotion, Office on Smoking and Health.

REFERENCES

1. U.S. Public Health Service (1964). *Smoking and Health. Report of the Advisory Committee to the Surgeon General of the Public Health Service.* Washington, D.C.: U.S. Department of Health, Education, and Welfare, Public Health Service, Centers for Disease Control.
2. Brandt A (1990). The cigarette, risk, and American culture. In: Burger E, ed. *Risk.* Ann Arbor, MI (USA): University of Michigan Press, pp. 155-176.
3. National Cancer Institute, National Institutes of Health (1997). *Changes in Cigarette-Related Disease Risks and Their Implication for Prevention and Control.* National Institutes of Health, NIH Publication No. 97-4213.
4. Doll R, Hill A (1950). Smoking and carcinoma of the lung: preliminary report. *Br Med J* **30:** 739-748.
5. McGinnis JM, Foege WH (1993). Actual causes of death in the United States. *JAMA* **270:** 2207-2212.
6. National Center for Health Statistics (1998). *SEER Cancer Statistics Review, 1973-1995.* Bethesda, MD, (USA): National Cancer Institute.
7. United States Environmental Protection Agency (1992) Respiratory Health Effects of Passive Smoking and Other Disorders. Washington, D.C.: Office of Research and Development.
8. Doll R, Peto R (1976). Mortality in relation to smoking: 20 years' observations on male British doctors. *Br Med J* **2:** 1071-1081.
9. Heineman E, Zahm SH, McLaughlin J, *et al.* (1995). Increased risk of colorectal cancer among smokers: results of a 26-year follow-up of U.S. veterans and a review. *Int J Cancer* **59:** 728-738.
10. Doll R (1996). Nature and nurture: possibilities for cancer control. *Carcinogenesis* **17:** 177-184.
11. Doll R, Peto R (1981). *The Causes of Cancer. Quantitative Estimates of Avoidable Risks of Cancer in the United States Today.* New York, NY (USA): Oxford University Press.
12. U. S. Department of Health and Human Services (1989*). Reducing the Health Consequences of Smoking: 25 Years of Progress. A Report of the Surgeon General.* Rockville, Maryland: U.S. Department of Health and Human Services, Public Health Service, Centers for Disease Control, Center for Chronic Disease Prevention and Health Promotion, Office on Smoking and Health.
13. Peto R (1977). Epidemiology, multistage models, and short-term mutagenicity tests. In: Hiatt H, Watson J, Winsten J, eds. *Origins of Human Cancer, Book C, Human Risk Assessment.* Cold Spring Harbor, NY (USA)S: Cold Spring Harbor Laboratory.
14. Doll R, Peto R (1978). Cigarette smoking and bronchial carcinoma: dose and time relationships among regular smokers and lifelong nonsmokers. *J Epidemiol Comm Health* **32:** 303-313.
15. U. S. Department of Health and Human Services (1994). *Preventing Tobacco Use among Young People. A Report of the Surgeon General.* Atlanta, GA (USA): U.S. Department of Health and Human Services, Public Health Service, Centers for Disease Control, National

Center for Chronic Disease Prevention and Health Promotion, Office on Smoking and Health.

16. Escobedo L, Marcus S, Holtzman D, *et al.* (1993). Sports participation, age at smoking initiation, and the risk of smoking among U.S. high school students. *JAMA* **269:** 1391-1395.

17. Taioli E, Wynder E (1991). Effect of the age at which smoking begins on frequency of smoking in adulthood (letter). *N Engl J Med* **325:** 968-969.

18. Johnston LD, O'Malley P, Bachman J (1998). National survey results on drug use from the Monitoring the Future study, 1975-1997. *Volume I: Secondary school students.* (NIH Publication No. 98-4345) and *Volume II: College students and young adults.* (NIH Publication No. 98-4346). Rockville MD: National Institute on Drug Abuse.

19. U. S. Department of Health and Human Services (1990). *The Health Benefits of Smoking Cessation. A Report of the Surgeon General.* Rockville, Maryland: U.S. Department of Health and Human Services, Public Health Service, Centers for Disease Control, Center for Chronic Disease Prevention and Health Promotion, Office on Smoking and Health.

20. Fuchs C, Colditz G, Stampfer M, *et al* (1996). A prospective study of cigarette smoking and the risk of pancreatic cancer. *Arch Intern Med* **156:** 2255-2260.

21. Doll R, Peto R, Wheatley K, *et al.* (1994). Mortality in relation to smoking: 40 years' observations on male British doctors. *Br Med J* **309:** 901-911.

22. Centers for Disease Control and Prevention (1997). Cigarette smoking among adults--United States, 1995. *MMWR Morbid Mortality Wkly Rep* **46:** 1217-1220.

Chapter 2

Dietary Factors

David J. Hunter, M.B.B.S., Sc.D. and Walter C. Willett, M.D., M.P.H.
Harvard Center for Cancer Prevention; Channing Laboratory, Department of Medicine,
Brigham and Women's Hospital, and Harvard Medical School; Departments of Epidemiology
and Nutrition, Harvard School of Public Health, Boston MA

INTRODUCTION

Dietary differences have long been suspected as a cause of the large international variations in cancer rates. However, until the last two decades, there has been little scientific evidence with which to evaluate these suspicions. This is a field of active research, and many associations between particular foods and nutrients and specific cancers are controversial. These have been extensively reviewed in a report by the World Cancer Research Fund [1]. Nevertheless, broad consistency has emerged on a sensible "prudent" dietary pattern which, if adopted for many years, is likely to reduce personal risk of some cancers: a summary of the relations of most major foods and nutrients with the four major cancer sites in the U.S. is listed in the Summary Points at the end of this chapter.

1.   BREAST CANCER

Much attention has been focused on whether dietary fat increases breast cancer risk. Although breast cancer rates are higher in countries with higher average fat consumption, these countries tend to be more economically developed and the prevalence of established risk factors for breast cancer (such

17

G.A. Colditz et al. (eds.), Cancer Prevention: The Causes and Prevention of Cancer - Volume I, 17–23.
© 2000 *Kluwer Academic Publishers.*

as earlier onset of menstrual periods, lower number of children and later age at first birth) is also higher [2]. Higher average dietary fat intake may be a marker of relative national affluence, and these other breast cancer risk factors are more common in affluent countries.

Large prospective studies that have measured individual fat intakes of women and compared these with risk of breast cancer in the subsequent five to ten years have all reached the same conclusion: fat intake had little or no relation to breast cancer risk [3]. Updated analyses of these studies have examined the group of women whose fat intake was less than 20 percent of calories from fat (very low by Western standards) and observed no reduction in risk. In the largest of these studies, the Nurses' Health Study, a slight inverse association was observed between total fat intake and risk of breast cancer during 14 years of follow-up [4]. While these studies do not exclude the possibility that fat intake may relate to breast cancer many years later, or that fat intake during childhood or adolescence may be important, they do indicate that women in middle life who reduce dietary fat intake cannot expect to lower their breast cancer risk substantially in the decade after making this change.

A growing body of evidence suggests that excess energy intake (caloric intake) in relation to physical activity may be associated with breast cancer risk. Restricting total food intake in animal experiments is one of the best ways to reduce the incidence of cancer at many sites, including mammary cancer. Breast cancer rates around the world are positively correlated with average adult height, a surrogate for caloric balance during growth, and even in studies conducted in the U.S. and Europe, a weak positive association between height and breast cancer is apparent. The possibility that an abundance of calories during childhood and adolescence is deleterious for future breast cancer risk could explain much of the international variation in breast cancer risk, but does not unfortunately lead to obvious interventions - few parents would wish to stunt their daughters' growth. If lesser degrees of energy restriction, or increasing energy expenditure through exercise, could be linked to reduced breast cancer risk, then these may be practical interventions. Weight gain during adult life is associated with breast cancer risk [5], so reducing caloric intake and increasing physical activity in order to prevent or minimize weight gain is likely to be beneficial.

An intriguing possibility is that, while total dietary fat bears little relation to breast cancer risk, monounsaturated fats may actually be protective. Studies in Europe demonstrate that women who regularly consume or cook with olive oil (a rich source of monounsaturated fats) may be at lower risk than women in the same countries who use little olive oil [6, 7]. More research is needed before olive oil can be recommended for breast cancer prevention; however, it is worth noting that substituting monounsaturated fat for saturated fat has a favorable effect on blood lipid levels and is likely to reduce coronary heart disease risk.

In contrast to the lack of association with overall dietary fat, some studies have indicated that higher consumption of vegetables may be associated with a modest reduction in breast cancer risk of the order of about 20 percent [6, 8]. Some recent evidence [9, 10] suggests that this inverse association may be stronger in, or even limited to, premenopausal women. The particular vegetables or nutrients responsible for this possible association are unclear – carrots, broccoli, and cabbage all have their proponents. At this point, sensible advice would be to adopt the National Cancer Institute guidelines of at least five servings of vegetables and fruits per day, and to try and vary these vegetables and fruits from day to day.

A large body of evidence suggests that even moderate alcohol consumption can increase breast cancer risk: each daily alcoholic drink increases risk by about ten percent [11]. Recent studies show that alcohol increases the levels of estrogens in the bloodstream [12], which would be expected to increase breast cell division and increase cancer risk. Recommendations are complicated by the fact that modest alcohol consumption almost certainly decreases the risk of coronary heart disease (perhaps related to the same mechanism of increasing circulating estrogens, perhaps in part due to the effect of alcohol on lipids or blood clotting); the balance of risks and benefits for individual women is complex. The fewer heart disease risk factors a woman has, the more likely it is that avoiding regular alcohol consumption would be of overall benefit.

2. COLON CANCER

Colon cancer is infrequent in countries with low meat intake, and less frequent in Western populations (such as Seventh Day Adventists) with a vegetarian diet [13]. In follow-up studies, higher intake of red meat has been linked with colon cancer risk with reasonable consistency [14]. The specific factors in red meat responsible for this are unclear – candidates include an effect due to animal fat (which may increase turnover of the cells of the colonic epithelium), and/or carcinogens, which may be created during the high-temperature cooking of animal protein.

A protective effect of dietary fiber has been less consistently observed. Greater vegetable and fruit fiber intake has been associated with, in some studies, decreased risk whereas grain fiber has not been protective [15]. Again, benefits of higher cereal fiber intake for prevention of cardiovascular disease and diabetes have been observed repeatedly, so there is still good reason to consume starches in a whole grain form. Folic acid (found in green vegetables and in many multivitamin supplements) has been associated with decreased risk of both colon polyps (the precancerous lesion) and colon cancer itself. High alcohol intake, particularly when combined with low folic acid intake [16], may also increase risk of colon cancer; many studies have also linked alcohol intake to increased risk of rectal cancer. In the Nurses' Health Study [17], women consuming a multivitamin supplement for more than 15 years had less than half the risk of colorectal cancer compared to women who did not use supplements.

The summary of the evidence suggests that reducing red meat intake to less than one-two servings per week, and increasing the intake of vegetables (particularly green vegetables), and perhaps fruit, and taking a daily multivitamin supplement containing at least 400 µg of folate is likely to reduce colon cancer risk.

3.   LUNG CANCER

Cigarette smoking is the overwhelming cause of lung cancer. Numerous studies have shown with great consistency that among smokers, those who eat more vegetables, particularly green and yellow vegetables, are at lower risk of lung cancer [1]. However, a smoker consuming the largest tolerable amounts of vegetables is still at much higher risk of lung cancer than a nonsmoker, reinforcing the fact that diet can only modestly ameliorate, not abolish, the harmful effect of smoking. In addition, it should be borne in mind that the magnitude of the inverse association of vegetable intake with lung cancer may have been overestimated in at least some studies due to inadequate control of confounding by cigarette smoking.

There is little consensus about which specific nutrients in green and yellow vegetables are responsible for the anti-cancer action. A prominent candidate was beta-carotene, but in two randomized trials, risk of lung cancer was higher among those given beta-carotene supplements.

4.   PROSTATE CANCER

Relatively little is known about risk factors for prostate cancer in general, and the nutritional epidemiology of the disease is equally enigmatic. Two recent follow-up studies have observed an increased risk among men with higher meat consumption [18, 19]; however, too few studies are available to reach firm conclusions. Vitamin A intake has been associated with both decreased risk, and increased risk, and few data are available for fiber or alcohol. Higher intake of the antioxidant lycopene, found in tomatoes and tomato products, has been associated with lower risk of prostate cancer in several studies [20]. Given that prostate cancer is the most common cancer among men in the U.S., it is surprising that so few large studies of diet and prostate cancer have been done; ongoing studies should help clarify whether diet is related to prostate cancer.

5.   OTHER CANCER SITES

Alcohol, particularly in conjunction with smoking, increases risk of cancer of the esophagus, while vegetables and fruits appear to be protective. Similarly, vegetables and fruits have been quite consistently shown to reduce risk of stomach cancer, although a recent large prospective study failed to find this association [21]; in Asia, consumption of salted foods may partially account for higher rates of stomach cancer.

CONCLUSIONS

The role of diet in cancer causation is complex and difficult to unravel. Ample evidence does exist to make some recommendations recognizing that these will need to be refined and modified as further evidence accrues. Reducing red meat intake, and perhaps animal fat intake, increasing consumption of vegetables and fruits, and reducing alcohol intake is likely to reduce risk of cancer overall, although the amount of risk reduction is uncertain.

SUMMARY POINTS

Major dietary associations for the four major cancer sites in the U.S.

Breast Cancer
- Risk is increased with excessive weight gain during adult life.
- There is no apparent association with dietary fat intake in mid-life.
- Higher consumption of vegetables may be protective.
- Each alcoholic drink per day probably increases risk by about ten percent.

Colorectal Cancer
- High consumption of meat increases risk two-fold.
- There is a possible inverse association with vegetables.
- Benefit from higher cereal fiber intake is unlikely.
- Folic acid either from supplements or green vegetables may be protective.
- High alcohol consumption is a risk factor.

Lung Cancer
- Green and yellow vegetables are protective among smokers, but no dietary factor can abolish the effect of smoking.

Prostate Cancer
- Red meat is a possible risk factor.
- Lycopene, an antioxidant found in tomatoes and tomato products, may be protective.

RECOMMENDATIONS

- Eat a varied diet.
- Reduce consumption of red meat to once a week or less.
- Increase vegetable and fruit intake; five servings of fruit and vegetables per day is probably a minimum desirable intake.
- Do not blacken or char meat, chicken or fish.
- Do not consume excess alcohol.

SUGGESTED FURTHER READING

1. World Cancer Research Fund (1997) *Food, Nutrition and the Prevention of Cancer: A Global Perspective*. Washington, D.C.: American Institute for Cancer Research

REFERENCES

1. World Cancer Research Fund (1997) *Food, Nutrition and the Prevention of Cancer: A Global Perspective*. Washington, D.C.: American Institute for Cancer Research
2. Hunter DJ, Willett WC (1994) Diet, body build, and breast cancer. *Annu Rev Nutr* **14:** 393-418.

3. Hunter DJ, Spiegelman D, Adami HO, *et al.* (1996) Cohort studies of fat intake and the risk of breast cancer a pooled analysis. *N Engl J Med* **334**: 356-361.
4. Holmes M., Hunter D, Colditz G, *et al.* (1999) Association of dietary intake of fat and fatty acids with risk of breast cancer. *JAMA* **281**: 914-920.
5. Huang, Z, Hankinson SE, Colditz GA, *et al.* (1997) Dual effects of weight and weight gain on breast cancer risk. *JAMA* **17**: 1407-1411.
6. Trichopoulou A, Katsouyanni K, Stuver S, *et al.* (1995) Consumption of olive oil and specific food groups in relation to breast cancer risk in Greece. *J Natl Cancer Inst* **87**: 110-116.
7. La Vecchia C, Negri E, Franceschi S, *et al.* (1995) Olive oil, other dietary fats, and the risk of breast cancer. (Italy). *Cancer Causes Control* **6**: 545-550.
8. Hunter DJ, Manson JE, Colditz GA, *et al.* (1993) A prospective study of the intake of vitamins C, E and A and the risk of breast cancer. *N Engl J Med* **329**: 234-40.
9. Freudenheim J, Marshall J, Vena J, *et al.* (1996) Premenopausal breast cancer risk and intake of vegetables and fruits and related nutrients. *J Natl Cancer Inst* **88**: 340-348.
10. Zhang S, Hunter D, Forman M, *et al.* (1999) Dietary carotenoids and vitamins A, C and E and risk of breast cancer. *J Natl Cancer Inst* **91**: 547-556.
11. Smith-Warner SA Spiegelman D, Yaun SS, *et al.* (1998) Alcohol and breast cancer in women: a pooled analysis of cohort studies. *JAMA* **279**: 535-540.
12. Reichman ME, Judd JT, Longcope C, *et al.* (1993) Effects of alcohol consumption on plasma and urinary hormone concentrations in premenopausal women. *J Natl Cancer Inst* **85**: 722-727.
13. Willett W (1989) The search for the causes of breast and colon cancer. *Nature* **338**: 389-94.
14. Potter J (1992) Reconciling the epidemiology, physiology, and molecular biology of colon cancer. *JAMA* **268**: 1573-1576.
15. Fuchs C, Giovannucci E, Colditz G, *et al.* (1999) Dietary fiber and the risk of colorectal cancer and adenoma in women. *N Engl J Med* **340**: 169-76.
16. Giovannucci E, Stampfer MJ, Colditz GA, *et al.* (1993) Folate, methionine, and alcohol intake and risk of colorectal adenoma. *J Natl Cancer Inst* **85**: 875-884.
17. Giovannucci E, Stampfer MJ, Colditz GA, *et al.* (1998) Multivitamin use, folate, and colon cancer in women in the Nurses' Health Study. *Ann Intern Med* **129**: 517-524.
18. Le Marchand L, Kolonel LN, Wilkens LR, *et al.* (1994) Animal fat consumption and prostate cancer: a prospective study in Hawaii. *Epidemiology* **5**: 276-282.
19. Giovannucci E, Rimm EB, Colditz GA, *et al.* (1993) A prospective study of dietary fat and risk of prostate cancer. *J Natl Cancer Inst* **85**: 1571-79.
20. Giovannucci E (1999) Tomatoes, tomato-based products, lycopene and cancer: review of the epidemiologic literature. *J Natl Cancer Inst* **91**: 317-331.
21. Botterweck A, van den Brandt P, Goldbohm R (1998) A prospective cohort study on vegetable and fruit consumption and stomach cancer risk in the Netherlands. *Am J Epidemiol* **148**: 842-853.

Chapter 3

Obesity

Alison E. Field Sc.D. and Joaquin Barnoya, M.D.
*Channing Laboratory, Harvard Medical School and Brigham and Women's Hospital, Boston,
MA and Department of Nutrition, Harvard School of Public Health, Boston, MA*

INTRODUCTION

The terms overweight and obesity are used almost interchangeably in the scientific and lay literature. The two concepts are related, but not identical. Overweight refers to weighing more than a standard level for height and age; whereas, obesity refers to excessive body fat. Overweight individuals may have excessive stores of body fat; however, because muscle weighs more than fat, people who are highly active and have substantial muscle mass may weigh slightly more than the standard for their height despite low body fat. Thus people may be overweight, but not over-fat. Obesity, on the other hand, traditionally has been classified based on body fat stores.

Body fat can be measured by skinfold thickness at multiple sites, underwater weighing, and radiographic techniques (such as dual-energy X-ray absorptometry, CTscans, and MRI). These methods of measurement are labor intensive, expensive to collect, and require skilled collection personnel. Therefore in many large epidemiologic studies, as well as clinical practice, it is not been feasible to collect these types of data. Instead, weight and height, and occasionally body circumferences, are the only measures that are collected. Thus it is not surprising that in the epidemiologic literature, obesity has also been defined as weighing much more than the standard for height and age. The assumption has been that individuals who weigh much more than the standard for their height are very likely to have excessive body fat stores.

G.A. Colditz et al. (eds.), Cancer Prevention: The Causes and Prevention of Cancer - Volume I, 25–35.
© 2000 *Kluwer Academic Publishers.*

Body mass index (BMI), a formula that combines weight and height, is commonly used in epidemiologic studies assessing the relationship between weight and disease. BMI is computed as weight (in kilograms) divided by height (in meters) squared. The advantage of using BMI (kg/m^2) instead of weight in pounds or kilograms is that it accounts for height, an essential piece of information when evaluating weight. For example, a woman who weighs 145 pounds is overweight if she is 5 feet 4 inches, but a healthy weight if she is 5 feet 8 inches. The United States Department of Agriculture classifies BMIs as follows: <18.5 is underweight, 18.5 to 24.9 is normal weight, 25-29.9 is overweight, and ≥30 is obese. People who are obese are also overweight, thus some organizations, such as the World Health Organization [1], define overweight as a BMI ≥ 25. Overweight is further broken down into four levels: 25 to 29.9 is pre-obese, 30 to 34.9 is obese class 1, 35 to 39.9 is obese class II, and ≥40 is obese class III [1]. As can be seen in Figure 3.1, a woman who is 5 feet 4 inches and weighs 145 pounds would be considered to be pre-obese, whereas she would be considered to be in obese class I if she weighed 180 pounds.

Body weight and body composition are a function of genetics, health status, basal metabolic factors, dietary intake, physical activity, race, and hormonal factors. Changes over time in basal metabolic factors, hormones, dietary intake, and physical activity result in changes in body weight and composition. The onset (*i.e.,* childhood, adolescence, or adulthood) and duration of obesity, as well as weight change all may have an important impact on health.

Excessive weight is associated with the development of numerous chronic diseases, as well as mortality [2]. In the U.S., the prevalence of obesity has been increasing sharply among children and adults over the past three decades. According to the third National Health and Nutrition Examination Survey (NHANES), 32 percent of adults in the U.S. are overweight and an additional 22.5 percent are obese [3]; however, among African-Americans and Hispanics the prevalences are much higher. Approximately 67 percent of adult African-American and Hispanic women are overweight or obese, compared to 46 percent of white women.

Adults who are overweight are at increased risk of developing numerous types of cancer, including colon, breast (among postmenopausal women), endometrial, gastric, prostate, and renal cell. The racial differences in the prevalence of excessive weight may partially explain the elevated rate of certain cancers among African-Americans. Obesity is thought to increase risk of developing cancer primarily through its effect on hormones. However, certain cancers, such as renal cell carcinoma, are related to obesity through other, not well understood mechanisms.

Wt.	100	105	110	115	120	125	130	135	140	145	150	155	160	165	170	175	180
Ht.																	
5'0"	20	21	21	22	23	24	25	26	27	28	29	30	31	32	33	34	35
5'1"	19	20	21	22	23	24	25	26	26	27	28	29	30	31	31	33	34
5'2"	18	19	20	21	22	23	24	25	26	27	27	28	29	30	31	32	33
5'3"	18	19	19	20	21	22	23	24	25	26	27	27	28	29	30	31	32
5'4"	17	18	19	20	21	21	22	23	24	25	26	27	27	28	29	30	31
5'5"	17	17	18	19	20	21	22	22	23	24	25	26	27	27	28	29	30
5'6"	16	17	18	19	19	20	21	22	23	23	24	25	26	27	27	28	29
5'7"	16	16	17	18	19	20	20	21	22	23	23	24	25	26	27	27	28
5'8"	15	16	17	17	18	19	20	21	21	22	23	24	24	25	26	27	27
5'9"	15	16	16	17	18	18	19	20	21	21	22	23	24	24	25	26	27
5'10"	14	15	16	17	17	18	19	19	20	21	22	22	23	24	24	25	26
5'11"	14	15	15	16	17	17	18	19	20	20	21	22	22	23	24	24	25
6'0"	14	14	15	16	16	17	18	18	19	20	20	21	22	22	23	24	24
6'1"	14	14	15	15	16	16	17	18	18	19	20	20	21	22	22	23	24
6'2"	14	13	14	15	15	16	17	17	18	19	19	20	21	21	22	22	23
6'3"	12	13	14	14	14	16	16	17	17	18	19	19	20	21	21	22	22
6'4"	12	13	13	14	14	15	16	16	17	18	18	19	19	20	21	21	22

☐ (18.5-24.9) = normal weight
▨ (25-29.9) = overweight
■ (≥30) = obese
▨ (≤18.5) = underweight

Figure 3.1 BMI Chart.

1. HORMONES AND CANCER

Carcinogenesis involves cell multiplication coupled with loss of differentiation. Increased cell division raises the chance of DNA damage. Hormones are involved in cell multiplication, either favoring the process or inhibiting it, and therefore play a role in the development of cancer. However, not all tissues in the body respond to hormone stimulation or inhibition. Cancers that arise in the tissues that do respond to hormonal stimulation are considered to be "hormone dependent". These cancers arise from the reproductive tract where most of the hormones exert their effect. In women, breast, endometrial, ovarian, and cervical cancers are considered to be hormone dependent; whereas, prostate cancer is the primary example in men.

Hormone exposure varies with age. Androgens and sex hormone binding globulin (SHBG) gradually decline with age. The sex hormones that are not bound either to albumin or SHBG are the ones that are completely active [4]. Due to the decrease in SHBG, sex hormone (*i.e.,* estrogens and androgens) are more bioavailable in older adults. In women, menarche and menopause are associated with marked and fairly rapid hormonal changes, particularly in estrogen levels. Estrogens, the female sex hormone, which promote breast cell proliferation, increase substantially around menarche and remain elevated until the perimenopausal period. In premenopausal women estrogens are secreted from the ovaries and to a lesser extent by adipose tissue [5]. In postmenopausal women not taking estrogen replacement therapy, adipose tissue becomes the principal source of estrogens [6] by converting androstenedione, a hormone secreted by the adrenal gland, to estrone, which is a form of estrogen [7].

2.   OBESITY AND HORMONES AND CANCER

In women, there is a complex relationship between obesity and hormone levels. Premenopausal overweight women are more likely than leaner women to have anovulatory menstrual cycles, irregular or missing menstrual cycles, and suffer from polycystic ovarian syndrome. These three conditions are associated with low levels of circulating estrogens and high levels of circulating androgens.

However, among postmenopausal women not taking hormone replacement therapy, circulating estrogen levels are quite low. Among these women, those that are overweight or obese have higher levels of estrogens because of peripheral conversion in adipose tissue. Among women taking replacement estrogens, adipose tissue is not the primary source of estrogen and the levels are similar to premenopausal women.

2.1   Breast cancer

Among premenopausal women, overweight women are less likely to develop breast cancer [8]. The decrease in risk may be due to a higher prevalence of menstrual irregularities, and their associated low estrogen levels, in overweight women. The relation is quite different among postmenopausal women. Among postmenopausal women, obesity is associated with an increased risk of developing breast cancer. Adipose tissue is the primary source of estrogen among postmenopausal women who do not use hormone replacement therapy. Therefore, it is not surprising that the obesity-related increase in risk is restricted to women who do not use hormone replacement therapy [9]. Breast cancer is more common among post- than premenopausal women, therefore, it is it fair to say obesity promotes more breast cancers than it prevents.

2.2 Endometrial cancer

Endometrial cancer is the most common gynecological cancer in the U.S. and the fourth most common cancer overall in women. Women who are overweight are at increased risk of developing endometrial cancer [10]. The magnitude of the increase is not well known, but most estimates range from a doubling to tripling of risk for obese women compared to their leaner peers [11]. The association with excess weight is stronger in older women [12], thus estrogens, which increase the mitotic rate of endometrial cells thereby increasing the probability of DNA damage [13], may be the mechanism through which weight acts.

2.3 Ovarian cancer

There is limited data on the association between obesity and ovarian cancer. Ovarian cancer is frequently diagnosed at a late stage and has a high fatality rate, therefore results from case control studies may be biased due to including only women who were sufficiently healthy to survive past the interview data. Nevertheless, the results from primarily case control studies suggest that the risk of ovarian cancer increases with relative weight [14].

2.4 Prostate cancer

Prostate cancer is a common cancer in developed countries; however, there is great variation in the incidence of prostate cancer even among developed nations. In the Untied States, it is the leading cause of morbidity and second cause of mortality [15]. The recent "westernization" of Asian culture has resulted in a rise of prostate cancer incidence in Japan, thus suggesting an environmental influence in the etiology of the cancer [16]. Little is know about the relation between prostate cancer and obesity, another common disease in westernized cultures.

Andersson *et al.* [17] observed that obesity was more predictive of death from prostate cancer than the development of the cancer. Their results suggest that obesity may be predictive of developing a more aggressive type of prostate cancer. The majority of the tumors are slow growing, thus presenting clinicians with a dilemma on whether to treat patients since the treatments (*i.e.,* surgery, radiation, and/or chemotherapy) can themselves have adverse outcomes. If the tumor is slow growing and therefore unlikely to impair health, then the treatments may cause more harm than the patient would suffer from the cancer itself. Unfortunately, at present there have been few factors identified as predictive of death from prostate cancer. Identification of prognostic factors would enable clinicians to decide who should be treated because they have more aggressive tumors.

The scarce data that exists on the relation of obesity to the development of prostate cancer is controversial and inconclusive. Some studies have found a positive or weak association between obesity and prostate cancer [18], while others have not [19, 20]. There are several possible mechanisms through which obesity could influence the prostate gland. As stated earlier obesity, particularly central adiposity, leads to a state of hyperinsulinemia which is accompanied by a rise in insulin-like growth factor I (IGF-I). Similar to other cell lines, insulin acts as a mitogen and stimulates the proliferation of prostate adenocarcinoma cell lines [21]. The association between IGF-I levels and prostate cancer has been studied extensively. Among men in the Physicians' Health Study the risk of prostate cancer increased with IGF-I levels. Men in the highest quartile of IGF-I levels were four times more likely than men in the lowest quartile to develop prostate cancer [22].

Another hormone through which the obesity effect might be mediated is testosterone, an androgen secreted by the testes that stimulates the growth of the prostate gland. Androgens, like estrogens, are sex hormones. Sex hormones can be further classified as bound (to either SHBG or albumin) or free (*i.e.*, circulating unbound), which is more biologically active. In a prospective study, Gann and co-workers found that high levels of circulating testosterone and low levels of SHBG, which should result in higher levels of free testosterone, were associated with increased risks of prostate cancer [23].

3.   OBESITY AND NON-HORMONE RELATED CANCERS

In addition to increasing the risk of developing hormone-related cancers, obesity is also associated with the development of other types of cancer, such as renal cell, esophageal, stomach, and colon cancer.

3.1   Renal cell cancer

Kidney cancer is the twelfth most common type of cancer in the U.S., accounting for approximately two percent of all new cancers [24]. Smoking is the most established risk factor for renal cell cancer. However, there is considerable evidence that the risk of renal cell cancer rises with increasing body weight, particularly among women [25, 26]. Although the precise mechanism for the obesity effect is not known, it has been speculated that since the effect is stronger in women, the effect may be mediated by hormonal changes. In some laboratory animals, estrogens induce renal cancer; however, there is little data from humans to suggest that a hormonal etiology. An alternate hypothesis is that it is diuretics, which are used to treat obesity, that increase the risk for renal cell cancer. Therefore the obesity association may be a due to a treatment given to people who are obese, rather than a direct causal relation.

3.2   Esophagus and gastric cardia

Obesity has a known relationship with gastroesophageal reflux, a risk factor for esophogeal adenocarcinoma [27]. Therefore it is not surprising that obesity is associated with the risk of adenocarcinoma of the esophagus and gastric cardia. Obese adults are up to 16 times as likely as lean adults to develop this type of cancer [28]. The increasing prevalence of obesity, coupled with the strength of the association between obesity and adenocarcinoma of the gastric cardia may explain why the incidence of the tumor has been increasing dramatically in the recent past [27].

3.3   Colorectal cancer

Colon cancer is the third most common cancer in the U.S. Although success with treatment is good if the tumor is detected early, colon cancer is the third leading cause of cancer death in the U.S. among both men and women. Although there was a slight decline between 1991 and 1995 in the number of new cases per year during, it has been suggested that the decrease was the result of increased screening and polyp removal, resulting in preventing progression of polyps to invasive cancer [29].

Obesity and central adiposity, measured with waist-to-hip ratio (WHR), are related to colon cancer; however, the evidence on gender differences is conflicting. Among the 13,420 men and women in the NHANES I follow-up study, the risk of colon cancer associated with excess weight was similar in men and women [30]. Although other researchers have observed an increase in risk associated with weight only among men [31-33], the more recent data shows an elevated risk in women [34].

The mechanism by which obesity contributes to the development of colon cancer has not been completely elucidated. It has been proposed that the influence of excessive weight on colorectal cancer risk may be mediated by increased insulin-like resistance and hyperinsulinemia [35-37]. Insulin and insulin growth factor (IGF) are believed to have a growth promoting effect on colorectal cancer [33]. More recently it has been proposed that obesity might alter the risk of colon cancer through its effect on prostaglandin E_2 (PGE$_2$) synthesis [38]. It has been reported that human as well as experimental colonic tumor cells show an increased production of prostaglandins, particularly the E series. In their results, they showed that a change in BMI from 24.2 to 28.8 kg/m^2 was associated with a 27 percent increase in rectal mucosa PGE$_2$ concentration.

CONCLUSION

Obesity is a serious public health problem in the U.S. and other developed countries and is becoming a problem is developing countries as well. The prevalence of obesity in both children and adults in the U.S., as well other westernized countries, is rising rapidly, thus we can expect the rates of breast, colon, renal cell, ovarian, and endometrial cancers to rise over the next several decades.

Although the precise mechanism by which obesity promotes or initiates carcinogenesis has not been clearly elucidated, the data suggest that the effect of obesity is mediated by hormone levels. In men and postmenopausal women, adipose tissue is the principal source of estrogens since that is where androstenedione is converted to estrogen. Estrogens have stimulating growth effects that promote carcinogenesis in some cell lines. Thus the association between excessive weight and risk of various cancers may be due to the elevated estrogen levels that occur with obesity.

Another possible explanation for the association between obesity and specific types of cancer is that excessive weight, particularly when it is centrally located, is associated with the development of hyperinsulinemia. Insulin and insulin-like growth factor are associated with cell development and proliferation. Greater cell proliferation increases the chance of DNA damage, which in turn increases the risk of the development of cancer.

In addition to increasing the risk of developing certain cancers, obesity is associated with the development of cardiovascular disease, diabetes, and osteoarthritis. Not all overweight or obese people will develop one or more of these diseases, but their chances of doing so are much greater than their leaner peers. Despite the health risks of obesity and the societal pressures to be thin, most adult Americans are steadily gaining weight. With rare exceptions, obesity is a preventable disease. To prevent the development of obesity, efforts must be made to increase physical activity, decrease inactivity, and modify dietary intake of children and adolescents. This will require societal changes that encourage activity. In addition, doctors should counsel their patients on the importance of maintaining a healthy weight and help their overweight patients lose weight and maintain the loss. Although cancer treatments have improved, cancer prevention should be the goal. By preventing the development of obesity, a substantial number of cancers could be avoided.

SUMMARY POINTS

- Adult women who are overweight or obese are more likely than their leaner peers to develop endometrial, ovarian, colon, and renal cell cancers. In addition, postmenopausal women who are obese are at increased risk of developing breast cancer.
- Among men, obesity is associated with an increased risk of developing colon and prostate cancers, two of the most common cancers in men.
- The prevalence of obesity is rising rapidly in developed countries, such as the U.S. Moreover, in developing countries as the societies become increasingly westernized, obesity is becoming a public health problem. As a result of these trends, the incidence of cancer of the breast, ovary, uterus, kidney, colon, and prostate should be expected to rise in much of the world.

RECOMMENDATIONS

- Maintain a healthy weight for one's height and avoid weight gain during adulthood by balancing the food consumed with the amount of physical activity.
- Try to prevent excessive weight gain and the development of obesity in children and adolescents by encouraging physical activity.

SUGGESTED FURTHER READING

1. National Institutes of Health, National Heart, Lung, and Blood Institute. Clinical (1998) *Guidelines on the Identification, Evaluation, and Treatment of Overweight and Obesity in Adults. The Evidence Report.* Bethesda, MD (USA): National Institutes of Health, National Heart, Lung, and Blood Institute.

REFERENCES

1. World Health Organization (1998) Obesity: Preventing and managing the global epidemic. In: *Report of a WHO Consultation on Obesity.* Geneva, Switzerland: World Health Organization.
2. Willett WC, Dietz WH, Colditz GA (1999) Guidelines for healthy weight. *N Engl J Med* **341:** 427-434.
3. Flegal KM, Caroll MD, Kuczmarski RJ, *et al.* (1998) Overweight and obesity in the U.S.: prevalence and trends, 1960-1994. *Int J Obesity* **22:** 39-47.
4. Risch H (1998) Hormonal etiology of epithelial ovarian cancer, with a hypothesis concerning the role of androgens and progesterone. *J Natl Cancer Inst* **90:** 1774-1786.
5. Stoll BA (1996) Obesity and breast cancer. *Int J Obesity* **20:** 389-392.
6. Sitteri PK (1987) Adipose tissue as a source of hormones. *Am J Clin Nutr* **45**(Suppl 1): 277-282.
7. Greenwald P, Sherwood K, McDonald SS (1997) Fat, caloric intake and obesity. Lifestyle risk factors for breast cancer. *J Am Diet Assoc.* **97**(Suppl):S24-S30
8. Peacock SL, White E, Daling JR, *et al.* (1999) Relation between obesity and breast cancer in young women. *Am J Epidemiol* **149:** 339-346.
9. Huang Z, Hankinson SE, Colditz GA, *et al.* (1997) Dual effects of weight and weight gain on breast cancer risk. *JAMA* **278:** 1407-1411.
10. Shoff SM, Newcomb PA (1998) Diabetes, body size, and risk of endometrial cancer. *Am J Epidemiol* **148:** 234-240.
11. Grady D, Ernster VL (1996) Endometrial Cancer In: Schottenfeld D, Fraumeni JF, eds. *Cancer Epidemiology and Prevention* New York, NY (USA): Oxford Press.
12. Tornberg SA, Carstensen JM (1994) Relationship between Quetelet's index and cancer of the breast and female genital tract in 47,000 women followed for 25 years. *Br J Cancer* **69:** 358-361.
13. Key TJ (1995) Hormones and cancer in humans. *Mutat Res* **333:** 59-67.
14. Farrow DC, Weiss NS, Lyon JL, *et al.* (1989) Association of obesity and ovarian cancer in a case-control study. *Am J Epidemiol* **129:** 1300-1304.
15. Ross RK, Schottenfeld D (1996) Prostate Cancer In: Schottenfeld D, Fraumeni JF, eds. *Cancer Epidemiology and Prevention* New York, NY (USA): Oxford Press.
16. Muir CS, Nectoux J, Staszewski J (1991) The epidemiology of prostatic cancer. Geographical distribution and time-trends. *Acta Oncol* **30:** 133-140.
17. Andersson SO, Wolk A, Bergstrom R, *et al.* (1997) Body size and prostate cancer: a 20-year follow-up study among 135006 Swedish construction workers. *J Natl Cancer Inst* **89:** 385-389.
18. Cerhan J (1997) Association of smoking, body mass, and physical activity with risk of prostate cancer in the Iowa 65+ Rural Health Study (U.S.). *Cancer Causes Control* **8:** 229-238.
19. Mills PK, Beeson WL, Phillips RL, *et al.* (1989) Cohort study of diet, lifestyle, and prostate cancer in Adventist men. *Cancer* **64:** 598-604.
20. Giovannucci E, Rimm EB, Stampfer MJ, *et al.* (1997) Height, body weight, and risk of prostate cancer. *Cancer Epidemiol Biomarkers Prev* **6:** 557-63.
21. King GL, Kahn CR (1981) Non-parallel evolution of metabolic and growth-promoting functions of insulin. *Nature* **292:** 644-646.
22. Chan JM, Stampfer MJ, Giovannucci E, *et al.* (1998) Plasma insulin-like growth factor-I and prostate cancer risk: A prospective study. *Science* **279:** 563-566.

23. Gann PH, Hennekens CH, Ma J, *et al.* (1996) Prospective study of sex hormone levels and risk of prostate cancer. *J Natl Cancer Inst* **88:** 1118-1126.
24. McLaughlin JK, Blot WJ, Devesa SS, *et al.* (1996) Renal Cancer In: Schottenfeld D, Fraumeni JF, eds. *Cancer Epidemiology and Prevention* New York, NY (USA): Oxford Press.
25. Mellemgaard A, Engholm G, McLaughlin JK, *et al.* (1994) Risk factors for renal-cell carcinoma in Denmark. III. Role of weight, physical activity, and reproductive factors. *Int J Cancer* **55:** 66-71.
26. Lindblad P, Wolk A, Bergsrtöm R, *et al.* (1994) The role of obesity and weight fluctuations in the etiology of renal cell carcinoma: a population-based case-control study. *Cancer Epidemiol Biomarkers Prev* **3:** 631-639.
27. Vaughn TL, Davis S, Fristal A, *et al.* (1995) Obesity, alcohol, and tobacco as risk factors for cancers of the esophagus and gastric cardia: adenocarcinoma versus squamous cell carcinoma. *Cancer Epidemiol Biomarkers Prev* **4:** 85-92.
28. Lagergren J, Bergstrom R, Nyren O (1999) Association between body mass and adenocarcinoma of the esophagus and gastric cardia. *Ann Intern Med* **130:** 883-890.
29. American Cancer Society (1999) *Cancer Facts & Figures - 1999.* Atlanta, GA (USA): American Cancer Society, Inc.
30. Ford ES (1999) Body mass index and colon cancer in a national sample of adult US men and women. *Am J Epidemiol* **15:** 390-398.
31. Giovannucci E, Colditz GA, Stampfer MJ (1996) Physical activity, obesity, and risk of colorectal adenoma in women (United States). adenoma in women 1996. *Cancer Causes Control* **7:** 253-63.
32. Le Marchand L, Wilkens LR, Kolonel LN *et al.* (1997) Associations of sedentary lifestyle, obesity, smoking, alcohol use, and diabetes with the risk of colorectal cancer. *Cancer Res* **57:** 4787-4794.
33. Giovannucci E, Ascherio A, Rimm EB, *et al.* (1995) Physical Activity, obesity, and risk for colon cancer and adenoma in men. *Ann Intern Med* **122:** 327-334.
34. Martinez ME, Giovannucci E, Spiegelman D, *et al.* (1997) Leisure-time, physical activity, body size, and colon cancer in women. Nurses' Health Study Research Group. *J Natl Cancer Inst* **89:** 948-955.
35. La Vecchia C, Negri E, Decarli A, *et al.* (1997) Diabetes Mellitus and colorectal cancer risk. *Cancer Epidemiol Biomarkers Prev* **6:** 1007-1010.
36. Kono S, Honjo S, Todoroki I, *et al.* (1998) Glucose intolerance and adenomas of the sigmoid colon in Japanese men (Japan). *Cancer Causes Control* **9:** 441-446.
37. Ma J, Pollak MN, Giovannucci E, *et al.* (1999) Prospective study of colorectal cancer risk in men and plasma levels of insulin-like growth factor (IGF)-I and IGF-binding protein-3. *J Natl Cancer Inst* **91:** 620-625.
38. Martinez ME, Heddens D, Earnest DL, *et al.* (1999) Physical Activity, body mass index and prostaglandin E_2 levels in rectal mucosa. *J Natl Cancer Inst* **91:** 950-953.

Chapter 4

Physical Activity

Howard D. Sesso, Sc.D. and I-Min Lee, M.B.B.S., Sc.D.
Division of Preventive Medicine, Department of Medicine, Brigham and Women's Hospital and Harvard Medical School, Boston, MA, and Department of Epidemiology, Harvard School of Public Health, Boston, MA

INTRODUCTION

There is general consensus that physical activity improves health and the quality of life [1]. Among its many benefits, higher levels of physical activity are associated with decreased risks of coronary heart disease, stroke, hypertension, diabetes, and fractures from osteoporosis. Over the past decade or so, there also has been accumulating evidence from the epidemiologic literature that physical activity may decrease the risk of developing certain site-specific cancers.

Therefore, it is unfortunate that Americans are highly sedentary. National data from the Behavioral Risk Factor Surveillance System indicate that about 30 percent of all adults do not engage in any leisure-time physical activity at all [1]. Further, this proportion has not changed much since the mid-1980s. Women tend to be more inactive than men, those older are less active than those younger, while blacks are more inactive than whites. If we additionally include adults who do engage in physical activity, but only sporadically or on an irregular basis, we observe an alarming statistic: almost 60 percent of American adults do no physical activity at all, or engage in it only irregularly, during their leisure-time [2].

The challenge to health professionals in the United States, then, is to motivate sustained increases in the level of physical activity. This should lead to reductions in the risk of many chronic diseases, including cancer. In this chapter, we argue the case for cancer. First, we discuss potential biologic mechanisms through which physical activity might act to prevent

37

G.A. Colditz et al. (eds.), Cancer Prevention: The Causes and Prevention of Cancer - Volume I, 37–47.
© 2000 *Kluwer Academic Publishers.*

cancer from developing. We then examine whether the epidemiologic data support a role of physical activity in preventing cancer. Next, we review some important methodological issues when assessing physical activity in studies of cancer. Finally, we conclude with some recommendations for future research and public health.

1.   PLAUSIBLE MECHANISMS FOR REDUCED CANCER RISK

From a biologic perspective, the hypothesis that physical activity decreases cancer incidence is highly plausible and can be supported by several lines of evidence. First, moderate amounts of physical activity appear to enhance immune function [3]. Following a bout of such exercise, investigators have observed increases in the number of circulating immune system cells, such as natural killer cells, cytotoxic T-lymphocytes, and cells of the monocyte-macrophage system. Additionally, increased function of immune system cells has been noted after moderate physical activity; *e.g.,* increased cell proliferation in response to mitogens, enhanced cytolytic ability of natural killer cells, and increased synthesis of cytokines and immunoglobulins. People who engage in moderate physical activity also may be at lower risk of developing upper respiratory tract infections, compared with those who are sedentary [4]. Since the immune system is responsible for regulating susceptibility to and severity from neoplastic processes, enhancement of the immune system by physical activity potentially could result in lower incidence of cancer.

Other biologic mechanisms support a role in physical activity in decreasing the risk of certain site-specific cancers. For colon cancer, investigators have postulated that physical activity may speed up transit within the intestinal tract [5]. The resulting shorter transit time may decrease contact between carcinogens, co-carcinogens, or promoters in the fecal stream and, thus, potentially reducing the risk of colon cancer. However, the data are not entirely consistent in showing that physical activity reduces transit time in the colon [6].

A third postulated mechanism hypothesizes that physical activity can, via altered levels of reproductive hormones, favorably influence the risk of developing reproductive cancers such as breast and prostate cancer. Young girls who participate in intensive athletic training, such as ballet dancing, experience a delay in the onset of menarche [7]. Even lesser amounts and intensity of physical activity may be associated with change in hormonal characteristics. For example, in one study, high school girls expending 600 kcal/week or more in physical activity (which can be achieved by a 1 to 1.5

hour gym class where exercise is sustained) were more likely to experience cycles that were anovulatory, compared with their less active counterparts [8]. Adult female athletes also are more likely to experience lower levels of estrogen and progesterone than sedentary women [9]. As with adolescent girls, even moderate levels of physical activity in adults, equivalent to walking seven to nine miles a week, may be associated with lower levels of female reproductive hormones [10]. Since lower levels of circulating estrogens are associated with lower risk of breast cancer [11], physical activity appears to have the potential to reduce breast cancer incidence. In men, an analogous situation exists. Among highly trained male athletes, basal levels of testosterone are lower than levels seen in sedentary men [12]. Since testosterone is necessary for the development of prostate cancer, physical activity may reduce the incidence of this cancer by decreasing testosterone levels.

Finally, physically active people weigh less and carry less body fat [1]. For cancers such as colon cancer and postmenopausal breast cancer, where obesity increases risk, physical activity may prevent the occurrence of these cancers through its favorable influence in helping to maintain normal body weight.

2.   PHYSICAL ACTIVITY AND COLON CANCER

Of the epidemiologic studies of physical activity and cancer, colon cancer has been most commonly studied. At least 30 such studies have been conducted to date [1, 13]. The data from these investigations consistently show an inverse association between physical activity and colon cancer risk, in men and in women. However, studies have been conducted primarily in white populations, with little data on minorities. Comparing those most active with those most sedentary, the median relative risks observed were 0.6 in studies where leisure-time or total physical activity was assessed, and 0.7 where occupational physical activity was assessed. Stated in another way, the data indicate that physical activity is associated with a 30 to 40 percent decrease in risk of colon cancer.

While the evidence for an inverse association is strong, details regarding the relation remain unclear. Few studies have examined issues such as: How much physical activity is needed? Does risk decrease linearly with higher levels of activity? How intense should the activity be? How frequently should activity be carried out? When should one be physically active in order to accrue benefit, at younger or older ages?

In the Harvard Alumni Health Study, investigators tried to quantify the amount of physical activity required [14]. They observed that men who consistently expended 1000 kcal/week or more had about half the risk of developing colon cancer compared with those more sedentary. This amount of energy expenditure can be achieved by moderate intensity activity, such as brisk walking, for 30 minutes a day, five days a week. In the Nurses' Health Study, investigators observed that women expending >21 MET-hours of physical activity a week also had about half the risk of colon cancer compared with those expending <2 MET-hours a week [13]. For a 55 kg women, 21 MET-hours is about equivalent to 1200 kcal/week, which can be achieved by brisk walking, 30 minutes a day, six days a week. Thus, the current physical activity recommendation that prescribes at least 30 minutes of moderate-intensity physical activity, such as brisk walking, on most days of the week [15] appears to be sufficient to decrease colon cancer risk in men and women.

If we were to assume that the relation is causal, the prevalence of physical inactivity is 60 percent, and that those who are active have a 40 percent lower risk of colon cancer, then approximately 29 percent of colon cancer occurring in the United States is attributable to physical inactivity.

3.   PHYSICAL ACTIVITY AND RECTAL CANCER

Many of the studies that investigated the association of physical activity with colon cancer risk also examined rectal cancer as a separate outcome [1]. The data regarding rectal cancer are as consistent as the data for colon cancer. However, they collectively indicate, instead, that physical activity is unrelated to the incidence of rectal cancer. Since the colon and the rectum are anatomically contiguous, it appears somewhat paradoxical that the associations for the two cancers are different. Some investigators have postulated that physical activity may shorten transit time within the colon, without materially affecting transit time in the rectum, since the rectum is only intermittently filled with fecal material.

4.   PHYSICAL ACTIVITY AND BREAST CANCER

While the postulated biologic mechanisms supporting an inverse association between physical activity and breast cancer are promising, the evidence from epidemiologic studies has yielded inconclusive results. Studies to date have reported a wide range of relative risks for physical activity in relation to breast cancer risk, from a 58 percent reduction in risk to an approximate 3-fold increase in risk among the most active women [16]. Not only is the overall physical activity/breast cancer relation unclear, details regarding this association remain unelucidated. For example, the critical time period for physical activity in the etiology of breast cancer remains uncertain. In addition, there may be important differences in the impact of physical activity on premenopausal and postmenopausal breast cancer, which have different etiologies and risk factor profiles. Yet only a few studies have examined physical activity levels at different time periods in relation to breast cancer risk. Bernstein *et al.* [17] observed that physical activity throughout a woman's reproductive years more strongly protected against premenopausal breast cancer than physical activity during the ten years after menarche. Recently, Rockhill *et al.* [18] found no link between physical activity, in late adolescence or in the recent past, and breast cancer risk among younger, premenopausal women. The association of physical activity and postmenopausal breast cancer risk has been equally puzzling; for example, data from the College Alumni Health Study yielded inverse results [19], while the Framingham Heart Study yielded positive results [20].

Methodological issues may have contributed to the inconsistency of findings in the epidemiologic literature. Because case-control studies have observed inverse associations more consistently than cohort studies, some investigators have suggested that recall bias in case-control studies may explain, in part, the inconsistencies observed [16]. Additionally, many studies have not assessed physical activity using instruments that have been tested for reliability and validity [16]. Well-designed and conducted studies are necessary to clarify the potential for physical activity to reduce breast cancer risk.

5. PHYSICAL ACTIVITY AND PROSTATE CANCER

Despite plausible biologic mechanisms supporting the hypothesis that physical activity can prevent the development of prostate cancer, findings from epidemiological studies of physical activity and prostate cancer remain inconclusive. Studies have yielded a broad range of risk estimates, suggesting an inverse association, no association, or positive association. Prospective data from 47,542 middle-aged men in the Health Professionals Follow-up Study reported no overall association between physical activity and risk of prostate cancer, but found that men expending >25 MET-hours/week had a 54 percent lower risk of metastatic prostate cancer compared to those expending 0 MET-hours/week [21]. The Harvard Alumni Health Study observed an inverse association for incident prostate cancer only among men with consistently high levels of physical activity (≥4000 kcal/week) compared to men with consistently low levels of physical activity

(<1000 kcal/week) [22]. In contrast, Whittemore *et al.* [23] conducted a large population-based case-control study in North America and found no association between physical activity and prostate cancer risk regardless of ethnicity. Comparing men in the highest *vs.* lowest tertiles of hours per day spent in activities other than sitting, reclining, or sleeping, the odds ratios of prostate cancer were 1.2 for blacks, 0.9 for whites, 0.7 for Chinese-Americans, and 0.8 for Japanese-Americans. Finally, data from the Iowa 65+ Rural Health Study indicated that men classified in the "very active" category of physical activity had a 60 percent increased risk of prostate cancer compared to men classified as "inactive" [24].

Few studies have reported significant dose-response trends [1], whereas comparisons of the most *vs.* least active men have suggested a possible inverse association in several studies. Therefore, a greater threshold level of physical activity may be necessary to lower the risk of prostate cancer. Because incidence rates for prostate cancer remain high, even small reductions in prostate cancer risk by increased physical activity may have an enormous public health benefit in terms of attributable risk.

6. PHYSICAL ACTIVITY AND CANCER OF OTHER SITES

The relationship between physical activity and other types of cancer, including endometrial, testicular, lung, pancreatic, and others, remains largely unstudied and unresolved [1]. For each of these site-specific cancers, some epidemiologic studies have suggested that physical activity may reduce the risk of cancer, yet data remain sparse. These other cancers warrant additional research in either case-control or large-scale prospective designs to ensure adequate case counts.

7. METHODOLOGICAL ISSUES IN ASSESSING PHYSICAL ACTIVITY

Most epidemiological studies on physical activity and the risk of cancer rely upon summary measurements of physical activity. The assessment of physical activity is always threatened by potential measurement errors, which in turn may attenuate the results of a study. Physical activity may be separated into occupational, leisure-time, and sedentary components. Many studies on physical activity and the risk of cancer tend to examine certain components of physical activity, but not others.

Within each component of physical activity, the specific type, intensity, and duration of energy expenditure may have differential effects on, for example, cardiovascular disease morbidity and mortality [1]. These more detailed aspects of physical activity measurement have yet to be fully explored in cancer prevention studies. For example, whereas an overall benefit of physical activity on colon cancer appears likely, the specific kinds of physical activity that may be most beneficial remain unclear. The intensity of physical activity, defined as either light (*e.g.,* bowling), moderate (*e.g.,* brisk walking), or vigorous (*e.g.,* running), may also have different effects on risk of different site-specific cancers.

Physical activity is a dynamic behavior that changes over time; several studies have demonstrated age-specific patterns of energy expenditure throughout a lifetime [1, 2]. Longitudinal studies must incorporate multiple measurements of physical activity to examine not only baseline levels in relation to cancer risk, but also changes in relation to cancer risk. Similarly, because cancer tends to progress over the course of years or decades, physical activity assessments over longer time periods may need to be considered.

These differences in the measurement and quantification of physical activity suggest that an overall assessment of physical activity on cancer risk may not be sufficient. Physical activity may not exhibit a dose-response relationship for a site-specific cancer; rather, a particular threshold level may be required. These measurement issues for physical activity in cancer research have important implications on subsequent public policy: Is the beneficial quantity or intensity of physical activity attainable, and by whom?

Table 4.1 Summary of epidemiologic evidence on physical activity and cancer.

Cancer	Epidemiologic Evidence
Colon	Physically active men and women have a 30 to 40% decreased risk, compared to those who are sedentary. Preliminary evidence suggests that physical activity equivalent to 30 minutes of moderate-intensity physical activity, such as brisk walking, on most days of the week is sufficient to decrease colon cancer risk.
Rectal	Data suggest no association with physical activity.
Breast	Biologically plausible for physical activity to reduce risk, but epidemiologic evidence does not consistently support a reduced risk with physical activity.
Prostate	Biologically plausible for physical activity to reduce risk, but findings from epidemiological studies of physical activity and prostate cancer remain inconclusive.
Other Cancers	Few data are available; additional research is warranted.

CONCLUSION

Physical activity is a modifiable aspect of behavior throughout an individual's lifetime and, thus, has important potential in the primary prevention of cancer. Several plausible biological mechanisms have been put forward in support of a beneficial effect between increased physical activity and the risk of several site-specific cancers.

Numerous case-control and cohort studies have investigated whether physical activity reduces the risk of developing cancer. The evidence to date strongly indicates that increased levels of physical activity reduce the risk of colon cancer in both men and women. In contrast, physical activity is not associated with the risk of rectal cancer, for reasons not entirely clear. Epidemiological evidence continues to build in support of physical activity in the primary prevention of breast cancer; however, findings to the contrary have also been reported. Studies have been inconsistent regarding the association between physical activity and risk of prostate cancer, with beneficial effects of physical activity possibly limited to those men at the highest activity levels. Finally, data on other site-specific cancers remain too limited to provide any conclusions.

Since individual patterns of physical activity may differ in terms of not only quantity, but also with regard to its type, intensity, and duration, future research needs to better define the appropriate levels and kinds of physical activity required to reduce the risk of selected site-specific cancers. The Centers for Disease Control and Prevention and the American College of Sports Medicine recommend that every adult should accumulate 30 or more minutes of moderate-intensity physical activity on most, preferably all, days of the week [2]. Yet 60 percent of American adults remain inactive [2]. Given the tremendous public health burden of cancer, even a moderate benefit from increased levels of physical activity may have important implications. Continued epidemiologic research must be balanced with continued efforts to promote physical activity in all individuals.

SUMMARY POINTS

- Physical activity has been established to decrease risk of chronic diseases, such as cardiovascular disease. In recent years, there also has been accumulating evidence that physical activity may reduce the risk of certain cancers.
- Biologically, there are several plausible mechanisms to support the hypothesis that physical activity can decrease the incidence of cancer.

- Based on the epidemiologic data to date, higher levels of physical activity are associated with decreased risk of colon cancer. Men and women who are physically active have about a 30 to 40 percent decrease in risk compared with those sedentary. While the data are sparse, it appears that at least 30 minutes of moderate-intensity physical activity, such as brisk walking, on most days of the week should be sufficient to decrease colon cancer risk.
- The epidemiologic data are inconsistent regarding whether physical activity decreases risk of breast cancer in women, or prostate cancer in men.
- Few data are available regarding the association of physical activity and other site-specific cancers.
- Americans are far too sedentary. It is important for public health professionals to motivate sustained increases in current levels of physical activity, since this will reduce the risk of many chronic diseases, including colon cancer. Given certain assumptions detailed above, some 29 percent of all colon cancer occurring in the United States are attributable to physical inactivity.

RECOMMENDATIONS

- Despite strong evidence for an association between increased levels of physical activity and a reduced risk of colon cancer, studies should clarify which specific type, frequency, intensity, and duration of activities may be most beneficial. The seemingly contradictory lack of an association between physical activity and rectal cancer needs to be better understood in terms of the underlying biology.
- Research needs to clarify whether physical activity reduces the risk of breast cancer and prostate cancer. The timing of a physically active lifestyle throughout life, as well as assessing whether physical activity has differential effects on premenopausal or postmenopausal breast cancer risk, needs to be better understood. For prostate cancer, it remains unclear whether a dose-response or threshold pattern of effect exists.
- Other site-specific cancers have been less well studied in relation to physical activity. Studies tend to be limited by the lower incidence of such cancers. Therefore, studies utilizing either case-control or large-scale prospective designs that ensure adequate statistical power to detect any effect present should be initiated.
- Americans should engage in at least 30 minutes of moderate intensity physical activity, such as brisk walking, on most days of the week.

SUGGESTED FURTHER READING

1. U.S. Department of Health and Human Services (1996) *Physical Activity and Health: A report of the Surgeon General.* Atlanta, GA: U.S. Department of Health and Human Services, Centers for Disease Control and Prevention, National Center for Chronic Disease Prevention and Health Promotion.
2. Pate RR, Pratt M, Blair SN, *et al.* (1995) Physical activity and public health: A recommendation from the Centers for Disease Control and Prevention and the American College of Sports Medicine. *JAMA* **273:** 402-407.
3. Pereira MA, FitzerGerald SJ, Gregs EW, *et al.* (1997) A collection of Physical Activity Questionnaires for health-related research. *Med Sci Sports Exerc* **29**(Suppl): S1-205.

REFERENCES

1. U.S. Department of Health and Human Services (1996) *Physical Activity and Health: A Report of the Surgeon General.* Atlanta, GA: U.S. Department of Health and Human Services, Centers for Disease Control and Prevention, National Center for Chronic Disease Prevention and Health Promotion.
2. Anonymous (1993) Prevalence of sedentary lifestyle: Behavioral Risk Factor Surveillance System, United States, 1991. *MMWR Morb Mortal Wkly Rep* **42:** 576-579.
3. Hoffman-Goetz L, ed. (1996) *Exercise and Immune Function.* Boca Raton, FL (USA): CRC Press.
4. Nieman DC (1994) Physical activity, fitness, and infection. In: Bouchard C, Shephard RJ, Stephens T, eds. *Physical Activity, Fitness, and Health: International Proceedings and Consensus Statement.* Champaign, IL (USA): Human Kinetics Publishers, pp. 796-813.
5. Oettlé GJ (1991) Effect of moderate exercise on bowel habit. *Gut* **32:** 941-944.
6. Coenen C, Wegener M, Wedmann B, *et al.* (1992) Does physical exercise influence bowel transit time in healthy young men? *Am J Gastroenterol* **87:** 292-295.
7. Frisch RE, Wyshak G, Vincent L (1980) Delayed menarche and amenorrhea in ballet dancers. *N Engl J Med* **303:** 17-19.
8. Bernstein L, Ross RK, Lobo RA, *et al.* (1987) The effects of moderate physical activity on menstrual cycle patterns in adolescence: implications for breast cancer prevention. *Br J Cancer* **55:** 681-685.
9. Loucks AB, Mortola JF, Girton L, *et al.* (1989) Alterations in the hypothalamic-pituitary-ovarian and the hypothalamic-pituitary-adrenal axes in athletic women. *J Clin Endocrinol Metab* **68:** 402-411.
10. Cauley JA, Gutai JP, Kuller LH, *et al.* (1989) The epidemiology of serum sex hormones in postmenopausal women. *Am J Epidemiol* **129:** 1120-1131.
11. Hankinson SE, Willett WC, Manson JE, *et al.* (1998) Plasma sex steroid hormone levels and risk of breast cancer in postmenopausal women. *J Natl Cancer Inst* **90:** 1292-1299.
12. Wheeler GD, Wall SR, Belcastro AN, *et al.* (1984) Reduced serum testosterone and prolactin levels in male distance runners. *JAMA* **252:** 514-516.

13. Martinez ME, Giovannucci E, Spiegelman D, *et al.* (1997) Leisure-time physical activity, body size, and colon cancer in women. *J Natl Cancer Inst* **89**: 948-955.
14. Lee I-M, Paffenbarger RS Jr, Hsieh C-c (1991) Physical activity and risk of developing colorectal cancer among college alumni. *J Natl Cancer Inst* **83**: 1324-1329.
15. Pate RR, Pratt M, Blair SN, *et al.* (1995) Physical activity and public health: a recommendation from the Centers for Disease Control and Prevention and the American College of Sports Medicine. *JAMA* **273**: 402-407.
16. Gammon MD, John EM, Britton LA (1998) Recreational and occupational physical activities and risk of breast cancer. *J Natl Cancer Inst* **90**: 100-117.
17. Bernstein L, Henderson BE, Hanisch R, *et al.* (1994) Physical exercise and reduced risk of breast cancer in young women. *J Natl Cancer Inst* **86**: 1403-1408.
18. Rockhill B, Willett WC, Hunter DJ, *et al.* (1998) Physical activity and breast cancer risk in a cohort of young women. *J Natl Cancer Inst* **90**: 1155-1160.
19. Sesso HD, Paffenbarger RS Jr, Lee I-M (1998) Physical activity and breast cancer risk in the College Alumni Health Study (United States). *Cancer Causes Control* **9**: 433-439.
20. Dorgan JF, Brown C, Barrett M, *et al.* (1994) Physical activity and the risk of breast cancer in the Framingham Heart Study. *Am J Epidemiol* **139**: 662-669.
21. Giovannucci E, Leitzmann M, Spiegelman D, *et al.* (1998) A prospective study of physical activity and prostate cancer in male health professionals. *Cancer Res* **58**: 5117-5122.
22. Lee I-M, Paffenbarger RS Jr, Hsieh C-C (1992) Physical activity and risk of prostatic cancer among college alumni. *Am J Epidemiol* **135**: 169-179.
23. Whittemore AS, Kolonel LN, Wu AH, *et al.* (1995) Prostate cancer in relation to diet, physical activity, and body size in blacks, whites, and Asians in the United States and Canada. *J Natl Cancer Inst* **87**: 652-661.
24. Cerhan JR, Torner JC, Lynch CF, *et al.* (1997) Association of smoking, body mass, and physical activity with risk of prostate cancer in the Iowa 65+ Rural Health Study (United States). *Cancer Causes Control* **8**: 229-238.

Chapter 5

Occupation

David C. Christiani, M.D., M.P.H. and Richard R. Monson, M.D.
Department of Environmental Health, Harvard School of Public Health, Boston, MA

INTRODUCTION

Occupational epidemiology studies have played an important role in identifying causes of human cancer. Most of the chemicals classified as carcinogens by the International Agency for Cancer Research (IARC) were first identified in the occupational setting. Occupational investigations have been informative because exposures in the workplace are often heavy and prolonged in contrast to other resources of chemical exposures.

Reviews conducted since 1970 by the International Agency for Research on Cancer (IARC) indicate that most of the exposures that have been judged to cause cancer in humans have occurred in the workplace [1]. In the workplace, people are likely to be exposed to a broad spectrum of carcinogens at high concentrations; therefore, epidemiologists and physicians are more likely to identify these cancer-causing agents. In contrast, it has been estimated that six to ten percent of cancer (and at most 15 percent) in men and one percent of cancer in women (and no more than five percent) can be attributed to occupational factors [2]. This apparent discrepancy relates to the quantity and quality of information available on human carcinogens as well as the fact that most of us have minimal exposure to potentially carcinogenic chemicals in the workplace.

Clearly, tobacco smoke is the single factor known to have caused the highest proportion of cancer. Next, a wide variety of exposures to chemicals in the workplace have been identified as causing a variety of cancers. Tobacco and many workplace exposures are relatively strong causes of cancer. The rate of cancer among people exposed to these agents has been ten to 100 times the rate in unexposed people. Other causes of cancer in

49

G.A. Colditz et al. (eds.), Cancer Prevention: The Causes and Prevention of Cancer - Volume I, 49–56.

humans, while possibly present among a larger proportion of the population, are likely to be weak and thus difficult to identify.

Table 5.1 Occupational agents, mixtures, and processes judged by IARC to be human carcinogens[a]

Substance or process	Sites of cancer	Year[b]
Aluminum production	Lung, bladder	1981
Aflatoxins	Liver	1993
4-Aminobiphenyl	Bladder	1955
Arsenic and certain arsenic compounds	Lung, skin	1822[d]
Asbestos	Gastroinstestinal tract, mesothelioma of pleura and peritoneum, lung, larynx	1935
Auramine manufacture	Bladder	1954
Benzene	HLS[c]	1964
Benzidine	Bladder	1895[d]
Beryllium and beryllium compounds	Lung	1979
Bis(chloromethyl) ether and chloromethyl methyl ether	Lung	1973
Boot and shoe manufacture and repair	Nasal cavity	1970
Cadmium and cadmium compounds	Lung	1976
Chromium and certain chromium compounds	Lung	1948
Coal gasification	Lung	1936
Coal tars and pitches	Skin	1875
Coke production	Lung	1971
Ethylene oxide	HLS[c]	1979
Furniture and cabinet making	Sinus, larynx	1987
Hematite mining (underground)	Lung	1956
Iron and steel founding	Lung	1977
Isopropanol		
Magenta (manufacture of)	Bladder	1895[d]
Mineral oils, treated and mildly treated	Skin	1922
Mustard gas	Pharynx, lung	1955
2-Naphthylamine	Bladder, HLS[c]	1954
Nickel and nickel compounds	Nose and nasal sinus	1933
Painting	Lung	1976
Radon	Lung	1879[d]
Rubber industry	Bladder, HLS[c]	1954
Shale oils	Skin	1876
Silica	Lung	1986
Soots	Skin	1775
Sulfuric acid mist	Nasal cavity, larynx, lung	1952
Talc containing abestiform fibers	Lung	1979
TCDD[e]	All cancer	1997
Vinyl chloride	Liver	1974
Wood dust	Nasal cavity	1972

[a]   Substances updated in later reviews are not included
[b]   Year suggested to be carcinogenic
[c]   Hematopoietic and lymphatic cancers
[d]   Year refers to work environment rather than to specific compound
[e]   -2, 3, 7, 8 - Tetrachlorodibenzo-*para*-dioxin

1.   EVALUATION OF EXPOSURES

The designation of a substance as a human carcinogen is a matter of collective scientific judgement. The reviews conducted by IARC are based on a comprehensive evaluation of the current scientific literature relating to chemical, physical, or biological exposures in humans and in other animals. Each year, one or more working groups meet in Lyon, France, to consider the scientific information available on exposures with carcinogenic potential. Since 1977, these working people have designated exposures according to their potential for carcinogenicity in humans [3]. The designations are as follows:

The agent (mixture) is:

Group 1 – Carcinogenic to humans;

Group 2A – Probably carcinogenic to humans;

Group 2B - Possibly carcinogenic to humans;

Group 3 – Not classified as to its carcinogenicity to humans;

Group 4 – Probably not carcinogenic to humans.

Each of the above designations takes into account information from epidemiologic studies in humans and, to a lesser extent, from experimental studies in laboratory animals. In order for an agent to be judged as belonging to Group 1, as a rule there must be sufficient evidence of information relating to humans based on epidemiologic studies. Group 2A indicates limited evidence for humans and sufficient evidence for animals. Group 2B indicates evidence in humans together with sufficient evidence in animals or limited evidence in both humans and animals. Group 3 implies lack of carcinogenicity in both humans and animals. Finally, all other exposures fall into Group 4.

In 1979, the first comprehensive list of exposures judged to cause human cancer was published by IARC [3-5]. Table 5.1 is based on this report and lists the substances present or processes that occur in the workplace, together with the cancer caused and the year that each was suggested by the IARC to be a carcinogen. Several of these agents or exposures had been suspected to be carcinogenic before 1900, and only two were initially identified after 1970. It should be noted that the year an agent was first thought to be a carcinogen is somewhat arbitrary; other dates have been suggested [6].

Many of the exposures listed in Table 5.1 are associated with an increased cancer risk of ten times or greater. The estimated risk increase depends, of course, on the level of duration of exposure to a working population as well as on the availability of reliable data. For example, shoe workers exposed to benzene-containing glues may have had a leukemia risk that was ten to 100 times the risk in the general population; however, no epidemiologic data are available. In contrast, the Pliofilm Cohort in Ohio, on which the primary epidemiologic study of people occupationally exposed to benzene was based, had an increased risk of leukemia of about 3.4 [7].

Many of the agents listed in Table 5.1 are *relatively* weak human carcinogens with an increased risk no higher than about five times. For some of these agents, for instance, ethylene oxide (EtO), epidemiologic evidence by itself was not sufficient to categorize them as Group 1 carcinogens; the mechanism of action of EtO was also used to make the final judgement.

One agent-ionizing radiation has not been evaluated by IARC but is clearly a human carcinogen [8]. Watch-dial painters in the early part of this century used radium-containing paint to make the dial glow in the dark. The painters, mostly women, would twirl the brush on their tongue to make a point on the brush. The radium that they ingested *via* this route was concentrated in their bones, and osteogenic sarcoma was an unfortunate but relatively common result. Also, radiologists who practiced in the early 20th century had an elevated rate of leukemia as a result of their occupational exposure to radiation.

Table 5.2 lists occupational exposures that to date have been classified by IARC as Group 2A – probable human carcinogens. These agents represent a mixture of chemical compounds. These agents represent a mixture of chemical compounds and manufacturing processes or more general exposures. Each has been brought to our attention only recently as being possibly carcinogenic. All of these agents, if they are in fact carcinogenic to humans, are relatively weak causes of the cancers listed. There is legitimate question as to whether sufficient epidemiologic information can be collected to provide an unambiguous judgement of causality.

2.   IMPROVEMENTS IN INDUSTRIAL HYGIENE

Almost all of the agents listed in Table 5.1 are substances or processes to which humans have been exposed in the workplace for many decades and, in some cases, even centuries. People have been exposed to these carcinogens at relatively high levels even in the second half of this century. Before 1900, little attention was given to the possibility that an agent in the workplace caused cancer or indeed any chronic disease. As long as a worker could function in an environment that may have been filled with dusts, mists, and gases, the primary concern was economic gain, often for the employer. During the first half of the 20th century, attention gradually was drawn to the possibility that exposure in the workplace may lead to chronic disease and cancer [9]. However, a lack of acute toxicity still served as the indicator that the workplace was safe. Only since World War II have industrial hygiene and epidemiology developed into professions that consider the possible long-term dangers of exposure in the workplace. In the United States, the Occupational Safety and Health Act in 1970 brought official notice to workers management that continuing vigilance was needed to prevent cancer among industrial workers [10]. Unfortunately, many improvements in workplace hygiene have not accompanied the rapid change in the industrializing nations of the world. Rapid industrialization, urbanization, and globalization have led to the introduction of carcinogens and export into the workplaces of these countries [11-13].

Table 5.2 Occupational agents, mixtures, and processes judged by IARC from 1979 through 1998 to be probable human carcinogens

Substance or process	Site(s) of cancer	Year[a]
Acrylamide	Uncertain	1994
Acrylonitrile	Lung	1978
Art glass	Lung	1993
1,3 Butadiene	HLS[b]	1987
Creosotes	Skin, scrotum	1987
Diesel exhaust	Lung	1983
Epichorhydrin	Lung	1999
Ethylene dibrimide	Lung	1999
Formaldehyde	Nose and nasopharynx	1982
Glass manufacture	Lung	1987
Hairdresser or barber	Bladder	1961
Nonarsenical pesticides, spraying of	Lung	1979
Petroleum refining, occupational exposure	Skin, HLS[b]	1982
Polychlorinated biphenyls	Liver, skin	1974
Styrene oxide	HLS[b]	1994
Tetrachloroethylene	Uncertain	1995
Trichloroethylene	Uncertain	1995

CONCLUSIONS

It is hoped that no worker will develop cancer because of current occupational exposures in developed countries. Ideally, known carcinogens or carcinogenic processes have been contained so that worker exposure is kept to a minimum, and no new carcinogens will be introduced into the workplace. The combination of reduction of exposure to known carcinogens will be introduced into the workplace. In the U.S., the combination of reduction of exposure to known carcinogens or carcinogenic processes have been contained so that worker exposure is kept to a minimum, and no new carcinogens and minimization of introduction of new carcinogens will likely lead to the inability of epidemiologists to identify new carcinogens from classic case-control or cohort studies, because the risks involved will be very low. Rather, continued vigilance or surveillance will be based on monitoring of physiologic change in workers or by evaluation of markers of genetic damage in cells [13]. (See Chapter 22 on Prevention of Work-related Cancers).

SUMMARY POINTS

- Body surfaces that have direct contact with carcinogenic agents in the workplace are at the highest risk for developing cancer. These surfaces include the skin and nasal passages and the main internal body surface, the lung and urinary bladder.
- Overall, six to ten percent of cancer in men is likely to be caused by occupational exposures [2]. For women, the percentage is probably no more than one percent. It is estimated that in men 15 percent of lung cancer and ten percent each of skin and bladder cancers are occupationally caused.

RECOMMENDATIONS

- Employees should know the name and chemical composition of all substances with which they work.
- Employees should get a copy of the Material Safety Data Sheet (MSDS), and review the information on toxicity and cancer potential.
- The work environment should be designed so as to prevent exposure to toxic substances.
- Employees should be required to wear personal protective equipment where indicated.

SUGGESTED FURTHER READING

1. Vineis P, Cantor K, Gonzales C, Lynge E, Vallyathan V (1995) Occupational cancer in developed and developing countries. *Int J Cancer* **62**: 655-60.
2. National Research Council (1990) Health *Effects of Exposure to Low Levels of Ionizing Radiation. BEIR V.* Washington, DC: National Academy Press.
3. Hamilton A (1943) *Exploring the Dangerous Trades: An Autobiography.* Boston, MA (USA): Little, Brown.
4. Monson RR (1990) *Occupational Epidemiology,* 2nd Edition. Boca Raton, FL (USA): CRC Press.
5. Siemiatycki J (1991) *Risk Factors for Cancer in the Workplace.* Boca Raton, FL (USA): CRC Press.

REFERENCES

1. Tomatis L (1998) The contribution of the IARC Monographs Program to the identification of cancer risk factors. *Ann NY Acad Sci* **534**: 31-8.
2. Leigh JP, Markowitz SB, Fahs M, *et al.* (1997) Occupational injury and illness in the United States. Estimates of costs, morbidity, and mortality. *Arch Intern Med* **157**: 1557-1568.
3. IARC (1979) *Chemicals and Industrial Processes Associated with Cancer in Humans.* Lyon, France: IARC Monographs, Volumes 1-20.
4. IARC (1987) *IARC Monographs on the Evaluation of Carcinogenic Risks to Human. Overall Evaluations of Carcinogenicity : An Updating of IARC. Monographs Volumes 1 to 42.* Lyon, France: IARC, Supplement 7.
5. IARC (1987-1998) *IARC Monographs on the Evaluation of Carcinogenic Risks to Humans.* Lyon, France, Volumes 43-70.
6. Vineis P, Cantor K, Gonzales C, *et al.* (1995) Occupational cancer in developed and developing countries. *Int J Cancer* **62**: 655-60.
7. Rinsky RA, Smith AB, Hornung R, *et al.* (1987) Benzene and leukemia. An epidemiologic risk assessment. *N Engl J Med* **316**: 1044-50.
8. National Research Council (1990) *Health Effects of Exposure to Low Levels of Ionizing Radiation. BEIR V.* Washington, DC: National Academy Press.
9. Hamilton A (1943) *Exploring the Dangerous Trades. An Autobiography.* Boston, MA (USA): Little, Brown & Co.
10. Bingham E (1992) The occupational safety and health act. In: Rom WN, ed. *Environmental and Occupational Medicine.* Boston, MA (USA): Little, Brown & Co. pp. 1325-31.
11. Magrath I, Litvak J (1993) Cancer in developing countries: opportunity and challenge. *J Natl Cancer Inst* **85**: 862-874.
12. Pearce N, Matos E, Vainio H, *et al.*, eds. (1994) *Occupational Cancer in Developing Countries.* Lyon, France: IARC.

13. Siemiatyeki J (1995) Future etiologic research in occupational cancer. *Environ Health Perspect* **103:** 209-215.

Chapter 6

Genetic Susceptibility

Frederick P. Li, M.D. and David J. Hunter, M.B.B.S., Sc.D.
Adult Oncology, Dana-Farber Cancer Institute, Boston, MA; Channing Laboratory, Department of Medicine, Brigham and Women's Hospital and Harvard Medical School; Harvard Center for Cancer Prevention and Departments of Epidemiology and Nutrition, Harvard School of Public Health, Boston, MA

INTRODUCTION

Technological advances in recent years have led to an explosion in knowledge of human genetics. In studies of cancer, laboratory investigators have shown that alterations in specific genes cause the transformation of a normal cell into a cancer cell. These neoplastic cells accumulate, overgrow surrounding tissues, and eventually spread to other anatomic sites. Mutations in multiple genes are required to produce the common forms of cancers [1].

1.   FAMILIAL AGGREGATION

The human genome is comprised of three billion nucleotides (building blocks) that encode genetic information. Within the genome are perhaps 60,000 to 100,000 genes that are in the nucleus of every human cell. Each gene (made up of many nucleotides) carries the instructions for building one or more proteins that do the work of the cell. Until molecular technology became available to analyze these sub-microscopic units, understanding of the fundamental structure of the human genome was not possible.

Even before the advent of modern molecular biology, epidemiologists had shown that cancers tend to aggregate in families. In striking family pedigrees in which many members have cancer, the pattern of cancer occurrence is consistent with inherited susceptibility through a single mutant gene. Carriers of mutations in certain genes experience a lifetime probability of cancer

G.A. Colditz et al. (eds.), Cancer Prevention: The Causes and Prevention of Cancer - Volume I, 57–62.

development that approaches 100 percent. Furthermore, familial aggregation has been found in virtually every form of cancer in humans, including tumors classified as carcinomas, sarcomas, brain tumors and leukemia/lymphomas. Some of this aggregation may be due to shared exposure to carcinogens, the rest is presumably due to inherited susceptibility. In general, a person who has a parent or sibling with cancer at young age has about a two-fold or higher risk of developing that cancer (Table 6.1). In some affected kindreds, susceptibility is extended to include several tumor types and organ sites. For example, members of families with dominantly inherited multiple endocrine neoplasia (type 1), develop tumors of the pituitary, parathyroid, adrenal, pancreatic islet cells and other endocrine tissues [2].

Table 6.1 Cancer risk and familial aggregation of genes

- Inherited genetic mutations cause a proportion of most cancer types.
- It is estimated that 5 to 50 percent of most types of cancer are due to highly penetrant defects in single genes.
- Increase in risk is associated with family history of the major cancer sites.

Site	Relationship	Approximate Increase in Risk
Breast	Mother <40 at diagnosis	Two-fold
	Mother >70 at diagnosis	50%
	Sister	Two-fold
Colon	One parent or sibling	70%
	Two parents or sibling	Three-fold
Prostate	Father	50%
	Brother	Two-fold
Lung	One parent or sibling	Two-fold

2.   INHERITED SUSCEPTIBILITY

In the last two decades, collaborations between laboratory scientists and epidemiologists have led to the discovery of a series of inherited cancer susceptibility genes. The retinoblastoma gene, called RB1, predisposes to a tumor of the retina in young children and, subsequently, to a variety of second cancers in adolescence and adulthood. RB1 was discovered in 1986 through cytogenetic and molecular analyses of unusual retinoblastoma patients with large chromosome deletions and families with multiply affected relatives [3]. Inherited susceptibility genes have now been found for many forms of cancer, including melanoma, breast cancer, colon cancer and kidney cancer.

Striking family aggregates of cancer are relatively rare in the general population. At first glance, identification of genetic alterations that predispose to cancer in unusual families might seem to have little public health importance. However, Knudson noted in 1971 that hereditary and non-hereditary forms of any cancer may involve the same series of genetic alterations; the major difference is that one of the mutations has been transmitted from a parent in hereditary cases, whereas these same mutations have all been acquired during the lifetime of those with non-familial cancers [4]. The implication of the Knudson model is that cancer-associated genes identified through rare families are also involved in the genesis of cancer in non-hereditary cases. In fact, discoveries of genes involved in the development of several common cancers were made through analyses of rare families, and ample empirical evidence has been accrued in support of the Knudson model. For example, inherited mutations in the retinoblastoma gene account for fewer than 100 cases of the tumor annually in the U.S. However, RB1 mutations acquired post-conception are involved in the development of more than 100,000 cancers per year nationwide.

3. GENES AND CANCER RISK

To date, genes that predispose to cancer can be divided into three major classes. The oncogenes are altered forms of genes, called proto-oncogenes, that encode for growth factors, growth factor receptors, intracellular signal transducers and transcription regulators involved in cell division and other functions. In the mutant form, these genes signal cells to divide and accumulate inappropriately. A second class, tumor suppressor genes, function to arrest cells from proceeding through the cell cycle, particularly if the cellular DNA has been damaged. When tumor suppressor genes are lost or disabled, cells divide at abnormal rates often under the control of mutant oncogenes. Mutations in certain oncogenes and tumor suppressor genes also retard the normal process of cell death, leading to aggregations of altered cells that eventually form tumors. Recently a third class of genes, the DNA mismatch repair genes, have been found to be the inherited defect in most hereditary cancers of the colon and some other sites. Mutations in these genes impair the ability of cells to repair errors in single nucleotides (Table 6.2).

Table 6.2. Genes and cancer risk: Inherited mutations in these genes are associated with high risk of the cancers indicated

Cancer Type and Gene	Tumor Type	Gene Class
Familial breast cancer		
BRCA1	Breast, ovary	Tumor suppressor
BRCA2	Breast (female and male)	Tumor suppressor
PTEN	Breast (Cowden's syndrome)	Tumor suppressor
Familial adenomatous polyposis		
APC	Colon cancer	Tumor suppressor
Hereditary non-polyposis colon cancer		
HMSH2	Colon, endometrium, other	DNA mismatch repair
HMSH1	Colon, endometrium, other	DNA mismatch repair
HMSH6	Colon	DNA mismatch repair
PMS 1,2	Colon	DNA mismatch repair
Familial melanoma		
P16	Melanoma, other	Tumor suppressor
Brain		
NF-1	Neurofibromas	Tumor suppressor
NF-2	Schwannomas, meningiomas	Tumor suppressor
Thyroid		
RET	Thyroid, other endocrine	Oncogene
Kidney		
WT-1	Wilm's Tumor	Tumor suppressor
VHL	Renal carcinoma, other	Tumor suppressor
MET	Papillary renal cancer	Oncogene
Li-Fraumeni syndrome		
P53	Sarcomas, breast and brain	Tumor suppressor
Retinoblastoma		
RB1	Retinoblastoma, osteosarcoma	Tumor suppressor
Xeroderma Pigmentosum		
XPA to XPG, XPV	Basal and squamous cell carcinoma, melanoma	DNA repair

4.   INTERVENTION AND SURVEILLANCE

The identification of potent inherited susceptibility genes to cancer have created new opportunities for interventions to reduce morbidity and mortality (see recommendations). It may be helpful for particularly these cancer prone individuals to reduce exposures to environmental carcinogens involved in tumor promotion and progression. Researchers are seeking natural products and medicinal agents that can retard or prevent cancer development (chemoprevention), particularly in susceptible individuals. In addition, more intensive medical surveillance for early detection might be more cost-effective among high-risk groups. From the knowledge of molecular mechanisms of carcinogenesis, new therapeutic agents are being developed to target specific mutant genes.   On the other hand, genetic information can have adverse psychological, social and economic consequences. Currently, research is underway to identify means to use newly available genetic information in ways that maximize benefits and minimize risks [5]. Until we know more, genetic testing of members of the general population is premature.

Despite the major advances in studies of hereditary cancers, the field is still in its infancy. Potent single gene disorders that are highly predictive of cancer development are rare in the general population, and account for less than ten percent of the total cancer burden. In contrast, every person carries multiple genes that are involved in the absorption, transport, metabolic activation, detoxification and excretion of environmental agents, including environmental carcinogens.   A defined dose of an environmental carcinogen may have profoundly different effects on cancer risk, depending on the individual's genetic constitution. For example, sunlight is known to cause skin cancer, one of the most common forms of cancer in humans. However, skin cancers are much more common in whites than in blacks, whose genetically endowed skin pigment minimizes absorption of harmful ultraviolet radiation.

CONCLUSIONS

To date, our knowledge of these complex genetic systems remains rudimentary. Ongoing research is attempting to define genetic factors that influence individual response to environmental carcinogens. The combined knowledge of environmental carcinogenesis from epidemiological studies and host susceptibility factors from laboratory studies will enhance the ability to identify additional causes of cancer in humans and target high-risk individuals for early interventions.

RECOMMENDATIONS

- Know if any close relatives (parents, brothers and sisters, children) have been diagnosed with cancer and let a health care provider know this information.
- Follow guidelines for screening for the major cancers, particularly for those who have a family history
- Because one or two family members have been diagnosed with cancer one is not doomed to get cancer, particularly if the cancers occurred at different sites.

SUGGESTED FURTHER READING

1. Andrews LB, Fullarton JE, Holtzman NA, Motulsky AG, eds. (1994) *Assessing Genetic Risks: Implications for Health and Social Policy.* Washington, D.C.: National Academy Press. (A book on the potential and ethical dilemmas of genetic testing for a variety of diseases including cancer).

REFERENCES

1. Cavanee WK, White RL (1995) The genetic basis of cancer. *Scientific Am* **272**: 72-79.
2. Eng C, Stratton M, Ponder B, *et al.* (1994) Familial Cancer Syndromes. (A review of familial cancer syndromes in which many members of a family are diagnosed with cancer.) *Lancet* **343**: 709-713.
3. Friend SH, Bernards R, Rogelj S, *et al.* (1986) A human DNA segment with properties of the gene that predisposes to retinoblastoma and osteosarcoma. *Nature* **323**: 643-646.
4. Knudson AG (1971) Mutation and cancer: statistical study of retinoblastoma. *Proc Natl Acad Sci* **68**: 820-823.
5. Anonymous (1994) Statement on use of DNA testing for presymptomatic identification of cancer risk. National Advisory Council for Human Genome Research. *JAMA* **271**: 785.

Chapter 7

Infectious Agents

Nancy Mueller, Sc.D.
Department of Epidemiology, Harvard School of Public Health, Boston, MA

INTRODUCTION

There is substantial evidence that a number of infectious agents play a causal role in a variety of human malignancies. These cancers include lymphomas, as would be expected from animal models, as well as other surprisingly diverse sites including the liver, cervix, stomach, nasopharynx, bladder, skin (Kaposi's sarcoma), and bile duct. Most of the oncogenic agents involved are viruses [1]. These viruses include two herpesviruses, Epstein Barr virus (EBV) and human herpesvirus 8/ Kaposi's sarcoma virus (HHV-8) [2]; the so-called high-risk strains of human papillomaviruses (HPV) [3]; two hepatotropic viruses, hepatitis B virus (HBV) and hepatitis C virus (HCV) [4]; and the retrovirus human T-cell lymphotropic virus type I (HTLV-I) [5]. In addition, two chronic parasitic infections, the blood fluke *Schistosoma haematobium* and the liver fluke *Opisthorchis viverrini*, have long been thought to be human carcinogens, and recently a bacterium, *Helicobacteri pylori*, has been implicated [6].

1. BIOLOGICAL FEATURES OF ONCOGENIC INFECTIONS

Table 7.1 summarizes the major oncogenic infections. Several of these agents are quite prevalent infections, such as the oncogenic strains of HPV to which many sexually active persons have been exposed, as well as EBV and *H. pylori*. Others are relatively uncommon such as HTLV-I, which is micro-endemic in relatively isolated populations in southern Japan, the Caribbean,

G.A. Colditz et al. (eds.), Cancer Prevention: The Causes and Prevention of Cancer - Volume I, 63–73.
© 2000 *Kluwer Academic Publishers.*

and elsewhere; and the parasitic flukes. HCV is an example of an oncogenic infection found throughout the world, but at a very low prevalence. The epidemiological patterns of HHV-8 and HBV infections are more variable.

The public health impact of these agents is substantial. It has been estimated that about 15 percent of all incident cases of cancer worldwide are attributable to infections; this accounts for 23 percent of all malignancies in economically developing countries and seven percent in developed countries [7]. In addition, since these malignancies tend to occur relatively early in life, their impact as person-years of life lost is somewhat greater than for other carcinogenic exposures.

The evaluation of causality for these infectious agents as human carcinogens is difficult, given the long latency involved and the relative rarity of malignancy [8]. That being said, the International Agency for Research on Cancer (IARC) has completed a series of monographs that review the evidence for carcinogenicity in humans for each. The Working Groups concluded that for almost of the agents, there is "sufficient evidence" for classification as a human carcinogen, with HHV-8 being classified as "probably carcinogenic" to humans. These judgments have rested heavily on the epidemiological evidence.

The agents described in Table 7.1 share several biologic characteristics. Each either establishes latency normally upon infection – such as EBV, or has the capacity to become a persistent or chronic infection under certain conditions – such as HBV. EBV is transmitted primarily via saliva between persons – often through kissing. Once a person is infected via close contact with a carrier who is shedding virus, the EB viral genome persists in conjunction with the host DNA in a sub-set of B-lymphocytes and in the oropharynx for the remainder of his or her life. Almost all adults have experienced infection with EBV and are thus carriers of these viral genes. The prevalence of pharyngeal EBV shedding among carriers is about 20 percent [9]. In contrast, HBV is an example of a conditionally chronic infection as detected by the presence of the HB surface antigen in an individual's blood. Most – but not all – HBV infections are cleared by an effective immune response. It is well documented that when HBV infection is acquired very early in life, a chronic infection is more likely to be established. The modification of risk for a virus-associated malignancy by the age (and probably dose) of infection with the agent is a common theme [1].

For each of these agents, the occurrence of malignancy is a relatively uncommon sequela of infection. This observation underscores the importance of host immunity in control of these latent or chronic infections. When host cellular immunity is severely compromised; for example, by chemotherapy for organ transplantation or by infection with the human immunodeficiency virus (HIV), the risk of malignancy secondary to the loss of control of latent viral infections is substantial [10].

The mechanisms of oncogenesis are fairly well understood for some infections, while for others they are not clearly defined. It has been shown that several of the viruses have evolved effective strategies to interfere with cell cycle control and induce transformation of infected cells. For example, in HPV-16 (the prototypic high-risk strain) infection, the viral product E6 inactivates the p53 tumor suppressor protein by inducing its rapid degradation. Similarly, the E7 protein binds with the tumor suppressor retinoblastoma protein (pRB), resulting in inactivation and degradation. E7 also activates cyclin-dependent kinase 2, which is involved in the transition from the G_1 to the S phase of the cell cycle. In HPV-associated cervical cancer, E6 and E7 are usually selectively expressed [11]. Similar viral protein - host gene interactions have been described for the EBV [12]. In HTLV-I infection, the product of the regulatory gene tax transactivates a number of host oncogenes, while down-regulating the expression of the DNA repair-enzyme gene for β-polymerase [5]. In contrast, the mechanisms by which HBV, HCV, *H. pylori,* and the oncogenic flukes induce malignancy are not at all defined, although a role for chronic inflammation with local tissue damage is often cited. A common feature of the natural history of these oncogenic infectious agents is that risk of malignancy is associated with a chronic or increased level of replication, raising the probability of secondary genetic damage to the target tissues via continued cell turnover.

Table 7.1 The major oncogenic infections, the major associated malignancies, and the estimated proportion attributable to the infection [Parkin and Pisani]

Agent	Malignancy	Estimated Proportion
Viruses		
EBV	Hodgkin's disease	35-50%
	Non-Hodgkin's lymphoma	10-15%
	Nasopharyngeal carcinoma	>95%
HBV	Hepatocellular carcinoma	35-50%
HCV	Hepatocellular carcinoma	20-30%
HHV-8	Kaposi's sarcoma	100%
HPV	Cervical cancer	>95%
HTLV-1	Adult T-cell leukemia/lymphoma	>95%
Bacteria		
H. pylori	Gastric carcinoma	42%
	Gastric lymphoma	75%
Parasitics		
S. haematobium	Bladder cancer	4%
O. viverrini	Cholangiocarcinoma	<5%

2.   VIRUS-ASSOCIATED MALIGNANCIES

2.1   Lymphomas

There are several well-described viral-associated lymphomas. The first example is HTLV-I and adult T-cell leukemia/lymphoma. Upon infection, HTLV-I establishes latency via integration of the reverse-transcribed DNA provirus into a sub-set of T-lymphocytes. No free virus is found in the non-cellular component of the blood.   Thus, transmission occurs through contaminated blood exposure, from mother-to-child primarily via breast milk, and through prolonged sexual exposure to an infected partner.   The risk of lymphoma in HTLV-I carriers is strongly related to having sustained a very early infection, and male carriers are at greater risk than females [5].

A second example is the EBV and Burkitt's lymphoma, a B-cell malignancy that occurs primarily in children. The detection of monoclonal EBV genome (or viral gene products) in Burkitt's cells, is characteristic of almost all cases of Burkitt's lymphoma occurring among African children, and in about 20 percent of the disease elsewhere. Again, very early infection with EBV appears to be important, and the risk is substantially greater in boys. The co-existence of holoendemic malaria is a strong risk factor [2].

The EBV is also clearly involved with about 35 to 50 percent of cases of Hodgkin's disease – as indexed by detection of monoclonal viral genome within the malignant Reed-Sternberg cells. Hodgkin's disease occurs most commonly in young adults - particularly those whose childhood social environment would foster susceptibility to "late" (post-adolescent) infection with the EBV [13].   Of note, late infections with many "childhood" infections including the EBV (seen clinically as infectious mononucleosis) can also be quite severe. In fact, history of infectious mononucleosis is an established risk factor for young adult Hodgkin's disease. Paradoxically, EBV-positive Hodgkin's disease occurs more commonly at the extremes of age, and is less common among young adults. Untangling this paradoxical relationship of EBV and the risk of Hodgkin's disease is the focus of current research [14].

2.2   Hepatocellular carcinoma

Hepatocellular carcinoma can be caused by chronic infection with either HBV or HCV [4]. Both viruses appear to act via chronic hepatitis, causing repeated cycles of cell death and regeneration. Hepatocellular cancer generally occurs in the presence of cirrhosis. In parallel, excessive alcohol consumption likely contributes to the risk of hepatocellular cancer in HBV and HCV carriers.

Chronic HBV infection is more common among Asian populations, and to a lesser degree among sub-Saharan Africans. In addition to blood-borne and perinatal exposure, the virus can be transmitted from a chronic carrier to household members and sexual contacts. As noted above, the risk of becoming chronically infected is strongly linked to early age at infection when cellular immunity is not fully established. With improvement in living standards with economic development, the prevalence of chronic HBV infection decreases rather rapidly, while that for seropositivity indicating past infection decreases more slowly. Following the institution of immunization of high-risk infants in Taiwan, there has been a reduction in HBV-associated hepatocellular cancer in the treated cohort [15]. Treatment of chronic HBV infection with interferonα and anti-viral agents is sometimes effective in clearing the infection, which would also reduce the risk of subsequent cancer.

HCV was identified in 1989 as the cause of much of what was termed "non-A-non-B" hepatitis". HCV is primarily transmitted by blood exposure, with the risk of sexual and perinatal transmission apparently quite low. The virus is worldwide in distribution with a low prevalence of infected persons of about one to two percent. The recent increase of hepatocellular carcinoma in the United States likely reflects the spread of HCV with the expansion of intravenous drug use during the 1960s. Rates of HCV infection are somewhat higher in parts of Japan and other Asian populations, in the Middle East, and in parts of Africa. The epidemiology and natural history of HCV infection is not well described. It appears that the risk of development of a chronic HCV infection following initial infection is high, about 85 percent in adults. The comparable rates for infection among children are not known. Current data suggest that among those with chronic HCV infection – as evidenced by the detection of viral RNA in blood, about 60 to 80 percent will develop chronic hepatitis, of whom 20 to 40 percent will subsequently develop cirrhosis. The proportion of those with HCV-induced cirrhosis that will develop hepatocellular carcinoma is estimated to be three to six percent a year [16]. Recent studies of combination anti-viral and interferon α chemotherapy for clearing the chronic HCV infection have been promising, and may reduce the risk of malignancy.

2.3   Cervical cancer

The HPVs comprise a large family of related strains that are highly adapted to infect various epithelial surfaces throughout the body. These viruses are extremely prevalent and are transmitted primarily by direct contact. The HPVs can cause benign warts and in some cases, malignancy. The evidence linking several of the sexually transmitted types to cervical cancer is now well-established [3]. In fact, assays for detection of the high-risk HPVs are likely to become part of routine cervical screening. Essentially all sexually active women have been exposed to genitally transmitted HPV infections. Factors related to infection with the high-risk strains include a woman's, as well as her partners', history of sexual exposure. The probability that HPV infections persist and if so, for how long varies among individuals [17]. The age at which a woman becomes sexually active appears to play a role, as cervical cancer risk is increased when early sexual exposure precedes the full maturation of the cervix. Not surprisingly, these same genital HPV infections are also implicated in other anogenital cancers [3]. It is likely that these and other sub-types may prove to be involved in malignancy of other infected sites including the upper respiratory tree and skin.

2.4   Nasopharyngeal carcinoma

Nasopharyngeal carcinoma commonly arises in a region of the nasopharynx rich with lymphoreticular tissue [2]. It is most commonly seen in persons of southern Chinese origin [18], suggesting that genetic factors are important in its etiology. The EBV is strongly implicated in the occurrence of nasopharyngeal carcinoma, with the detection of EBV genome or gene products in virtually all cases of the non-differentiated sub-type [2]. Viral clonality has been demonstrated in pre-cancerous lesions. It is likely that early infection with EBV is important as well as exposure to highly salted food in infancy.

2.5   Kaposi's sarcoma

Kaposi's sarcoma is a rare malignancy of endothelial spindle cells, which characteristically appears as multiple pigmented lesions of the skin and occasionally of the internal organs. The epidemiology of Kaposi's sarcoma includes the "classic type" involving elderly men of Mediterranean and eastern European origin, the "endemic type" occurring in Africa, and the "epidemic type" occurring in AIDS and in other immune suppressed patients [2].

The detection in 1994 of a new herpesvirus from a Kaposi's sarcoma lesion biopsy taken from an AIDS patient, and the demonstration of the viral genome in multiple biopsy series of cases confirmed the long-held suspicion of a viral etiology. HHV-8 appears to be transmitted primarily by sexual contact, and the risk of malignancy among carriers is strongly modified by co-existing immune suppression. The natural history of this infection, its persistency, and its oncogenic mechanisms are not well defined. It is likely that genetic factors related to immune function are associated with increased risk of the malignancy among HHV-8 carriers. Like its distant cousin the EBV, HHV-8 carries a number of genes whose products interfere with regulation of the cell cycle [2].

3. OTHER INFECTION-ASSOCIATED MALIGNANCIES

3.1 Gastric cancer

There is substantial evidence that chronic *H. pylori* infection is involved in the development of gastric adenocarcinoma and in some cases of gastric lymphoma [6]. This is most evident for the strains that carry the CagA gene, which produces a potent inflammatory cytotoxin. Transmission of this bacterium appears to occur via fecal-oral or oral-oral routes. The infection colonizes the gastric mucosa, but can be cleared with appropriate anti-biotic treatment. The epidemiological evidence that stomach cancer rates generally vary inversely with level of economic development supports the role of early infection in pathogenesis [19]. The development of malignancy is thought to be secondary to chronic gastritis, which may often be asymptomatic. The pathogenic pathway proceeds through atrophy, intestinal metaplasia, dysplasia, to adenocarcinoma [20]. A diet high in fruits and vegetables and low in salt intake appears to be protective for gastric cancer. Several intervention trials are now underway to evaluate the efficacy of eradicating the infection with antibiotics in high-risk populations.

3.2 Bladder cancer

Infection with *S. haematobium,* a parasitic blood fluke, is an established cause of bladder cancer [6]. *S. haematobium* mature and live in the veins that drain the urinary bladder of humans, with an intermediary reproductive phase in susceptible snails via eggs shed in urine and feces. The adult worms can live up to 30 years in an infected host. Risk of infection is dependent on skin or oral exposure to contaminated freshwater in endemic areas. This is a widespread infection in Africa, the eastern Mediterranean region, Turkey, and India. The infection is curable with appropriate drugs. Most of the pathogenesis of the infection is secondary to the chronic irritation of the copious egg production; these can survive for up to three weeks in bladder epithelium. Risk of bladder cancer is associated with heavy long term infection.

3.3   Choliangiocarcinoma

Infection with *O. viverrini*, a parasitic liver fluke, is an established cause
of bile duct carcinoma [6]. *O. viverrini* establish a chronic infection within
the smaller intrahepatic bile ducts of infected humans. Its life cycle includes
a reproductive stage in susceptible snails, infected via eggs shed through
fecal contamination, followed by an infective stage in fish. Transmission to
humans occurs with ingestion of raw contaminated fish. The fluke can live
for up to 25 years in an infected host. Again, pathogenesis is secondary to
the chronic irritation of eggs in the bile duct tissue. Infection with *O.
viverrini* is treatable, and the cycle can be broken by changes in dietary
patterns. Again, the risk of developing choliangiocarcinoma among carriers
includes heavy infection of long duration.

3.4   Public Education and Policy Development

Measures to reduce the burden of cancer from these infections fall into
two categories: the primary prevention of infection itself, and secondary
prevention of progression among carriers of these infections. Primary
prevention of infection itself by vaccination appears to be achievable for
HBV infection to a large extent. In many high-risk areas that are
economically developed, as well as much of the western world, vaccination
programs for newborns are in place. The development of candidate HPV
vaccines is now underway, but is not in the foreseeable future for the other
infections.

The most important policy to reduce the burden of these oncogenic
infections is to eliminate infection by contaminated blood. This is essential
for the reduction of the transmission of HCV, HTLV-I, HBV, and HIV (a
strong contributing factor to the development of virus-induced
malignancies). The screening of blood products for these agents is now
commonly done in many parts of the economically developed world. Much
more worrisome and highly controversial is the control of self-selected
exposure to injectable drugs (or other percutaneous exposure such as
tattooing) with contaminated needles. Policies to reduce this route of
exposure include education of children and young adults to prevent the use
of intravenous drugs; and for users, availability of drug treatment and needle
exchange programs.

Measures to reduce and control sexually transmitted diseases –
particularly by barrier methods – as discussed in Chapter 19, is a necessary
but not sufficient measure for primary prevention of several of these
infections including HPV, HHV-8, HBV; to a lesser extent HTLV-I and
HCV; and the contributing infection of HIV. Again effective education

programs for children and young adults to postpone sexual activity and increase safer sex practices are indicated.

Much less controversial are education programs to improve hygiene, particularly among young children, and their caretakers. Simple hand washing, for example, is a proven measure that we tend to overlook. Yet the declining rates of gastric cancer that have been documented throughout the world likely reflect the delay in age of infection with *H. pylori* with better living conditions and improved hygiene in the past century. In the endemic areas for *S. haematobium* and *O. viverrini*, behavioral interventions to reduce exposure to contaminated freshwater and to raw fish (respectively) will reduce primary infections, among other control measures. There is little to be done - and reason not to - to prevent EBV infection. Prudence suggests that parents and caretakers of young children should try to minimize very early exposure – via oral kissing or pre-chewing of food.

In terms of secondary prevention of progression to cancer, a policy of screening for HBV and HCV chronic carriers is necessary in order to determine if treatment is appropriate and to offer counseling for reduction of alcohol consumption. Policies for treatment for *H. pylori* infection need to be established. The availability of Pap screening with appropriate follow-up and treatment for sexually active women clearly reduces the incidence of invasive cervical cancer. In the endemic areas for *S. haematobium* and *O. viverrini*, appropriate drug treatment must be available.

CONCLUSIONS

The impact of these infections on the burden of cancer in the United States is becoming increasingly evident as they are largely responsible for the cascade of opportunistic malignancies accompanying the AIDS epidemic. Although the HIV is not in itself oncogenic, by damaging host immune control of latent infections, it contributes to the carcinogenesis of the oncogenic viruses – particularly EBV and HHV-8. In global terms, the burden is heaviest among populations in developing countries, reflecting the impact of very early infection with these agents on subsequent risk of cancer. Some of the burden can be reduced by primary prevention such as by universal HBV vaccination. Some can be reduced by secondary prevention, such as treatment for HCV infection. Those policies involving sexual behavior and the use of injectable drugs are controversial, and their adoption for the control of HIV infection in the United States has been contentious. It is somewhat ironic that such policies also play a role in cancer control.

SUMMARY POINTS

- Several infectious agents are known to play a causal role in the development of cancer.
- The age at infection and the host immune competency influence the risk of cancer.
- Primary prevention of infection can be achieved by a number of interventions including protection against sexual and blood-borne transmission.
- Secondary prevention for the development of malignancy can be achieved in some cases by medical intervention.

RECOMMENDATIONS

- Implement effective public policies for the prevention of HIV infection as a means for reducing the spread of oncogenic infections;
- Insure HBV vaccination for infants and regular Pap smearing for sexually active girls and women;
- Insure the availability of treatment (when medically appropriate) and counseling to reduce alcoholic consumption for HBV and HCV carriers;
- Develop guidelines for the treatment of *H. pylori* infection.

SUGGESTED FURTHER READING

1. Evans AS, Kaslow R, eds. (1997) *Viral Infections of Humans: Epidemiology and Control.* Fourth edition New York: Plenum Publishers.
2. IARC Working Group on the Evaluation of Carcinogenic Risks to Humans (1994) *Hepatitis Viruses.* Volume 59. Lyon, France: IARC.
3. IARC Working Group on the Evaluation of Carcinogenic Risks to Humans (1994) *Schistosomes, Liver Flukes and* Helicobacter Pylori . Volume 61. Lyon, France: IARC.
4. IARC Working Group on the Evaluation of Carcinogenic Risks to Humans (1995) *Human Papillomaviruses.* Volume 64. Lyon, France: IARC.
5. IARC Working Group on the Evaluation of Carcinogenic Risks to Humans (1996) *Human Immunodeficiency Viruses and Human T-cell Lymphotropic Viruses.* Volume 67. Lyon, France: IARC.
6. IARC Working Group on the Evaluation of Carcinogenic Risks to Humans (1997) *Human* Epstein-Barr *Virus and Kaposi's Sarcoma Herpesvirus/Human Herpesvirus 8.* Volume 70. Lyon, France: IARC.

REFERENCES

1. Mueller N, Evans AS, London T (1996) Viruses. In: Schottenfeld D, Fraumeni JF Jr., eds. *Cancer Epidemiology and Prevention.* Second Edition. New York, NY (USA): Oxford University Press, pp. 501-31.
2. IARC Working Group on the Evaluation of Carcinogenic Risks to Humans. (1997) *Epstein-Barr Virus and Kaposi's Sarcoma Herpesvirus/Human Herpesvirus 8.* Volume 70. Lyon, France: IARC.
3. IARC Working Group on the Evaluation of Carcinogenic Risks to Humans (1995) *Human Papillomaviruses.* Volume 64. Lyon, France: IARC.
4. IARC Working Group on the Evaluation of Carcinogenic Risks to Humans (1994) *Hepatitis Viruses.* Volume 59. Lyon, France: IARC.
5. IARC Working Group on the Evaluation of Carcinogenic Risks to Humans (1996) Human Immunodeficiency Viruses and Human T-Cell Lymphotropic Viruses. Volume 67. Lyon, France: IARC.
6. IARC Working Group on the Evaluation of Carcinogenic Risks to Humans (1994) *Schistosomes, Liver Flukes and* Helicobacter Pylori. Volume 61. Lyon, France: IARC.
7. Parkin DM, Pisani P, Muñoz N, *et al.* (1999) The global burden of infection associated cancers. In: *Cancer Surveys Volume 33: Infections and Human Cancer.* (In press)
8. Evans AS, Mueller NE (1990) Viruses and cancer-causal associations. *Ann Epidemiol* **1:** 71-92.
9. Evans AS, Mueller NE (1997) Epstein-Barr virus and malignant lymphomas. In: Evans AS, Kaslow R, eds. *Viral Infections of Humans: Epidemiology and Control.* Fourth Edition. New York, NY (USA): Plenum Publishers, pp. 985-933.
10. Mueller N (1999) Overview of the epidemiology of malignancy in immune-deficiency. *JAIDS* **21**(Suppl 1): S5-S10.
11. Alani RM, Münger K (1998) Human papillomaviruses. *Sci Med* **5:** 28-35.
12. Spender LC, Cannell EJ, Hollyoake M, *et al.* (1999) Control of cell cycle entry and apoptosis in B lymphocytes by Epstein-Barr virus. *J Virol* **73:** 4678-4688.
13. Mueller N (1996) Hodgkin's disease. In: Schottenfeld D, Fraumeni JF, Jr., eds. *Cancer Epidemiology and Prevention.* Second Edition. New York, NY (USA): Oxford University Press, pp. 893-919.
14. Mueller NE (1997) Epstein-Barr virus and Hodgkin's disease: an epidemiological paradox. *Epstein-Barr Virus Report,* pp. 1-2.
15. Chang M-H, Chen C-J, Lai M-S, *et al.* (1997) Universal hepatitis B vaccination in Taiwan and the incidence of hepatocellular carcinoma in children. *N Engl J Med* **336:** 1855-1859.
16. Okuda K (1997) Hepatitis C virus and hepatocellular carcinoma. In: Okuda K, Tabor E, eds. *Liver Cancer.* New York, NY (USA): Churchill Livingston, pp. 39-50.
17. Herrero R, Muñoz N (1999) HPV and cancer. In: *Cancer Surveys. Volume 33: Infections and Human Cancer.* (In press).
18. de-Thé G, Ho JHC, Muir CS (1997) Nasopharyngeal carcinoma. In: Evans AS, Kaslow R, eds. *Viral Infections of Humans: Epidemiology and Control.* Fourth Edition. New York, NY (USA): Plenum Publishers, pp. 935-967.
19. Fuchs CS, Mayer RJ (1995) Gastric carcinoma. *N Engl J Med* **333:** 32-40.
20. Telford JL, Covacci A, Rappouli R, Ghiara P (1997) Immunobiology of Helicobacter pylori infection. *Curr Opin Immunol* **9:** 498-503.

Chapter 8

Reproductive Factors and Cancer Risk

Stacey A. Missmer, M.Sc. and Susan E. Hankinson, Sc.D.
Channing Laboratory, Department of Medicine, Brigham and Women's Hospital and Harvard Medical School, Boston, MA and Department of Epidemiology, Harvard School of Public Health, Boston, MA.

INTRODUCTION

Reproductive factors have been evaluated in relation to cancer development at several major sites including the breast, ovary, endometrium, cervix and colon. Reproductive factors are generally considered to be characteristics specifically related to reproduction (*e.g.,* parity, age at first birth, lactation) or that mark a change in a woman's reproductive capacity (*e.g.,* age at menarche, menopause) but may also include factors such as *in utero* exposures.

Most of these factors are associated with substantial hormonal changes. Menarche marks the beginning of menstruation (and ovulation), and each pregnancy is associated with large increases in circulating hormones, particularly estrogens. Menopause marks the end of menstruation and is associated with substantial decreases in estrogen levels and increases in gonadotropin levels compared to premenopausal women. It is because of these hormonal changes, and the resulting established or possible effects on a number of tissues, that reproductive factors have been hypothesized to influence cancer risk.

In the last decade, epidemiologic research has improved our understanding of the effect of reproductive choices such as childbirth, breast feeding, gynecologic surgeries, and induced abortion, as well as the biologic implications of pre- and perinatal exposures.

G.A. Colditz et al. (eds.), Cancer Prevention: The Causes and Prevention of Cancer - Volume I, 75–86.

1.   BREAST CANCER

Nulliparity, late age at first birth, early age at menarche and late age at menopause all have been consistently associated with an increase in breast cancer risk [1]. For each of these factors, the breast cancer risk tends to increase (or decrease) incrementally throughout the range of the variable so that there is no single high risk or low risk group. For example, risk tends to increase with increasing age at menopause from before 40 years of age to after 50 years of age.

In general, these reproductive factors are modestly related to risk of breast cancer. Women who have a first birth after age 30 years have a 50 to 100 percent higher risk of breast cancer relative to women who had their first child by age 20. Women who have menarche by age 12 have only a 20 to 30 percent higher breast cancer risk compared to women who had menarche at age 14 years. The relationship is somewhat stronger for age at menopause, with a relative risk of approximately 2.0 for menopause after age 54 *vs.* before age 45 [2].

The relationship between parity and breast cancer risk is more complex. Relative to nulliparous women, breast cancer risk is actually increased for one to two decades after giving birth, perhaps because of the increased exposure to circulating steroid hormones during pregnancy or to growth of the mammary tissue in preparation for lactation [2]. After this time, however, breast cancer risk is greater in nulliparous women as compared to parous women (RR = 1.1-2.0) [3]. This delayed (but long lasting) reduction in risk may be related to hormone-induced changes in the epithelial cells of the breast that result in their decreased susceptibility to carcinogens [2]. Also, there appears to be a very modest, incremental decrease in risk with increasing parity and with births that are spaced more closely together relative to those that are spaced further apart [2]. Overall, the reduction in risk associated with parity outweighs the initial increase in risk, as the reduction occurs later in life when a woman's absolute breast cancer risk is much higher.

Findings for the relationship between lactation and breast cancer risk have been less consistent; generally, no association or an inverse association (primarily among premenopausal women) has been reported [4]. In a large, population-based case-control study of parous women residing in four U.S. states, a lower risk of breast cancer was observed among premenopausal women who had breastfed relative to similar women who had never breast fed (OR = 0.78, 95% CI = 0.66-0.91). However, no effect of breast feeding was found among postmenopausal women (OR = 1.04, 95% CI = 0.95-1.14). This relationship persisted when duration of lactation was evaluated, with an inverse relationship between duration and risk of breast cancer among premenopausal women (test for trend $p < 0.001$) but no discernible trend among postmenopausal women ($p = 0.51$) [4]. Of the 32 studies published through 1998, only about half found a statistically significant decrease in risk with increasing duration of lactation, with the strongest effect noted in women with very high parity [2]. Additional assessments that include more precise characterization of the breastfeeding itself (*e.g.,* exclusive breast *vs.* bottle supplemented feeding) are needed.

Although the associations are modest, these reproductive factors are thought to account for a substantial part of the difference in breast cancer rates observed internationally as the contrast between countries for each of these factors is larger than that generally observed within a single country. For example, the average age at menarche is 12 or 13 years in the U.S. and other developed countries compared to a mean age of about 17 years in rural China.

The precise mechanisms underlying these associations are as yet unknown. One or more estrogens, or other growth factors, are hypothesized to increase risk by promoting cell division and thereby increasing the possibility of genetic errors [2]. Given this, an early age at menarche and a late age at menopause would result in a longer lifetime exposure to higher estrogen levels and thus a greater breast cancer risk. In addition, the hormonal changes associated with pregnancy may lead to differentiation of the breast tissue that increases the length of the cell cycle phase during which DNA is repaired. Over the long run, these changes may decrease the tissue's susceptibility to carcinogens [2].

Abortion, whether spontaneous or induced, and its relationship to breast cancer risk has been a controversial topic during the past decade. While it is hypothesized that the hormonal profile of a women who chooses to terminate a viable pregnancy would differ from that of a pregnancy that ends in miscarriage, many epidemiologic studies have not distinguished between the two. In addition, studies differ by their choice of reference group – some using women who have never been pregnant and others using parous women who have never had an abortion, all in comparison to women who previously had an abortion. Exposure assessment also is complicated by the legal changes and social stigma surrounding induced abortion and the inability to detect many spontaneous abortions [5].

In 1996, a meta-analysis of 25 individual studies of the relationship between induced abortion and breast cancer was conducted [6]. The overall odds ratio for women who had ever had an induced abortion compared to women who had never had an induced abortion was 1.3 (95% CI = 1.2-1.4). However, 24 of the 25 studies in this analysis were case-control studies where accuracy of recall or reporting of these events may vary between case and control groups, leading to a biased relative risk. Prospective analyses circumvent this potential problem. In a very large and well-conducted prospective study with 28.5 million woman-years, contributed by a cohort of Danish women for whom induced abortion information was available through the Danish National Registry of Induced Abortion no association was found between induced abortion and breast cancer risk (multivariate RR = 1.00, 95% CI = 0.94-1.06). Risk was not modified by number of induced abortions or full-term pregnancy (either before or after induced abortion) [7]. These data provide substantial evidence against any important association between abortion and subsequent breast cancer risk.

There has also been growing interest in the effect of the intrauterine environment on breast cancer risk, as several maternal and fetal conditions influence the level of *in utero* estrogen exposure. For example, it is known that twin gestations exhibit higher estrogen levels than do singleton pregnancies. A recent case-control study among women under age 55 indicated that the risk of breast cancer among twins was higher than that among singleton births (RR = 1.6, 95% CI = 1.0-2.7), especially in dizygotic twins (RR = 2.1) [8]. It is also known that pre-eclampsia is marked by low estrogen levels while the perinatal conditions of jaundice and prematurity are correlated with high estrogen levels. In one study, the risk of breast cancer was decreased in those women whose mothers had pre-eclampsia (OR = 0.41, 95% CI = 0.22-0.79), while those who as infants were jaundiced or <33 weeks gestation were at significantly increased risk (OR = 2.2, 95% CI = 1.3-3.7; OR = 4.0, 95% CI = 1.5-10.8, respectively) [9]. Finally, in several, but not all studies, a positive association between birthweight, a marker of higher *in utero* hormone levels, and breast cancer risk has been reported [10]. Although the data remain limited and not entirely consistent, increasing evidence suggests some influence of *in utero* exposures on subsequent breast cancer risk.

Table 8.1 Reproductive risk factors for breast cancer

Reproductive factor	Approximate strength of relative risk
Menarche at <12 years *vs.* 14	1.2-1.3
First birth at >30 years *vs.* <20	1.5-2.0
Lactation ever *vs.* never (premenopausal women)	0.6-0.9
Menopause at >54 years *vs.* <45	1.8-2.2

2.   OVARIAN CANCER

Most ovarian cancers arise from epithelial cells that make up the external surface of the ovary. Ovulation may increase ovarian cancer risk by subjecting these epithelial cells to repeated minor trauma (occurring when the ovum breaks through the surface epithelium during ovulation), increased cellular division (associated with repair of the surface epithelium after each ovulation) or exposure to hormone-rich fluid that surrounds the ovum [11]. This theory suggests that factors that decrease the number of ovulations (*e.g.* parity) would decrease ovarian cancer risk. High levels of gonadotropins, hormones secreted by the pituitary, also have been hypothesized to increase ovarian cancer risk. As pregnancy decreases gonadotropin levels and a late age at menopause would postpone exposure to high postmenopausal gonadotropin levels, each of these factors would be expected to reduce ovarian cancer risk according to this hypothesis.

By far the most consistent finding in epidemiologic studies of ovarian cancer has been the inverse association with parity [12-14]. A trend of increasing protection from this cancer with increasing parity has been observed in most studies. Generally, relative to nulliparous women, women who have one child have a 10 to 15 percent lower risk of ovarian cancer, and women who have had three or more children have a 30 to 50 percent lower risk of ovarian cancer [15].

Results have been much less consistent for age at first birth, age at menarche, age at menopause and lactation in relation to ovarian cancer risk. In a combined analysis of several European studies, nulliparous women and women having a first pregnancy after age 34 had a modestly higher risk of cancer compared to women who had their first child at an earlier age [13]. In a large Norwegian cohort study, the observed reduction in risk due to parity was greatest with higher age at last birth and shorter time since last delivery. Although not true of multiparous women, among women with only one child, older age at first birth decreased risk [16]. In contrast, in a U.S. pooled analysis of 12 case-control studies [12] and in a large prospective study [14], little association was noted. Given the data accumulated to date, age at first birth, at least in women <35 years, does not appear to have a substantial effect on ovarian cancer risk.

Although not as well-established as the relationship between parity and ovarian cancer there is more consistent support for a protective effect of lactation than for the other reproductive variables just reviewed. In a recent case-control study conducted in Australia (n = 824 cases, 855 community controls), a possible modest inverse association per month of lactation was observed among premenopausal women (OR = 0.98, 95% CI 0.95-1.01) but not among postmenopausal women (OR = 1.00, 95% CI = 0.99-1.01) [17]. A similar modest inverse association was reported in the pooled analysis of 12 case-control studies [12].

In most studies, little if any relationship has been observed between late age at menarche and ovarian cancer risk [12, 14]. However, in a case-control study conducted in China, age at menarche ≥18 years (later age at menarche than has been assessed in any developed country) was noted to be protective [18]. Overall, there appears to be little effect of age at menarche on ovarian cancer risk, at least within the range of ages that menarche typically occurs in Western societies. Similarly, no consistent association has been noted between age at menopause and ovarian cancer risk; in most studies, age at menopause has generally been found to be either unrelated or positively related to risk.

Having had a tubal ligation has been consistently associated with a decrease in risk of ovarian cancer, although the magnitude of this reduction has varied substantially between studies (with relative risks ranging from 0.2 to 0.8). A strong inverse relationship was observed between tubal ligation and ovarian cancer risk after 12 years of follow-up of 121,700 women participating in the Nurses' Health Study (RR = 0.33, 95% CI = 0.16–0.64). This protective effect persisted even after excluding cases diagnosed in the first four years of follow-up, suggesting that the relative risk was not affected by detection bias. Within this cohort the risk of ovarian cancer was also decreased among women who had had a hysterectomy (RR = 0.67, 95% CI = 0.45-1.00) [19]. Similarly within an Australian case-control study, a 39 percent lower risk of ovarian cancer (95% CI = 0.46-0.85) was observed in women who had had a tubal ligation and a 36 percent lower risk in women who had had a hysterectomy (95% CI = 0.48-0.85) [20]. These gynecologic surgeries may decrease the risk of ovarian cancer development either by impeding the transport of carcinogenic substances into the peritoneal cavity, or by influencing ovarian blood flow thus altering exposure to pituitary gonadotropins and other hormones and decreasing the frequency of ovulation.

Table 8.2 Reproductive risk factors for ovarian cancer

Reproductive factor	Approximate strength of relative risk
Nulliparous *vs.* >2 children	1.4-1.8
Per month of lactation	0.9-1.0
Tubal ligation	0.3-0.9

3.   ENDOMETRIAL CANCER

The incidence of endometrial cancer has been closely linked to exposure to unopposed estrogen (*i.e.*, estrogen in the absence of progesterone) and as such is related to a number of reproductive variables [21, 22]. Late age at menopause is positively associated with this disease, presumably due to the longer period of exposure to high premenopausal estrogen levels. Early age at menarche has generally been found to increase endometrial cancer risk, although whether this association is independent of obesity (a known risk factor for endometrial cancer) is unclear. Similar to the epidemiology of breast cancer, parity appears to lower the risk of endometrial cancer. Only a handful of studies have evaluated the relationship between age at first birth and endometrial cancer and their findings have been rather inconsistent and generally do not support any substantial association.

The largest prospective study to evaluate the association between reproductive factors and risk of endometrial cancer is the Iowa Women's Health Study [23]. During 5 years of follow-up of a cohort of 24,848 postmenopausal women, with 167 incident cases, risk of endometrial cancer increased with increasing gravidity (test for trend $p < 0.0005$) with a relative risk of 0.49 (95% CI = 0.33-0.75) comparing women who had ever been pregnant to women who were never pregnant. Earlier age at menarche (test for trend $p < 0.005$) and older age at natural menopause (test for trend $p < 0.0005$) were also found to be linearly related to cancer risk. Neither age at first nor age at last pregnancy was associated with endometrial cancer risk.

Data are much more limited on the relationships between endometrial cancer and both abortion and miscarriage. In the Iowa Women's Health Study, an increased risk was observed among those who reported having had an induced abortion (RR = 2.5, 95% CI = 1.1-5.7), however this comparison had only six exposed cases. Among gravid women, the risk of endometrial cancer was lower among those who had had a miscarriage during the first or middle pregnancy (RR = 0.48, 95% CI = 0.28-0.85) but non-significantly higher among those who had had a miscarriage in their last pregnancy (RR = 1.34, 95% CI 0.79-2.26) relative to women who had never had a recognized miscarriage. The authors suggest that the latter finding may mark a progesterone deficiency [23]. These findings all require further confirmation.

4.   CERVICAL CANCER

The reproductive risk factors most consistently associated with an increase in risk of cervical cancer are having had multiple sexual partners and having an early age at first intercourse [24], factors that are primarily surrogates for infection with human papilloma virus (HPV), a well-established cause of cervical cancer. Of the 33 types of HPV that have been identified to date, types 16 and 18 have consistently been shown to be the infective agent in >90 percent of cervical cancer cases with observed relative risks ranging from 20 to 150 [25]. In several, but not all, studies where the number of sexual partners and age at intercourse could be accounted for in the analysis, high levels of parity were observed to independently increase disease risk [24]. This possible association may be related to the hormonal changes of pregnancy or to cervical trauma occurring during childbirth. Neither age at menarche nor age at menopause has been associated with cervical cancer risk.

Within the population of 1.3 million women born in Norway between 1935 and 1971, 2870 cases of cervical cancer were identified as of 1991. Among parous women, no effect of parity was noted, however, risk was decreased with later age at first birth (RR = 0.54, 95% CI = 0.46-0.62 comparing age >27 to <21 at first birth). The risk of cervical cancer among nulliparous women was similar to that of parous women with age at first birth of 24 [26]. These relationships continue to support the complicated sociodemographic relationship between sexual choices, risk of HPV infection, and progression to virally induced cervical cancer. In addition, the effect of age at first birth may not only represent patterns of sexual activity that increase the risk of HPV infection but also the action of HPV in the immature/adolescent as compared to the mature cervix.

5.   COLON CANCER

The observation that nuns were at higher risk of colon cancer relative to other women, in addition to gender differences in colon cancer incidence rates and tumor site distribution, first sparked interest in the relationships between reproductive factors (particularly parity) and colon cancer risk. Results of epidemiologic studies have been inconsistent however, such that, although a modest association between parity and colon cancer cannot be ruled out, no substantial association is likely to exist [27].

In the largest prospective study of these relationships with 501 cases who were diagnosed during 1,012,280 woman-years of follow-up, risk of colorectal cancer was not associated with either parity or age at menopause [28]. A trend of decreasing risk with increasing age at menarche was noted, however (RR for age at menarche ≥14 *vs.* ≤13 = 0.83, 95% CI = 0.64-1.08, test for trend $p = 0.01$). Among parous women, risk of colorectal cancer was higher if age at first pregnancy was ≥30 years compared to <24 years;

however, no association was observed with age at first birth in a number of other studies. Overall, to date, none of the reproductive factors have been consistently related to colon cancer.

6. OTHER FACTORS RELATED TO REPRODUCTION

Several other reproductive factors have been hypothesized to increase or decrease risk of specific cancers. Menstrual cycle length and regularity may be associated with risk of breast, endometrial and ovarian cancers, although relatively few studies have addressed these relationships and consistent findings have yet to emerge. In several, but not all, studies, men who have had a vasectomy had a relative risk of prostate cancer of 1.3 to 2.0 compared to men who did not have this procedure; this increased risk was generally observed only after an induction period of 10 to 20 years. Finally, *in utero* exposures have been considered as risk factors for prostate and testicular cancer. In several studies, men with higher birthweights, neonatal jaundice, and who had mothers who were older at delivery or did not have pre-eclampsia have been found to be at higher risk for prostate cancer. In contrast to *in utero* risk factors for breast cancer, premature delivery ($\leq$36 weeks gestation) may reduce the risk of prostate cancer. In the several studies of *in utero* exposures and testicular cancer, lower birthweight, higher maternal age, lower birth order, and maternal pregnancy symptoms of nausea and spotting have all been shown to increase risk; however, the effects may be modified by histologic type (seminomas *vs.* non-seminomas) [10].

CONCLUSION

Several reproductive factors have been consistently associated with risks of breast, ovarian, and endometrial cancers. Findings for age at menarche and menopause, parity and age at first birth in relation to risk of breast cancer have been extremely consistent, although the associations are generally modest in magnitude. A strong and consistent inverse association has been observed for both parity and tubal ligation and risk of ovarian cancer; relationships with other reproductive risk factors are less clear. The relationship between unopposed estrogen and endometrial cancer has been well established, however the association with parity and other reproductive factors bears further investigation. Reproductive factors generally do not appear to have an important role in the incidence of colon cancer. Factoring these reproductive exposures into an assessment of an individual's risk of cancer is important, however, with a few exceptions (*e.g.,* prevention of HPV infection for cervical cancer), their overall importance to cancer prevention efforts will be limited as most of the factors are not easily modifiable.

SUMMARY POINTS

- Late age at first birth, early age at menarche, late age at menopause, and nulliparity are each associated with an increase in breast cancer risk.
- Nulliparity increases the risk of ovarian cancer, while tubal ligation has been found to decrease risk.
- Although less well studied, nulliparity and late age at menopause appear to increase the risk of endometrial cancer.

RECOMMENDATIONS

- Reproductive history will influence cancer risk, this information should be factored into overall risk profile.
- An absence of reproductive risk factors to does not prevent breast cancer or cancer in general, because overall these factors are relatively weak predictors of risk.

SUGGESTED FURTHER READING

1. Harris JR, Lippman ME, Veronsei U, Willett WC (1992) Breast cancer. *N Engl J Med* (3 parts) **327**: 319-328, 390-398, 473-480.
2. Willett WC, Rockhill B, Hankinson SE, Hunter D, Colditz GA (1999) Non-genetic factors in the causation of breast cancer. In: Harris JR, Lippman ME, Morrow M, Osborne CK, eds. *Diseases of the Breast*, 2nd ed. Philadelphia, PA (USA): Lippincott-Raven Press.
3. Whittemore AS, Harris R, Itnyre J, and the Collaborative Ovarian Cancer Group (1992) Characteristics relating to ovarian cancer risk: collaborative analysis of 12 US case-control studies. IV. The pathogenesis of epithelial ovarian cancer. *Am J Epidemiol* **136**: 1212-1220.

4. Parazzini F, La Vecchia C, Bociolone L, Franceschi S (1991) The epidemiology of endometrial cancer. *Gynecol Oncol* **41:** 1-16.
5. Brinton LA (1992) Epidemiology of cervical cancer - overview. In: Muñoz N, Bosch FX, Shah KV, Meheus A, eds. *The Epidemiology of Cervical Cancer and Human Papillomavirus*. Scientific Publication No. 119. Lyon, France: International Agency for Research on Cancer, pp. 3-23.
6. Potter JD, Slattery ML, Bostick RM, Gapstur SM (1993) Colon cancer: a review of the epidemiology. *Epidemiol Rev* **15:** 499-545.

REFERENCES

1. Harris JR, Lippman ME, Veronesi U, *et al.* (1992) Breast cancer. *N Engl J Med* **327:** 319-328, 390-398, 473-480.
2. Willett WC, Rockhill B, Hankinson SE, *et al.* (1999) Non-genetic factors in the causation of breast cancer. In: Harris JR, Lippman ME, Morrow M, Osborne CK, eds. *Diseases of the Breast*, 2 ed. Philadelphia, PA (USA): Lippincott-Raven Press.
3. Kelsey JL, Bernstein L (1996) Epidemiology and prevention of breast cancer. *Annu Rev Public Health* **17:** 47-67.
4. Newcomb PA, Storer B, Longnecker MP, *et al.* (1994) Lactation and a reduced risk of premenopausal breast cancer. *N Engl J Med* **330:** 81-87.
5. Michels KB, Willett WC (1996) Does induced or spontaneous abortion affect the risk of breast cancer? *Epidemiology* **7:** 521-528.
6. Brind J, Chinchilli VM, Severs WB, *et al.* (1996) Induced abortion as an independent risk factor for breast cancer: a comprehensive review and meta-analysis. *J Epidemiol Community Health* **50:** 481-496.
7. Melbye M, Wohlfahrt J, Olsen JH, *et al.* (1997) Induced abortion and the risk of breast cancer. *N Engl J Med* **336:** 81-85.
8. Weiss HA, Potischman NA, Brinton LA, *et al.* (1997) Prenatal and perinatal risk factors for breast cancer in young women. *Epidemiology* **8:** 181-187.
9. Ekbom A, Hsieh C-C, Lipworth L, *et al.* (1997) Intrauterine environment and breast cancer risk in women: a population-based study. *J Natl Cancer Inst* **89:** 71-76.
10. Ekbom A (1998) Growing evidence that several human cancers may originate *in utero*. *Semin Cancer Biol* **8:** 237-244.
11. Whittemore AS, Harris R, Itnyre J (1992) Characteristics relating to ovarian cancer risk: collaborative analysis of 12 US case-control studies. IV. The pathogenesis of epithelial ovarian cancer. Collaborative Ovarian Cancer Group. *Am J Epidemiol* **136:** 1212-1220.
12. Whittemore AS, Harris R, Itnyre J (1992) Characteristics relating to ovarian cancer risk: collaborative analysis of 12 US case-control studies. II. Invasive epithelial ovarian cancers in white women. Collaborative Ovarian Cancer Group. *Am J Epidemiol* **136:** 1184-1203.
13. Negri E, Franceschi S, Tzonou A, *et al.* (1991) Pooled analysis of 3 European case-control studies: 1. Reproductive factors and risk of epithelial ovarian cancer. *Int J Cancer* **49:** 50-56.
14. Hankinson SE, Colditz GA, Hunter DJ, *et al.* (1995) A prospective study of reproductive factors and risk of epithelial ovarian cancer. *Cancer* **76:** 284-290.

15. Daly M, Obrams GI (1998) Epidemiology and risk assessment for ovarian cancer. *Semin Oncol* **25:** 255-264.
16. Albrektsen G, Heuch I, Kvale G (1996) Reproductive factors and incidence of epithelial ovarian cancer: a Norwegian prospective study. *Cancer Causes Control* **7:** 421-427.
17. Siskind V, Green A, Bain C, Purdie D (1997) Breastfeeding, menopause, and epithelial ovarian cancer. *Epidemiology* **8:** 188-191.
18. Shu XO, Brinton LA, Gao YT, *et al.* (1989) Population-based case-control study of ovarian cancer in Shanghai. *Cancer Res* **49:** 3670-3674.
19. Hankinson SE, Hunter DJ, Colditz GA, *et al.* (1993) Tubal ligation, hysterectomy, and risk of ovarian cancer. *JAMA* **270:** 2813-2818.
20. Green A, Purdie D, Bain C, *et al.* (1997) Tubal sterilisation , hysterectomy, and decreased risk of ovarian cancer. *Int J Cancer* **71:** 948-951.
21. Parazzini F, La Vecchia C, Bociolone L, *et al.* (1991) The epidemiology of endometrial cancer. *Gynecol Oncol* **41:** 1-16.
22. Elwood JM, Cole P, Rothman KJ, *et al.* (1977) Epidemiology of endometrial cancer. *J Natl Cancer Inst* **59:** 1055-1060.
23. McPherson CP, Sellers TA, Potter JD, *et al.* (1996) Reproductive factors and risk of endometrial cancer. *Am J Epidemiol* **143:** 1195-1202.
24. Brinton LA (1992) Epidemiology of cervical cancer - overview. In: Muñoz N, Bosch FX, Shah KV, Meheus A, eds. *The Epidemiology of Cervical Cancer and Human Papillomavirus.* Lyon, France: International Agency for Research on Cancer, IARC Scientific Publication No. 119, pp. 3-23.
25. Ngelangel C, Muñoz N, Bosch FX, *et al.* (1998) Causes of cervical cancer in the Philippines: a case-control study. *J Natl Cancer Inst* **90:** 43-49.
26. Bjorge T, Kravdal O (1996) Reproductive variables and risk of uterine cervical cancer in Norwegian registry data. *Cancer Causes Control* **7:** 351-357.
27. Potter JD, Slattery ML, Bostick RM, *et al.* (1993) Colon cancer: a review of the epidemiology. *Epidemiol Rev* **15:** 499-545.
28. Martinez ME, Grodstein F, Giovannucci E, *et al.* (1997) A prospective study of reproductive factors, oral contraceptive use, and risk of colorectal cancer. *Cancer Epidemiol Biomarkers Prev* **6:** 1-5.

Chapter 9

Socioeconomic Status

Ichiro Kawachi, M.D., Ph.D. and Kimberly Lochner, Sc.D.
Harvard Center for Society and Health and the Department of Health and Social Behavior, Harvard School of Public Health, Boston, MA

INTRODUCTION

For as long as health statistics have been collected, researchers have recognized that socioeconomic status (SES) is linked to health. Individuals higher on the socioeconomic hierarchy – whether measured by income, educational attainment, or occupational status – enjoy better health than those below [1]. Cancer is no exception. Who gets cancer and dies of the disease is not a matter of a random lottery, but is systematically patterned by one's position in the SES hierarchy.

In the United States, as well as in Europe, lower SES individuals have been shown to be at increased risk of overall cancer incidence. For example, based on data from the National Cancer Institute's Surveillance, Epidemiology, and End Results (SEER) Program in three U.S. cities (San Francisco-Oakland, Detroit, and Atlanta), cancer incidence for all sites combined was significantly higher for individuals with lower income (Figure 9.1) [2]. Among individual sites most consistently associated with low SES are cancers of the lung, cervix, and stomach [3]. Other cancer sites where there is some evidence that incidence rates are higher among low SES populations include cancers of the esophagus, oral cavity, larynx, liver, and bladder [3].

G.A. Colditz et al. (eds.), Cancer Prevention: The Causes and Prevention of Cancer - Volume I, 87–100.
© 2000 *Kluwer Academic Publishers.*

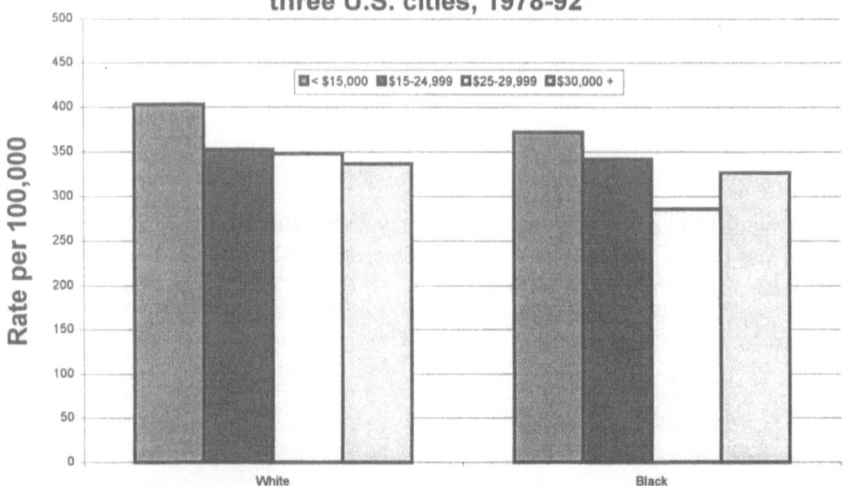

Age-adjusted cancer incidence rate (all sites combined) by race and income ages 25 and over, in three U.S. cities, 1978-92

Source: Bacquet et al., 1991

Figure 9.1

However, cancer is not a uniform disease and different sites have varying associations with SES. Notably, breast cancer incidence is higher among more affluent groups, as is melanoma [3]. Furthermore, for a number of cancer sites, there are nonexistent or inconsistent associations with SES, *e.g.*, cancers of the prostate, uterus, testis, rectum, bladder, kidney, pancreas, bone, connective tissues, malignant lymphomas and leukemias [3]. On the other hand, if lower SES is not always associated with increased incidence of cancer, it almost always related to poorer survival following the onset of cancer. The known relationships of SES to cancer incidence for several sites are summarized in Table 9.1. For a recent detailed review of the evidence linking SES to various cancer sites, the reader is referred to the International Agency for Research on Cancer (IARC) publication no. 138, *"Social Inequalities and Cancer"* (Kogevinas M, Pearce N, Susser M, Boffetta P, eds. [4]).

Table 9.1 Cancer sites associated with SES

	Association with low SES		Association with higher SES	
	Established	Probable	Established	Probable
Lung	X			
Cervix uteri	X			
Stomach	X			
Oral cavity		X		
Esophagus		X		
Liver		X		
Bladder		X		
Breast			X	
Melanoma			X	

1.   EXPLANATIONS FOR THE LINK BETWEEN SES AND CANCER

A number of possible explanations have been put forward to explain the links between SES and cancer. The UK Black Report on health inequalities [5] provides a convenient starting point for considering the various mechanisms linking lower SES to increased cancer risk. Following the framework of the Black Report, the four general classes of explanations are: social selection, access to health care, variations in lifestyles, and structural explanations.

Social selection, also referred to as the "drift hypothesis", posits that the association between lower SES and poor health status is the result of illness causing downward drift in one's socioeconomic position (rather than the reverse).   Earlier evidence on some forms of mental illness (*e.g.*, schizophrenia) suggested that patients with such illnesses do indeed tend to follow a downward trajectory in their socioeconomic circumstances [5]. On the other hand, there is scant evidence that the SES/cancer link can be explained by such a mechanism.   Moreover, the drift hypothesis cannot adequately account for the known link between level of educational attainment (which is set relatively early in life) and cancer incidence (which for the most part occurs in mid-life and beyond).

Unequal access to health care undoubtedly accounts for an important portion of the socioeconomic differential in cancer incidence and mortality, especially in a country like the United States where currently an estimated 43 million individuals are either uninsured or under-insured. Inequalities in access to cancer screening (*e.g.*, Pap smears and mammograms) have been widely documented [6]. Even the standards of medical treatment for those seeking care for established cancer have also been shown to be less adequate among the poor [4]. Indeed the provision of preventive and curative services for cancer seems to be governed by what Julian Tudor Hart [7] once famously termed "the inverse care law", *i.e.*, health care tends to be received in inverse proportion to need. Thus, women of low socioeconomic status have a higher than average risk of cervical cancer, yet have lower than average participation rates in screening. On the other hand, despite the urgent need to provide universal health care in the United States, it is important to recall that socioeconomic disparities in cancer have also been documented in most other countries including the UK and in Scandinavia, where uniform health care is ensured by single payer systems. In other words, the provision of adequate health care is unlikely to provide the "magic bullet" against socioeconomic disparities in cancer.

An important reason why medical care is unlikely by itself to solve the problem of health inequalities is because cancer (along with most other chronic diseases) is often the end-result of a series of risk behaviors accumulated over a lifetime. In other words, by the time a 70-year old patient presents to the oncology clinic with chronic cough, the disease (lung cancer) represents the end-stage of a process that began decades earlier – including early initiation into cigarette smoking, inadequate intake of vegetables, occupational exposure to diesel fumes, and so on. By this token, medical care can be likened to the proverbial ambulance waiting at the bottom of the cliff. Several cancer sites demonstrating the strongest SES gradient (lung, oral cavity, esophagus, and bladder) are caused by cigarette smoking, which itself has been shown to be more prevalent among lower SES groups. Nevertheless, it is a mistake to think of lifestyle behaviors as the primary pathway through which SES influences cancer risk. For one thing, "explaining" SES differentials in cancer *via* lifestyles automatically raises the question of why risk behaviors should themselves be patterned according to socioeconomic position.

This brings us to the final category of explanation, which the Black Report emphasized above others, *vis a vis,* "structural" explanations for health inequalities. Structural explanations include both the material circumstances and psychosocial factors (*e.g.,* stress) associated with lower position on the socioeconomic hierarchy. Researchers focusing on the link between the social structure and the distribution of disease have proposed that lower socioeconomic position is accompanied by inherently stressful life circumstances which may prompt health-damaging coping responses, such as cigarette smoking. For example, a survey of African-American adults residing in disadvantaged neighborhoods in the San Francisco area found that smoking behavior was likely to be influenced by exposure to chronic stressors – or daily hassles – such as "being concerned about getting credit", "being concerned about living in an unsafe area", or "not having enough money for food, clothing, or other necessities of life" [8]. Those scoring high on a daily "Hassles Index" were significantly more likely to report barriers to quitting, while the number of daily hassles was inversely related to level of income. These findings suggest that smokers may use nicotine as a coping mechanism against stress. Other examples of potentially health-damaging behavioral responses to stress include drinking to excess, curtailment of leisure-time physical activity, and reductions in the quality of the diet. Under such circumstances, a successful cancer prevention strategy needs to address the social context in which much of lifestyle behavior takes place – for example, by intervening at the level of communities and work-places to strengthen the resources (*e.g.,* social support) which enable individuals to overcome daily hassles. Simply putting out educational messages to alter individual behavior is unlikely to suffice.

Other researchers have viewed SES as a "fundamental" cause of disease, because higher social status embodies resources like knowledge, money, power, and prestige that can be used differently, in accordance with changing situations, to avoid risks for disease and death [9]. Despite persuasive evidence that socioeconomic differences in lifestyle behaviors do not arise in a vacuum, cancer prevention campaigns have all too often ignored this lesson. By assuming that personal choice and preferences play the primary role in differential cancer risks, such efforts lead to an under-socialized notion of cancer risk, as well as victim blaming.

For the remainder of the chapter, we shall focus on three emerging foci of research related to SES disparities. The three areas of investigation together represent a more sophisticated approach to understanding the link between SES and cancer risk across time and space. They include: (1) taking a lifecourse approach to cancer risk; (2) examining the influence of the social environment on cancer risk, including the effects of neighborhoods and workplaces; and (3) understanding the sociobiologic translation, *i.e.,* how social conditions "get under the skin" to produce biological effects that predispose to increased cancer risk.

2. EMERGING APPROACHES TO UNDERSTANDING SES DISPARITIES IN CANCER

2.1 Lifecourse effects on cancer risk

A lifecourse approach to disease causation is one that explicitly acknowledges the importance of either early life exposures, and/or the cumulative differential lifetime exposure to health-damaging physical and social environments. The approach can be contrasted to prevailing etiological models for chronic disease, which emphasize risk factors in adulthood [10].

In the area of cancer, two examples illustrate the growing attention being devoted to lifecourse effects. Infection with *Helicobacter pylori* has now been shown to increase the risk of stomach cancer by two to four-fold [11]. *H. pylori* is largely acquired during childhood, and is associated with poor living conditions, such as overcrowding and sharing a bed with parents [11]. The epidemiology of *H. pylori* infection fits with the well-established association between stomach cancer and low SES, as well as with the decline in stomach cancer incidence with a society's level of economic development.

In contrast to stomach cancer, the incidence of breast cancer is known to be higher among upper SES groups. While this reversal of the usual pattern can be partly explained by SES differentials in reproductive risk factors during adulthood (*e.g.,* later age at first pregnancy as well as lower parity among higher SES women), researchers have also begun to focus on the influence of early life factors. According to one current hypothesis, breast cancer risk may begin *in utero,* with the level of fetal exposure to estrogens determining subsequent risk [12]. Two perinatal factors have been examined as proxy measures of *in utero* exposure to estrogens: high birthweight (indicating high exposure) and history of pre-eclampsia during pregnancy (indicating low exposure). Although the evidence is not entirely consistent, the higher birthweight of babies born to women of higher SES may partly account for their excess risk of breast cancer.

As useful as it is to consider early life influences on the *biological* mechanisms underlying the SES/cancer link, it is equally important to keep in mind the relevance of the lifecourse perspective in terms of the accumulation of *social* disadvantage. Hence, many resources and skills that the affluent take for granted are often unavailable to those growing up in disadvantaged households. For example, the skills and knowledge required to put together a successful job or college application, or to navigate the complicated series of steps required to purchase a home, might be lacking in households where there is no prior experience in accomplishing these tasks. The lifecourse perspective thus forces us to consider the transgenerational accumulation of social disadvantage. In other words, the *history* of how individuals and families got to where they are on the socioeconomic ladder matters. Even if social policies could remedy the disparities in current income between poor and non-poor households, policymakers would still need to address the lingering disparities in human, cultural, and social capital accumulated over a lifetime.

2.2 The contributions of neighborhood and workplace environments on cancer risk

Virtually all individual risk behaviors take place within a social context. This realization has spurred the search for the characteristics of social environments – such as neighborhoods and workplaces –that either promote or damage health [13]. To return to the example of cigarette smoking, it is now recognized that smoking initiation is influenced not only by individual factors (such as knowledge of the hazards of smoking, and attitudes towards risk), but also by the physical and social characteristics of the neighborhoods in which children grow up. One highly visible feature of the physical environment related to the risk of smoking initiation among lower SES children is the placement of cigarette billboards, which have been shown to be more prevalent in low-income neighborhoods [14]. Additionally, a recent study of advertising on top of taxicabs in the city of Boston found that cabs serving less affluent neighborhoods were twice as likely to carry cigarette advertisements compared with their counterparts in more affluent neighborhoods [15]. More affluent neighborhoods by contrast are more likely to take active steps to ban cigarette vending machines or pass local ordinances to restrict smoking in area restaurants.

Turning to the social environment in neighborhoods, so-called "contagion" models of health behavior suggest that a youth's risk of smoking initiation is much greater when the prevalence of smoking among peers is high, and cigarette use appears to be a normative behavior – both features that characterize socioeconomically deprived neighborhoods. It is perhaps not surprising then that several multi-level studies have found an increased risk of smoking as a result of residing in deprived neighborhoods over and above the risks associated with low *individual* socioeconomic status [16].

Poorer quality diet – especially inadequate intake of fresh fruits and vegetables – and lack of physical activity are both associated with increased cancer risk [4]. Both risk "behaviors" are more common in deprived neighborhoods, though not necessarily because lower SES people "choose" these lifestyles, but often because the options to exercise healthy choices are simply unavailable where they live. Thus, stores in lower SES neighborhoods are not as well stocked with fresh produce; residents are also less likely to have access to both private and public transport to get to the nearest supermarket. There are fewer recreational facilities within lower SES neighborhoods, and citizens may be deterred from exercising through fear of crime [13]. On the other hand, deprived neighborhoods are disproportionately more likely to be served by liquor stores and fast food outlets [17].

Like neighborhoods, the workplace can also be considered a type of social environment that may lead to differential exposure to cancer risk according to socioeconomic status. The most obvious example is exposure to occupational carcinogens, which is estimated to account for about 4 percent of total human cancers in industrialized countries [18]. According to the International Agency for Research on Cancer (IARC), thirteen industries or occupations are currently classified as posing a carcinogenic risk. Notably, these risks are disproportionately concentrated among blue-collar, manufacturing occupations, *e.g.,* coke production (lung cancer), dye/pigment manufacture (bladder cancer), rubber manufacture (bladder cancer, leukemia), and so on.

In addition to increased risk through exposure to occupational carcinogens, research has increasingly turned towards aspects of the *psychosocial* work environment that may directly or indirectly affect cancer risk. Of the various approaches to characterizing the psychosocial work environment, the job-strain model developed by Robert Karasek and colleagues has received the most attention [19]. According to Karasek's model, any workplace psychosocial environment can be characterized along two dimensions: the level of psychological demands imposed by the job and the amount of control that the worker is able to exercise over aspects of the job. The combination of high demands and low control (termed "high strain") on the job has been hypothesized to elicit a physiological stress response, and eventually lead to deleterious health consequences. Notably, high strain work environments tend to be disproportionately concentrated in lower SES occupations (*e.g.,* assembly line workers, various forms of "service"-sector jobs). Considerable evidence supports the predictive value of this model for the risk of cardiovascular disease [19], though data on cancer are still lacking. Nonetheless, studies have shown that men and women in high strain jobs tend to smoke more, thus raising the possibility of indirect effects on cancer risk [20].

2.3   Stress and cancer – the sociobiologic translation

Health inequalities mirror the disparities in underlying social conditions. The notion that individuals who are lower on the SES hierarchy "embody" their adverse life circumstances through their excess burden of premature disease has led researchers to focus on the physiological processes by which social conditions "get under the skin" to produce ill health [21]. The notion that features of social organization/hierarchy influence individual biology and subsequent disease risk has been referred to as the sociobiologic translation [22]. Recently, the term "allostatic load" has been introduced to describe the cumulative wear and tear on the body's endocrine, immune, and physiological systems induced by repeated exposure to adverse life events and stress [21].

A leading hypothesis in the field of psychoneuroimmunology conjectures that stress can influence the onset and progression of cancer by altering immune function -- including reduced lymphocyte proliferative response to mitogen stimulation, reduced natural killer cell cytotoxicity, as well as changes in the production of cytokines -- all of which reduce the functioning of the organism's immune surveillance system [23]. Although evidence of clinically significant alterations in immune functioning as a direct result of stress is still lacking, animal models suggest the antitumor cytotoxicity of CD8 and NK lymphocytes and the localized inflammatory response mediated by CD4 lymphocytes may influence tumor growth and metastasis [23]. Additional indirect evidence of an association between stress and cancer is provided by the finding that the availability of social support (which buffers the effect of stress and moderates stress-induced immunosuppression) has been consistently shown in both observational and intervention studies to increase cancer survival and reduce tumor recurrence [24].

Since socioeconomically disadvantaged individuals are more likely to experience stress, both in the form of negative life events (*e.g.,* illness of a family member, being laid off work) as well as chronic hassles (*e.g.,* economic hardship, exposure to violence), there is some plausibility to the notion that the low SES/cancer link may be mediated by stress-induced alterations in immune function. Additionally, lower SES individuals are more likely to be socially isolated and thus may not have access to social support to help them cope with the effects of stress.

Thus far, however, most of the epidemiological evidence linking stress to cancer has been in the realm of tumor progression, recurrence, and survival, whereas the evidence linking stress to cancer incidence remains unclear. Studying the role of psychological stress in the etiology of cancer is difficult because of the long latency period involved in tumor development and detection.

3. RACE OR SES?

In the United States, there has been a much greater focus on racial disparities in cancer risk, mortality, and survival than on socioeconomic disparities [25]. Excess cancer incidence rates among African-Americans have been consistently documented since the 1970s [2]. African-Americans have higher rates of cancer incidence overall compared to whites, as well as higher rates of cancers of the prostate, cervix, lung, and stomach [25]. "Race" as a variable concatenates a variety of exposures, including socioeconomic, cultural, and possibly biologic differences. For example, because of the overrepresentation of African-Americans among lower SES groups, race has often been used as a proxy for socioeconomic status in the United States. Importantly, several studies that gathered data on both race and SES have concluded that controlling for SES greatly reduces the disparities in cancer risk between blacks and whites [2]. Thus, Baquet *et al.* [2] found that age-adjusted cancer incidence rates were significantly higher among African-Americans for all sites combined compared to whites, but when the data were adjusted for SES, overall cancer incidence was actually slightly higher among whites (although African-Americans still had higher incidence rates for prostate and cervical cancer). Furthermore, SES disparities in cancer risk are evident *within* race groups [2]. Thus, the use of race as a proxy for SES may actually obscure our understanding of why African-Americans, as well as lower SES groups, are at increased risk for cancer.

CONCLUSION

Compared to the wealth of evidence linking SES to cardiovascular disease, our knowledge and understanding of socioeconomic inequalities in cancer risk have not progressed far beyond documenting the existence of disparities with descriptive statistics.

When SES is considered, etiologic studies have tended to treat it as a potential confounder to be controlled away. Seldom have investigators approached SES disparities in cancer as a thing to be studied in its own right. In other instances, analysts have myopically focused on individual "lifestyle" behaviors, such as smoking, diet, alcohol, and sexual behavior, to "explain" SES differences in cancer. However, the knowledge that certain risk behaviors among lower SES groups account for their higher incidence rates cannot "explain away" the important role that socioeconomic factors play in cancer risk [4]. Smoking as well as other individual "lifestyle" factors are not competing explanations for cancer risk, rather they are one set of proximate mechanisms by which SES influences cancer risk. The purpose of this chapter has been to provide a brief overview of the ways in which a more sophisticated notion of socioeconomic status can be applied to understand disparities in cancer risk. The future success of cancer prevention depends on our ability to tackle these socioeconomic disparities.

SUMMARY POINTS

- Socioeconomic disparities in cancer are large, persistent, and possibly widening.
- The cancer sites with established associations to low SES include cancers of the lung, cervix, and stomach.
- Smoking and other individual "lifestyle" factors are not competing explanations for cancer risk, rather they are one set of proximate mechanisms by which SES influences cancer risk.

RECOMMENDATIONS

- Further research on socioeconomic disparities in cancer risk should concentrate on three topical areas:
  - incorporating a lifecourse perspective on cancer risk;
  - understanding the influence of social environments (neighborhoods and workplaces) on cancer risk
  - elucidating the biologic processes by which social conditions "get under the skin" to produce differential cancer risk.
- Although there are large racial disparities in cancer risk, race should not be used as a proxy for socioeconomic status. The effects of race and socioeconomic status on cancer should be addressed separately.

SUGGESTED FURTHER READING

1. Kogevinas M, Pearce N, Susser M, Boffetta P, eds. (1997) *Social Inequalities and Cancer. IARC Scientific Publications* No. 138. Lyon, France International Agency for Research on Cancer.
2. Berkman LF, Kawachi I, eds. (2000) *Social Epidemiology.* New York, NY (USA): Oxford University.
3. Baquet CR, Horm JW, Gibbs T, Greenwald P (1991) Socioeconomic factors and cancer incidence among blacks and whites. *J Natl Cancer Inst* **83:** 551-557.

REFERENCES

1. Adler NE, Boyce T, Chesney MA, *et al.* (1994) Socioeconomic status and health. The challenge of the gradient. *Am Psychol* **49:** 15-24.

2. Baquet CR, Horm JW, Gibbs T, *et al.* (1991) Socioeconomic factors and cancer incidence among blacks and whites. *J Natl Cancer Inst* **83**: 551-557.
3. Faggiano F, Partanen T, Kogevinas M, *et al.* (1997) Socioeconomic differences in cancer incidence and mortality. In: Kogevinas M, Pearce N, Susser M, Boffetta P, eds. *Social Inequalities and Cancer.* IARC Scientific Publications No. 138. Lyon, France: International Agency for Research on Cancer, pp. 68-184.
4. Kogevinas M, Pearce N, Susser M, Boffetta P, eds. (1997) *Social Inequalities and Cancer.* IARC Scientific Publications No. 138. Lyon, France: International Agency for Research on Cancer.
5. Department of Health and Human Services (1980) *Inequalities in Health: Report of a Research Working Group.* London, UK: DHHS.
6. Segnan N (1997) Socioeconomic status and cancer screening. In: Kogevinas M, Pearce N, Susser M, Boffetta P, eds. *Social Inequalities and Cancer.* IARC Scientific Publications No. 138. Lyon: International Agency for Research on Cancer, pp. 369-376.
7. Hart JT (1971). The inverse care law. *Lancet* **1**: 405-412.
8. Romano PS, Bloom J, Syme SL (1991). Smoking, social support, and hassles in an urban African-American community. *Am J Public Health* **81**: 1415-1422.
9. Link BG, Phelan J (1995). Social conditions as fundamental causes of disease. *J Health Soc Behav* **(Spec No)**: 80-94.
10. Kuh D, Ben-Shlomo Y (1997). *A Lifecourse Approach to Chronic Disease Epidemiology.* Oxford, UK: Oxford University Press.
11. International Agency for Research on Cancer (1994) Infection with *Helicobacter pylori.* In: *IARC Monographs on the Evaluation of Carcinogenic Risks to Humans Volume 61. Schistosomes, Liver Flukes and* Helicobacter pylori. Lyon: IARC pp.177-240.
12. Trichopoulos D (1990) Hypothesis: Does breast cancer originate *in utero? Lancet* **335**: 939-940.
13. Macintyre S, MacIver S, Sooman A (1993) Area, class and health: Should we be focusing on places or people? *J Soc Pol* **22**: 213-234.
14. Hackbarth DP, Silvestri B, Cosper W (1995) Tobacco and alcohol billboards in 50 Chicago neighborhoods: market segmentation to sell dangerous products to the poor. *J Public Health Policy* **16**: 213-230.
15. Sesso H, Kawachi I (1997) Cigarette advertising on taxi cabs in Boston. *Tobacco Control* **6**: 128-130.
16. Diez-Roux AV, Nieto J, Muntaner C, *et al.* (1997) Neighborhood environments and coronary heart disease: a multilevel analysis. *Am J Epidemiol* **146**: 48-63.
17. Troutt D (1993) *The Thin Red Line: How the Poor Still Pay More.* San Francisco, CA (USA): Consumers Union, West Coast Regional Office.
18. Boffetta P, Westerholm P, Kogevinas M, *et al.* (1997) Exposure to occupational carcinogens and social class differences in cancer occurrence. In: Kogevinas M, Pearce N, Susser M, Boffetta P, eds. *Social Inequalities and Cancer. IARC Scientific Publications No. 138.* Lyon, France: IARC, pp. 331-341.
19. Karasek RA, Theorell T (1990) *Healthy Work.* New York, NY (USA): Basic Books.
20. Hellerstedt WL, Jeffrey RW (1997) The association of job strain and health behaviors in men and women. *Int J Epidemiol* **26**: 575-583.
21. McEwen BS (1998) Protective and damaging effects of stress mediators. *N Engl J Med* **338**: 171-179.
22. Tarlov AR (1996) Social determinants of health: the sociobiological translation. In: Blane D, Brunner EJ, Wilkinson RG, eds. *Health and Social Organization.* London, UK: Routledge.

23. Cohen S, Rabin BS (1998) Psychologic stress, immunity, and cancer. *J Natl Cancer Inst* **90:** 3-4.

24. Spiegel D, Kato PM (1996) Psychosocial influences on cancer incidence and progression. *Harv Rev Psychiatry* **4:** 10-26.

25. Freeman HP (1989) Cancer in the economically disadvantaged. *Cancer* **64**(Suppl): 324-334

Chapter 10

Environmental Pollution

Lucas M. Neas, Sc.D.
Epidemiology and Biomarkers Branch, Human Studies Division, National Health and Environmental Effects Research Laboratory, U.S. Environmental Protection Agency, Research Triangle Park, NC

INTRODUCTION

Environmental factors are generally recognized as an important determinant in the development of most cancers. When epidemiologists use the word "environmental" it is usually to contrast with the inherited or "genetic" risk of cancer. It thus encompasses a much broader range of exposures than the common use of the word to imply aspects of the "environment" such as industrial pollution. As defined by the epidemiologist, most "environmental" causes of cancer are related to personal behaviors (such as cigarette smoking, alcohol, exercise, and delayed childbearing), viral agents (such as human papilloma virus and Epstein Barr virus), occupational exposures (such as benzene, asbestos, and coke oven emissions), or dietary factors (such as nutritional status, nitrosamines and aflatoxins). Specific environmental risk factors including passive exposure to environmental tobacco smoke, indoor radon, ultraviolet radiation, and electric and magnetic fields are considered in other chapters. This chapter will focus on cancer risks posed by environmental pollutants such as air toxics, drinking water contaminants, pesticides and related organochlorine compounds.

G.A. Colditz et al. (eds.), Cancer Prevention: The Causes and Prevention of Cancer - Volume I, 101–110.
© 2000 *Kluwer Academic Publishers.*

1.   AIR TOXICS

The relative excess of cancer among urban populations has been the subject of scientific speculation since the European Renaissance. Descriptive studies over the last 20 years from Europe, Japan, and Australia have provided support for the hypothesis that urban air pollution is associated with an increased risk of lung cancer. Relative risks as high as 1.6 in men and 1.9 in women were observed in Norway, that is a 60 percent and 90 percent increase in lung cancer incidence respectively. These early descriptive studies often did not adequately consider potential confounders such as age of initiation of smoking and occupational exposures and had no direct measures of air pollution exposure.

Recent analytic epidemiologic studies of lung cancer and air pollution have controlled for the effects of cigarette smoking and occupation. Lifetime exposures to air pollution are estimated from direct, but short-term, measurements of particles, sulfur dioxide, or polycyclic aromatic hydrocarbons. Among 552,138 participants in an American Cancer Society study of 151 U.S. metropolitan areas, Arden Pope and colleagues found that lung cancer deaths were associated with air pollution measured as sulfate particles [1]. However, this association was very much weaker than the association of lung cancer deaths with active cigarette smoking. Among 6338 nonsmoking California Seventh-day Adventists, David Abbey and colleagues found that air pollution measured as either particles, sulfur dioxide, or nitrogen dioxide also was associated with an increase in lung cancer deaths [2].

Air pollution may also increase the effect of known respiratory carcinogens. Among nonsmokers, the risk of lung cancer is low in both urban and rural populations and the urban-rural differences are not consistent across multiple studies. In contrast, six cohorts and six case-control studies of the general population have found that urban smokers are at increased risk from the additional effects of urban exposure with relative risks ranging from 1.1 to 1.8. Several excellent technical reviews of the epidemiologic literature are available [3, 4].

What air pollutants could be responsible for an increased risk of lung cancer? Inventories of industrial emissions and direct chemical analyses of air samples have documented the presence in urban air of many compounds that are known to cause cancers in animals. Combustion products, principally polycyclic aromatic hydrocarbons, have long been considered as one agent responsible for the carcinogenic potential of outdoor air pollution. Industrial emissions, motor vehicle emissions, and consumer products contain benzene, formaldehyde, and other volatile organic compounds that are known carcinogens in both human and animal studies. Other exposures of concern include metal refineries (arsenic, cadmium and nickel) and ore processing wastes (asbestos and uranium).

Diesel exhaust particles are of particular concern since they are very common in areas with truck traffic, they contain many air toxics including polycyclic aromatic hydrocarbons, and they deposit on the peripheral airways. In a quantitative review of 23 cohort and case-control studies, Rajiv Bhatia and colleagues concluded that occupational exposures to diesel exhaust were consistently associated with increased risk of lung cancer [5]. Diesel exhaust's relative importance as a carcinogen at the much lower levels found in urban air remains an area of scientific uncertainty.

From these studies, the U.S. Environmental Protection Agency (EPA) [6] has estimated that the proportion of lung cancers due to air pollution is about one percent or about 1600 lung cancer deaths per year in the U.S. population. The vast majority of all lung cancers are due to the effects of active and passive exposure to cigarette smoke and to occupational exposures.

The 1990 amendments to the U.S. Clean Air Act identified 189 pollutants (later reduced to 188 by the removal of caprolactum) to be regulated as hazardous air pollutants (Table 10.1). The Clean Air Act requires the EPA to develop standards that require the application of stringent air pollution controls. Sources that emit ten tons/year or more of a listed toxic air pollutant must utilize the maximum achievable control technology. These standards will reduce air toxics emissions from chemical plants, oil refineries, manufacturers, coke ovens, steel mills, and other stationary sources by over one million tons per year. The EPA has also issued tighter standards for car and truck emissions, vehicle refueling, and cleaner gasoline. Since 1993, the EPA's Photochemical Assessment Monitoring Stations have been collecting data on eight volatile air toxics in more than 20 major urban areas. Soon a new network of speciation monitors for fine airborne particulate matter will provide measurements of 10 hazardous metals at over 50 locations.

On 14 September 1998, the EPA's administrator Carol Browner announced a new Integrated Urban Air Toxics Strategy to assess the residual risk to human health posed by the most hazardous air pollutants and the need for additional regulation. The draft strategy identified a subset of 33 compounds of greatest impact on the public in urban areas (Table 10.1). While some of these air toxics have non-cancer health effects such as neurotoxicity, most of these pollutants were listed because they are known or suspected animal carcinogens. The draft strategy identified 34 types of area sources that may be subject to new emission standards and the goal is to ensure that 90 percent of the air toxic emissions from these sources are addressed by the air toxics program. Emissions of air toxics from mobile sources such as cars and trucks will also be assessed and the draft strategy details a schedule for decisions by the EPA on the need for additional motor vehicle emission or fuel standards.

In summary, most epidemiologic studies can be considered as supportive or consistent with a modest role for urban air pollution in the causation of lung cancer, albeit a small role as compared with cigarette smoking or certain occupational exposures. Some epidemiologic studies have strongly suggested that diesel exhaust particles are human carcinogens, but additional research is needed to clarify this association. The EPA has initiated a program for assessing the residual risks of toxic air pollutants in urban areas and for controlling the emissions of these compounds.

Table 10.1 Hazardous air pollutants listed by the U.S. Environmental Protection Agency's Urban Air Toxics Program, 1999

Acetaldehyde	Ethylene dichloride	Trichlorethylene
Acolein	Ethylene oxide	Vinyl chloride
Acrylonitrile	Formaldehyde	Arsenic compounds
Benzene	Hydrazine	Cadmium compounds
Bis(2-ethylhexyl)phthalate	Methyl oxide	Chromium compounds
1,3-Butadiene	Methyl tert butyl ether	Coke oven emissions
Carbon tetrachloride	Methylene chloride	Lead compounds
Chloroform	Methylene diphenyl	Manganese compounds
1,4-para-Dichlorobezene	Propylene dichloride	Mercury compounds
1,3-Dichloropropene	Tetrachlorodibenzo-p-dioxin	Nickel compounds
Ethylene dibromide	Tetrachloroethylene	Polycyclic organic matter

2.   DRINKING WATER CONTAMINANTS

Drinking water may contain a number of contaminants including bacteria, viruses, nitrate, arsenic and other metals, organic chemicals, and radionuclides. Arsenic and radionuclides are natural contaminants, while industrial organic chemicals and nitrates contamination of drinking water is due to human activity. The chlorination of drinking water, especially water from surface supplies, is generally used to kill harmful bacteria, but chlorination of organic contaminants produces harmful disinfection by-products that are animal carcinogens at high doses. Fluoride is often added to drinking water to reduce dental caries.

Arsenic in drinking water from natural arsenic sources has been consistently associated with skin and internal cancers in numerous studies throughout the world [7]. Many of these studies have been conducted among Taiwanese patients with Blackfoot disease, a vaso-occlusive disorder caused by arsenic that serves as a biological marker of high exposure. Blackfoot disease patients have a consistently higher incidence of cancers of the skin, liver, lung, bladder and kidney compared with matched noncases. At the lower levels of exposure found in the U.S., epidemiological studies have not been able to demonstrate a significant association between drinking water arsenic and cancer. However, in a recent retrospective cohort study in Utah, drinking water arsenic showed a dose-related association with cancer of the prostate [8].

Nitrate contamination from agricultural, recreational, and residential sources is an important research area due to the increasing levels of nitrate in drinking water. In his review, Morris cited studies in China where high levels of nitrates in drinking water have been linked to increased risks of stomach and liver cancer and to the formation of N-nitroso compounds in human urine [9]. However, Cantor [7] stressed the lack of consistent results across numerous epidemiologic studies in more developed countries and the lack of individual level exposure assessment.

Disinfection by-products, such as trihalomethanes and haloacetic acids, are an unintended consequence of the chlorination of drinking water to control microbial pathogens. Disinfection by-products have been linked to increased risk of cancer of the bladder and rectum in a quantitative review of the epidemiological literature conducted by Robert Morris of the Medical College of Wisconsin [9]. Morris concluded that these epidemiological studies suggest that 5000 cases of bladder cancer and 8000 cases of rectal cancer per year in the U.S. may be associated with the consumption of chlorinated drinking water. In a separate review, Kenneth Cantor, National Cancer Institute, agreed that chlorination by-products were consistently associated with bladder cancer across six epidemiological studies, but he felt that the results were not as consistent for colon and rectal cancer [7]. Both reviewers mentioned the uncertainties of exposure assessment in epidemiological studies of drinking water when the specific chlorinated compounds that are responsible for the association are unknown. Both reviewers also found that drinking water fluoridation has repeatedly been studied with consistently negative results [7, 9].

The best means of reducing carcinogens in drinking water is the development and protection of our sources of drinking water. Arsenic contamination of ground water may be resolved by the development of new wells and distribution networks, while nitrate contamination may require greater regulatory efforts to protect water supplies. Disinfection by-products are a more problematic issue since the contamination is an unintended consequence of an extremely beneficial public health measure that protects us from water-borne diseases. Reduction of disinfection by-products through changes in water treatment must be balanced against any potential increase in the microbial contamination of drinking water.

The 1996 Safe Drinking Water Act Amendments require the EPA to develop rules to balance the risks of disinfection by-products with the risks of microbial pathogens. The Stage I Disinfectants and Disinfection By-products Rule announced in December 1998, sets new maximum contaminant levels for trihalomethanes and haloacetic acids. Large surface water systems must comply with the new standard in 2001, and ground water systems and small surface water systems must comply in 2003. The EPA's Office of Ground Water and Drinking Water has estimated that the new rule will result in a 24 percent reduction in the national average trihalomethane levels. A continuing effort in research and risk assessment will determine the needs for further regulations.

3.   PESTICIDES AND RELATED ORGANOCHLORINE COMPOUNDS

Aromatic organochlorines include chlorophenoxy pesticides (DDT and its metabolite DDE), combustion by-products such as polychlorinated dibenzo-p-dioxins (PCDDs) and dibenzofurans (PCDFs), and industrial products such as polychorinated biphenyls (PCBs) and polybrominated biphenyls (PBBs). These compounds are chemically stable over many decades, they are passed along the food chain, accumulate in fatty tissue, and are eliminated slowly from the body. Animal studies have shown that PCBs, and DDT are carcinogens at high doses. Phenoxy acid herbicides (2,4-D and 2,4,5-T) do not appear to be carcinogenic in experimental animals, but a potential contaminant of these herbicides (TCDD) is a known carcinogen.

Two recent reviews have reached similar conclusions regarding the role of pesticides in childhood leukemia. Shelia Zahm and Mary Ward of the National Cancer Institute concluded in their review of 17 case-control studies and one cohort study that the literature supported a possible role for pesticides in childhood leukemia [10]. After reviewing the same literature, Julie Daniels and colleagues at the University of North Carolina concluded that the leukemia association was more consistent among children whose parents had occupational pesticide exposures than among children with residential pesticide exposures [11]. Brain cancer, Wilms' tumor, Ewing's sarcoma, and germ cell tumors also have been linked to pesticides in epidemiological studies among children whose parents had occupational exposures. Both reviews cited the small sample sizes and the numerous difficulties of exposure assessment among children with residential pesticide exposures, which reduces the statistical power and precision of such epidemiologic studies.

Many aromatic organochlorines are capable of binding to estrogen receptors and are hormonally active in animals with either estrogenic or anti-estrogenic effects. For example, human studies have shown that breast-feeding women with higher DDE burdens have a decreased duration of lactation. While the observed hormonal effects are a thousand-fold less than with naturally occurring estrogens, these hormonal properties are of interest since estrogens are growth factors for tissues of the breast and uterus. At lower doses, the aromatic organochlorines may serve as tumor promoters to increase the rate by which a transformed cell grows into a clinically relevant tumor.

In a review of estrogen-related cancers in women, Adami and colleagues concluded that epidemiological studies present conflicting evidence regarding the association of aromatic organochlorine insecticides and breast and uterine cancer [12]. Recent trends and international, racial and socioeconomic patterns in breast and uterine cancer incidence do not match data on body burdens of organochlorines. One large occupational study of TCDD exposure was positive, but five larger studies (two of TCDD and three of PCBs) were convincingly negative. A study of breast cancer in Long Island, New York, was negative for proximity to hazardous waste sites or contaminated wells, but found an association with residence near industrial facilities among post-menopausal women. Measured levels of DDE were associated with breast cancer in a small (58 cases) case-control study, but the association was much weaker in a larger (150 cases) case-control study; both of these studies were negative for measured levels of PCB. In a recent nested case-control study within a prospective cohort of 7224 women, Dorgan and colleagues at the National Cancer Institute concluded that plasma levels of organochlorine pesticides and PCBs were not associated with breast cancer [13]. In another nested case-control study within a larger prospective cohort of 32,826 women, Hunter and colleagues at the Nurses Health Study found that plasma levels of DDE and PCBs actually were lower among the incident breast cancer cases than among the matched controls [14].

Pesticides are regulated by the U.S. EPA's Office of Pesticide Programs under the authority of two core statutes: the Federal Insecticide, Fungicide, and Rodenticide Act and the Federal Food, Drug, and Cosmetic Act. The 1996 Food Quality Protection Act amended these earlier laws to establish a tougher, health-based standard for pesticides used on food crops or animal feed. An important new aspect of the Act was the requirement that when setting new or revised tolerances for pesticide residues in food, the EPA administrator must explicitly consider the exposures and risks to infants and children, including *in utero* effects. The 1996 Act also requires the EPA to review by 2006 all existing pesticides to ensure that their tolerances for

residue in food meet the new standard. Pesticide residues in drinking water
are regulated by the U.S. EPA under the authority of the Safe Drinking
Water Act.

4.   SPECIAL ISSUES IN ENVIRONMENTAL CANCER

Air pollution, water pollution and pesticides share several similar
features. Exposures to these cancer risk factors are very common across
most developed and developing countries, but with very weak exposure
gradients. Aside from occupational exposures, most individuals share a
common low-level exposure to these environmental risk factors. Exposure
assessment in epidemiological studies is very difficult in the absence of a
biological marker for exposure and the differences in accumulated exposure
between the exposed and referent groups in such studies may be quite small
[10].

Another shared characteristic of these environmental risk factors for
cancer is the need for government regulations to control exposure. Unlike
behavioral or dietary risk factors where individuals may change their
accumulated risk by avoiding certain behaviors or foods, the ubiquitous
nature of air pollution, water pollution and pesticides requires collective
action to control exposures at their source. Governmental regulatory
decisions may be grounded on our limited scientific knowledge and
developed through the pragmatic application of impartial, health-based risk
assessment, but these decisions may also be subject to political, social and
economic influences and constraints. In a democracy, public support for
collective actions requires the involvement of informed citizens and their
elected representatives.

CONCLUSION

Environmental exposures via routes such as air and food contamination
may include known or suspected carcinogens. Current epidemiologic
research supports an association between urban air pollutants and cancers of
the respiratory system, but the evidence for an association of hormonally
active aromatic organochlorines appears to be inconclusive. In both cases,
the levels of exposures are typically much lower than with active cigarette
smoking, replacement estrogens, or occupational exposures, or even passive
exposures to environmental tobacco smoke and natural variations in estrogen

levels. Consequently, the risk associated with environmental exposures are generally several orders of magnitude less, but involve much larger populations and persons who are unwillingly subjected to the additional burden of these exposures. These topics are an area of very active research in which the contribution of improved techniques for exposure assessment and creative epidemiologic study designs should provide guidance to public health interventions.

SUMMARY POINTS

- Air pollution - Epidemiologic studies are supportive or consistent with a modest role for urban air pollution in the causation of lung cancer.
- Drinking water – Excessive exposure to arsenic in drinking water is clearly linked to skin and internal cancers, but the risks at low levels more typical of those in the U.S. deserve additional study. Chlorination by-products in drinking water have been associated with increased risk of bladder and rectal cancer, but fluoridation has not been associated with increased cancer risk.
- Pesticides and related organochlorine compounds – leukemia and certain tumors in children have been associated with occupational pesticide exposures of the parents, but the role of residential pesticide exposures in childhood cancer remains uncertain. Organochlorine pesticides and PCBs are not associated with breast cancer in several large prospective epidemiological studies.

SUGGESTED FURTHER READING

1. Silverman DT (1998) Is diesel exhaust a human lung carcinogen? *Epidemiology* **9**: 4-6.
2. Cantor KP (1994) Water chlorination, mutagenicity, and cancer epidemiology. *Am J Public Health* **84**: 1211-1212.
3. Goldman LR (1998) Chemicals and children's environment: what we don't know about risks. *Environ Health Perspect* **106**(Suppl 3): 875-880.

DISCLAIMER

The contents of this report are solely the responsibility of the author and do not necessarily represent the official views of the EPA. This article has been subject to the EPA's peer and administrative review and it has been approved for publication.

REFERENCES

1. Pope CA III, Thun MJ, Namboodiri MM, *et al.* (1995) Particulate air pollution as a predictor of mortality in a prospective study of U.S. adults. *Am J Respir Crit Care Med* **151:** 669-674.
2. Abbey DE, Nishino N, McDonnell WF, *et al.* (1999) Long-term inhalable particles and other air pollutants related to mortality in nonsmokers. *Am J Respir Crit Care Med* **159:** 373-382.
3. Cohen AJ, Pope CA III (1995) Lung cancer and air pollution. *Environ Health Perspect* **103**(Suppl 8): 219-224.
4. Katsouyanni K, Pershagen G (1997) Ambient air pollution exposure and cancer. *Cancer Causes Control* **8:** 284-291.
5. Bhatia R, Lopipero P, Smith AH (1998) Diesel exhaust exposure and lung cancer. *Epidemiology* **9:** 84-91.
6. U.S. Environmental Protection Agency (1990) *Cancer Risk from Outdoor Exposure to Air Toxins*. Vol. 1: *Final Report*. EPA-450/1/90/004a. Washington DC: U.S. Environmental Protection Agency.
7. Cantor KP (1997) Drinking water and cancer. *Cancer Causes Control* **8:** 292-308.
8. Lewis DR, Southwick JW, Ouellet-Hellstrom R, *et al.* (1999) Drinking water arsenic in Utah: A cohort mortality study. *Environ Health Perspect* **107:** 359-365.
9. Morris RD (1995) Drinking water and cancer. *Environ Health Perspect* **103**(Suppl 8): 225-231.
10. Zahm SH, Ward MH (1998) Pesticides and childhood cancer. *Environ Health Perspect* **106**(Suppl 3): 893-908.
11. Daniels JL, Olshan AF, Savitz DA (1997) Pesticides and childhood cancers. *Environ Health Perspect* **105:** 1068-1077.
12. Adami HO, Lipworth L, Titus-Ernstoff L, *et al.* (1995) Organochlorine compounds and estrogen-related cancers in women. *Cancer Causes Control* **6:** 551-66.
13. Dorgan JF, Brock JW, Rothman N, *et al.* (1999) Serum organochlorine pesticides and PCB's and breast cancer risk: results from a prospective analysis (USA). *Cancer Causes Control* **10:** 1-11.
14. Hunter DJ, Hankinson SE, Laden F, *et al.* (1997) Plasma organochlorine levels and the risk of breast cancer. *N Engl J Med* **337:** 1253-1258.

Chapter 11

Ultraviolet Light

Lydia M. E. Jones, M.D. and Martin A. Weinstock, M.D., Ph.D.
Deparment of Dermatology, Brown University, Providence, RI

INTRODUCTION

Ultraviolet radiation exposure has many adverse health effects, including benign and malignant disorders of the skin and other organs. The most common ultraviolet-associated malignancies are non-melanoma skin cancers, the majority of which are squamous cell and basal cell carcinomas. In the United States, these keratinocyte carcinomas are approximately equal in incidence to all other malignancies combined [1]. Malignant melanoma, also due in large part to ultraviolet exposure, is the least common of the three common types of skin cancer, although it is responsible for most skin cancer deaths.

1.   ULTRAVIOLET RADIATION

The solar spectrum at the earth's surface includes wavelengths between 290 and 3000 nm. The wavelengths implicated in sun-induced human skin reactions and cutaneous carcinogenesis generally range from 290 to 400 nm (the ultraviolet), and rarely, visible radiation (wavelengths 400 to 760 nm).

Ultraviolet radiation is produced both naturally by the sun and artificially by various types of lamps, and it is conventionally divided into A, B, and C bands. Ultraviolet A includes UVA_1 (340-400 nm) and UVA_2 (320-340 nm) wavelengths. Upon exposure to UVA radiation, which is invisible to the human eye, human skin may exhibit erythema (redness) which is of maximum intensity at 10 to 12 hours. Skin may also exhibit an immediate pigment darkening reaction, the extent of which varies according to the

G.A. Colditz et al. (eds.), Cancer Prevention: The Causes and Prevention of Cancer - Volume I, 111–122.
© *2000 Kluwer Academic Publishers.*

amount of melanin pre-existing in the skin as well as the exposure dose. Ultraviolet A may cause sunburn, but it is 1000 to 10,000 times less efficient in doing so than UVB or UVC [2]. Ultraviolet B (UVB) includes the wavelengths 290 to 320 nm. This is the radiation spectrum which most efficiently produces erythema and sunburns in human skin in response to ultraviolet exposure. Ultraviolet B-induced erythema is of maximum intensity at 20 to 24 hours post-exposure. It also stimulates melanin synthesis in the skin, which is responsible for the delayed and prolonged tanned appearance of exposed skin. Ultraviolet C (UVC) comprises the wavelengths 200 to 290 nm. Ultraviolet C does not reach the earth's surface due to absorption by the stratospheric ozone layer. As a result, human UVC exposure arises from artificial sources, including germicidal and mercury arc lamps. Artificially induced UVC radiation results in erythema of normal skin, reaching maximal intensity in six to eight hours. The atmospheric ozone layer screens out all of the UVC and a substantial proportion of the UVB that reaches it from the sun.

2.   BASAL CELL CARCINOMA

Basal cell carcinoma (BCC) is the most common malignancy in Caucasians. Approximately 80 percent arise in the head and neck region, the most consistently sun-exposed area of the body. Basal cell carcinomas occur in non-sun-exposed areas as well [13]. Basal cell cancers do arise in non-white races, although less commonly than squamous cell carcinomas. Among African-Americans, up to nearly 90 percent of BCCs are located on sun-exposed body regions [3]. The location and age of diagnosis of most of these basal cell carcinomas are consistent with the causal role of ultraviolet light.

Environmental, host, and genetic factors contribute to an individual's risk of developing basal cell carcinoma. Ultraviolet exposure during childhood and adolescence (ages 0 to 19 years) has been the most closely linked external risk factor, more so than cumulative ultraviolet exposure, although more investigation is needed before definitive conclusions can be drawn [5]. The mechanism of ultraviolet-induced damage to the basal cell layer is incompletely known. A mechanism similar to that involved in the pathogenesis of squamous cell cancer is plausible and may involve primarily ultraviolet B exposure.

Host factors associated with increased risk include a background of Celtic, English, or Scandinavian descent, fair skin, blue eyes, red or blond hair, and inability to tan, as with the development of squamous cell carcinoma. A childhood history of frequent or blistering sunburns is also associated with increased risk. A personal history of previous basal cell carcinomas is an additional risk factor: almost half of the patients with one basal cell carcinoma will have a second independent primary within five years. Basal cell carcinoma has been reported in non-sun-exposed areas as well, such as the genitalia [14].

Basal cell carcinomas have been identified in burn, vaccination, and other scars, as well as in chronic extremity ulcers. Fewer than 1 percent of BCC arise from pre-existing scars, and most of these are in regions which are exposed to sunlight, suggesting a role for ultraviolet light, in addition to other mechanisms which have yet to be fully elucidated [6].

Genetic factors also affect the risk of developing BCC. Gorlin syndrome, also known as basal cell nevus syndrome, is a condition in which individuals develop many basal cell cancers throughout life, beginning as early as childhood. These patients may also have other cutaneous and skeletal abnormalities. *Xeroderma Pigmentosum* (XP) is a disorder with a genetic defect of DNA repair mechanisms and susceptibility to ultraviolet induced damage and carcinogenesis, which may be manifest by the eruption of both squamous cell and basal cell carcinomas in early childhood [2].

Underlying immunosuppression from the presence or treatment of other malignancies, such as leukemia or lymphoma, and immunosuppression following solid organ transplantation are also documented risk factors for BCC development, however, the risk increase is significantly lower than that for SCC development.

Exposure to chemical carcinogens, such as trivalent arsenic and radiation therapy have been associated with an increased risk of basal cell carcinoma [15, 16].

3.   SQUAMOUS CELL CARCINOMA

Squamous cell cancer (SCC) of the skin is a tumor of malignant keratinocytes of the epidermis which tends to be more aggressive than basal cell carcinoma, and more likely to metastasize to other body areas. This is the second most common malignancy in Caucasians, accounting for 20 percent of skin cancers. In non-white races, it is the most common skin cancer. Though most SCC develop in sun-exposed areas, they may also arise within areas of chronic inflammation or scarring. In individuals with dark skin, they do not have a tendency to occur in sun-exposed areas [1, 3].

Established causes of cutaneous SCC include environmental, host, and genetic factors. Sun exposure is the most important avoidable cause of SCC. SCC has been linked to cumulative sun exposures, and recent exposures appear to be important factors in its development, as well as past exposures. In this aspect it appears to differ from both BCC and melanoma.

Psoralen and ultraviolet A (PUVA) is a therapy which has been used for decades for patients with psoriasis, mycosis fungoides, and other dermatoses. This therapy involves ingestion or application of a strongly photosensitizing compound (psoralen), and subsequent exposure to intense UVA radiation. Studies indicate that this is carcinogenic and immunosuppressive, particularly with long-term therapy (greater than 100 treatments) and at doses of $250j/cm^2$ or greater [4].

Several host factors contribute to the risk of developing non-melanoma skin cancer. These include skin color (light skin is more susceptible), inability to tan, susceptibility to sunburn, and light color of skin and hair. The rates of squamous cell carcinoma are greater than ten times higher in white than in black individuals. Among whites, those with red hair have a risk of developing skin cancer which is three times greater than those with black hair [5]. Underlying diseases, which result in suppression of the immune system, increase the risk of developing squamous cell cancer through impairment of the individual's ability to detect and reject tumors. Iatrogenic immunosuppression of organ transplant recipients frequently results in particularly high multiplicity of cutaneous SCC, and those SCCs have a relatively poor prognosis. Leukemia and lymphoma also have been linked to increased SCC risk. The risk for developing non-melanoma skin cancer is 40 percent at 20 years after renal transplant and is greater than 40 percent at seven years following cardiac transplantation according to some reports [9-11]. This risk varies substantially with latitude of residence.

The presence of burn scars and ulcers predisposes an individual to squamous cell cancer development. Approximately two percent of squamous malignancies arise within burn scars [6].

A history of previous squamous cell carcinoma has proven to be an additional risk factor, as with basal cell carcinoma.

Several genetic disorders predispose individuals to an increased risk of developing cutaneous malignancy. These include *Xeroderma Pigmentosum*, albinism, and *Epidermodysplasia Verruciformis*. *Xeroderma Pigmentosum* (XP) is a genetic disease associated with abnormal DNA repair. It is a rare autosomal recessive disorder manifest by extreme sensitivity to ultraviolet light, abnormal skin pigmentation, premature skin aging, and the early development of many ultraviolet-induced skin cancers. Patients with XP have a 1000-fold increased risk of developing non-melanoma skin cancer [2].

Human papillomavirus infection has also been associated with non-melanoma skin cancer. Certain HPV types (particularly 16 and 18) have been associated most closely with SCC, mostly when it occurs in the genital tract, perianal area or on the fingers. The association between HPV and SCC in other distributions is less clear. *Epidermodysplasia Verruciformis* is a disorder of generalized human papillomavirus infection (HPV) manifest by multiple flat warts with a tendency to develop into squamous cell carcinoma [8]. In immunosuppressed populations, such as renal transplant recipients, HPV infection may play a significant role in cutaneous malignancy [7].

Albinism is a genetic disorder of melanin production resulting in white skin and hair and ocular changes. The decrease in or absence of melanin predisposes the individual to skin cancer.

Other factors associated with non-melanoma skin cancer development include exposure to arsenic, and to a smaller degree, polycyclic and aromatic hydrocarbons, soot, coal tar, paraffin, creosol, asphalt, and diesel oils [12].

4.   MALIGNANT MELANOMA

Malignant melanoma is the third most common cancer of the skin. It derives from melanocytes, which are the pigment producing cells of the skin. Malignant melanoma has several causes. Ultraviolet exposure appears to be responsible for most cases. Early, intense and intermittent sun exposure, rather than cumulative exposure is most important. A history of multiple severe, painful sunburns is associated with malignant melanoma. Traits including the size, type, and multiplicity of nevomelanocytic nevi on the skin, skin complexion, eye and hair color, facultative skin color, and ethnic heritage have been identified as risk factors. A family history of melanoma, immunosuppression and photochemotherapy with psoralens and UVA radiation also appear to have a causal role [17].

Sun exposure is the major avoidable risk factor for malignant melanoma development. Intense, intermittent sun exposure is strongly associated with melanoma, and individuals with a history of multiple painful sunburns during childhood have a greater risk of developing malignant melanoma than those without such a history. Residence during the childhood years in regions with intense sunlight exposure is an important risk factor. These factors demonstrate the importance of ultraviolet exposure during childhood [18].

Ultraviolet exposure from artificial sources is of great interest in the study of malignant melanoma. Recreational and cosmetic use of artificial UV lamps and beds has become increasingly popular. In North America, an estimated 25 million individuals use these annually. Artificial ultraviolet sources emit varying proportions of both UVA and UVB. Ultraviolet A emission from tanning lamps, however, may be two to three times greater than that from the sun. Artificial UVA exposure may even enhance the skin's response to subsequent UVB. This has yet to be fully clarified. A causal association between ultraviolet exposure and malignant melanoma has not been proven. Some studies find no statistically significant association, and some find a positive association and suggest a dose-response relationship. The latter studies contain many limitations which make the conclusions difficult to interpret and reliably accept [17, 19, 30].

Risk enhancing host factors are numerous. Celtic, Scandinavian, Australian, or Canadian heritage may significantly increase an individual's risk of developing a melanoma. Light complexion, facultative skin color with an early and easy burning reaction to sunlight, red or blond hair color, and numerous ephelides as a child are reproducibly identified as significant host factors. Blue, gray, or green eye color has been implicated in some studies and not in others. The presence of multiple large nevi, is one of the most significant host factors which enhances the risk of MM development, and the risk increases with increasing number of nevi [21]. Personal history of melanoma substantially increases (about eight to nine-fold) the risk of subsequent such cancers. A history of a first-degree relative with melanoma also substantially increases the risk [17].

Iatrogenic risk factors may play a role in malignant melanoma. Photochemotherapy with psoralens and UVA radiation (PUVA) as used for the treatment of psoriasis, mycosis fungoides, and other dermatologic conditions is a suggested etiologic factor. PUVA induces abnormal melanocytic proliferations and abnormal pigmentation of the skin and is carcinogenic. One study which followed PUVA patients for a period of fifteen years after therapy identified an increased risk of malignant melanoma in this population and suggested a dose-response relationship. The presence of confounding factors is omitted in this study, posing limitations to interpretation. Additional studies are needed to fully elucidate the etiologic role of PUVA therapy [22]. Immunosuppression in kidney and heart transplant recipients produces an elevated risk of developing malignant melanoma relative to the immunocompetent population [23].

5.   OTHER CUTANEOUS MALIGNANCIES

Squamous cell carcinoma, basal cell carcinoma, and malignant melanoma are the most common cutaneous malignancies, and their association with ultraviolet radiation has been extensively studied in efforts to understand their etiology and to determine the optimal methods of prevention. Ultraviolet radiation may play an etiologic role in the development of two other neoplastic conditions of the skin, atypical fibroxanthoma and Merkel cell carcinoma. Atypical fibroxanthoma is an uncommon neoplasm of the skin that most commonly arises in actinically damaged skin of elderly individuals. Ultraviolet B radiation induced DNA mutations and p53 mutations have been implicated [24].

Merkel cell carcinoma (MCC) is an uncommon aggressive malignancy of the neuroendocrine system which commonly arises in the head and neck region. A relationship to ultraviolet radiation and to immunosuppression is suggested, but a definite causal relationship has not been proven [26].

6. NONCUTANEOUS MALIGNANCIES

The relationship between ultraviolet radiation and cutaneous malignancies has been extensively studied and has been well delineated in certain types of skin cancer, particularly the non-melanoma skin cancers. The role of the ultraviolet light in the pathogenesis and development of other malignancies is uncertain, and requires further investigation. Cancers of the lymphoreticular system, breast, colon, and prostate, in particular, have been suggested to be linked in some way to UV radiation.

Non-Hodgkin's lymphoma (NHL) is a malignancy of the lymphatic tissues with an uncertain etiology. Various chemicals and immunosuppressive medications, and blood transfusions have been associated with this disease. A role for ultraviolet light has also been postulated. Though no definitive causal relationship has been found for any of these factors, it is evident that each of these exposures impairs the immune system. Ultraviolet light may do so by altering antigen presentation to the immune cells, influencing the expression of specific immunologically active substances, and altering cellular immunity in the manners previously described [26].

Breast cancer is a common malignancy affecting women of various ages. Genetic, endocrinologic, and environmental factors have been identified in the development of breast cancer. There is a suggested relationship between breast cancer mortality and differences in the amount of incident ultraviolet light in different areas of the United States [27]. The significance of these variations and associations remains to be determined. Colon and prostate cancers also have uncertain associations with ultraviolet exposure [28-30].

Though squamous cell and basal cell carcinomas, and malignant melanomas, as well as less common cutaneous malignancies, have well documented associations with ultraviolet radiation, cancers of several other organs may be associated with this radiation spectrum through postulated mechanisms which are shared and unique. Ultraviolet-induced immunosuppression and UV-induced DNA damage are important in cutaneous malignancy development and may be so in non-Hodgkin's lymphoma. Ultraviolet exposure may conceivably play a protective role and reduce the risk of colon and prostate cancers through the production of vitamin D or vitamin D precursors or derivatives. All of these hypotheses are highly speculative.

7.   PRIMARY PREVENTION

Since most skin cancers in general and melanomas in particular are attributable to ultraviolet light exposure, prevention is a key public health priority. Although sun exposure is not the only cause of any skin cancer, it remains the most important avoidable cause. Hence primary prevention has been the focus of many public health campaigns. Worldwide efforts in this regard have recently been reviewed [31].

The first major effort was the Australian "Slip!Slop!Slap!" campaign, which was recently adopted by the American Cancer Society (ACS). The slogan refers to slip on a shirt, slop on the sunscreen, and slap on a hat. Avoidance of intense exposures with shade, particularly in recreational areas, and avoiding the scheduling of activities when solar intensities are greatest have been emphasized in many campaigns. Protection of the skin with clothing and sunscreens has also been widely recommended. The focus on protection during the hours when the ultraviolet radiation (particularly the shorter wavelengths) is its most intense has led to the "shadow rule", *i.e.,* protection is most important when your shadow is shorter than you are. Additional information on the United States campaigns is available from the ACS, as well as the American Academy of Dermatology, the Centers for Disease Control and Prevention, and the Skin Cancer Foundation.

Two technological innovations in widespread use are likely to impact skin cancer incidence rates: sunscreen lotions and tanning lamps. For both, evaluation of their impact is complicated by their relatively recent widespread use that has deprived us of good observational data for the cancers with long lag periods, particularly melanoma. The nature of both has also been evolving. For sunscreens, the initial products were quite weak, their substantivity and photostability were poorly documented, and they protected against the shorter wavelengths of ultraviolet radiation only. For tanning lamps, the spectral distribution and typical patterns of use have both changed over time, although the nature of these changes has not been well documented. Both are associated with economic forces associated with their use that complicate the public discussion and evaluation.

Considerable controversy has surrounded the effectiveness of sunscreen lotion use for the prevention of skin cancer. Sunscreen lotions do not protect against all wavelengths of ultraviolet light equally, so both the quantity and composition of the ultraviolet exposure are changed by their use. Also, some have questioned whether these lotions allow for increased exposure to certain wavelengths because of their particular efficacy at preventing the most prominent acute consequence of excessive sun exposure, the sunburn, and hence their ability to allow wearers to increase sun exposure times. These issues have been addressed in detail elsewhere, and appear to be overblown. Existing evidence strongly supports the use of sunscreen lotions for skin cancer prevention [32]. Further evidence in this regard awaits publication of evidence from randomized trials, which is expected in the near future.

No such trial is underway for tanning lamps. The existing epidemiologic data has been summarized elsewhere. Those data suggest but do not prove that tanning lamp exposure increases melanoma risk [33].

8.   EARLY DETECTION

Because melanoma is responsible for the most deaths among skin cancers, public health campaigns have also focused (and in many cases, primarily focused) on reducing its case fatality. Since localized melanoma is more than 95 percent curable if excised when it is less than 1mm in thickness, but less than 50 percent curable if excised when greater than 4 mm in thickness, early detection is critical. Campaigns have generally encouraged early recognition by publicizing checklists or the "ABCD rule" [34]. The latter refers to Asymmetry, irregular Border, multiple Colors, and large Diameter. Both the checklists and the ABCD rule have their shortcomings [35]. Other algorithms have more recently been proposed to address these shortcomings [36]. These particularly address the importance of changes in size, shape, and color of spots on the skin.

Early detection campaigns generally involve education of health care providers and the general public. The former are encouraged to perform complete skin examinations, and the latter to perform regular thorough skin self-examinations. Formal screening has been a controversial concept in skin cancer [37, 38]. Limited evidence has been published that supports skin self-examination as a useful strategy for reducing mortality [39]. A large randomized community intervention trial of an early detection effort is underway.

9.   CONCLUSION

All individuals exposed to sunlight receive ultraviolet radiation. Geographic location and individual recreation and occupation behaviors determine the extent of exposure. Specific host factors, including skin color, skin type, hair color, and eye color, determine the skin's response to ultraviolet exposure. Certain cutaneous malignancies, squamous cell and basal cell carcinomas and malignant melanoma, have been definitively linked to UV exposure. Ultraviolet radiation is a suggested etiologic factor in other cutaneous neoplasias: atypical fibroxanthoma and Merkel cell carcinoma. Given the definitive role of UV radiation in the pathogenesis of cutaneous malignancies, protection against the potentially harmful effects of UV exposure involves several simple behaviors and should be pursued.

RECOMMENDATIONS

- Stay out of the sunlight from 10 AM to 4 PM.
- Wear hats, long-sleeve shirts, and SPF 15 sunscreens or higher.
- Avoid getting sunburned.
- Do not use sun lamps or tanning booths.

SUGGESTED FURTHER READING

1. Gallagher RP, Hill GB, Bajdik CD, *et al.* (1995) Sunlight exposure, pigmentary factors, and risk of nonmelanocytic skin cancer. II. Squamous cell carcinoma. *Arch Dermatol* **131:** 164-169.
2. Grossman D, Leffell DJ (1997) The molecular basis of non-melanoma skin cancer: new understanding. *Arch Dermatol* **133:** 1263-1270.
3. Weinstock MA (1995) Overview of Ultraviolet Radiation and cancer: what is the link? How are we doing? *Environ Health Perspect* **103:** 251-254.
4. Gallagher RP, Hill GB, Bajdik CD, *et al.* (1995) Sunlight exposure, pigmentary factors, and risk of nonmelanocytic skin cancer: I. Basal cell carcinoma. *Arch Dermatol* **131:** 157-163.

REFERENCES

1. Miller DL, Weinstock MA (1994) Nonmelanoma skin cancer in the United States: incidence. J *Am Acad Dermatol* **30:** 774-778.

2. Grossman D, Leffell DJ (1997) The molecular basis of non-melanoma skin cancer new understanding. *Arch Dermatol* **133:** 1263-1270.
3. Halder RM, Bang KM (1988) Skin cancer in blacks in the United States. *Dermatol Clin* **6:** 397-405.
4. Stern RS, Lange R (1988) Nonmelanoma skin cancer occurring in patients treated with PUVA five to ten years after first treatment. *J Inv Dermatol* **91:** 120.
5. Gallagher RP, Hill GB, Bajdik CD, *et al.* (1995) Sunlight exposure, pigmentary factors, and risk of nonmelanocytic skin cancer: II. squamous cell carcinoma. *Arch Dermatol* **131:** 164-169.
6. Phillips TJ, Salman SM, Bhawan J, Rogers GS (1998) Burn scar carcinoma - diagnosis and management. *Dermatol Surg* **24:** 561-565.
7. Euvrard S, Chardonnet Y, Pouteil-Noble C, *et al.* (1993) Association of skin malignancies with various and multiple carcinogenic and noncarcinogenic human papillomaviruses in renal transplant recipients. *Cancer* **72:** 2198-2206.
8. Majewski S, Jablonska S (1995) *Epidermodysplasia Verruciformis* as a model of human papillomavirus-induced genetic cancer of the skin. *Arch Dermatol* **131:** 1312-1318.
9. Liddington M, Richardson AJ, Higgins RM, *et al.* (1989) Skin cancer in renal transplant recipients. *Br J Surg* **76:** 1002-1005.
10. Hartevelt MM, Bavinck JN, Kootte AM, *et al.* (1990) Incidence of skin cancer after renal transplantation in The Netherlands. *Transplantation* **4:** 506-509.
11. Espana A, Redondo P, Fernandez AL, *et al.* (1995) Skin cancer in heart transplant recipients. *J Am Acad Dermatol* **32:** 458-465.
12. Brookes P, ed. (1980) Chemical Carcinogens. *Br J Med Bull* **36:** 1.
13. Gallagher RP, Ma B, McLean DI, *et al.* (1990) Trends in basal cell carcinoma, squamous cell carcinoma, and melanoma of the skin from 1973 through 1987. *J Am Acad Dermatol* **23:** 413-421.
14. Miller ES, Fairley JA, Neuberg M (1997) Vulvar basal cell carcinoma. *Dermatol Surg* **23:** 207-209.
15. Wong SS, Tan KC, Goh CL (1998) Cutaneous manifestations of chronic arsenicism: review of seventeen cases. *J Am Acad Dermatol* **38:** 179-185.
16. Dinehart SM, Anthony JL, Pollack SV (1991) Basal cell carcinoma in young patients after irradiation from childhood malignancy. *Med Pediatr Oncol* **19:** 508-510.
17. Weinstock MA (1998) Issues in the epidemiology of melanoma. *Hematol Oncol Clin North Am* **12:** 681-698.
18. Holly EA, Aston DA, Cress RD, Ahn DK, Kristiansen JJ (1995) Cutaneous melanoma in women: II. phenotypic characteristics and other host-related factors. *Am J Epidemiol* **141:** 934-942.
19. Osterlind A, Tucker MA, Stone BJ, Jensen OM (1988) The Danish case-control study of cutaneous malignant melanoma II. Importance of UV-light exposure. *Int J Cancer* **42:** 319-324.
20. Swerdlow AJ, Weinstock MA (1998) Do tanning lamps cause melanoma? An epidemiologic assessment. *J Am Acad Dermatol* **38:** 89-98.
21. Elwood JM, Williamson C, Stapleton PJ (1986) Malignant melanoma in relation to moles, pigmentation, and exposure to fluorescent and other lighting sources. *Br J Cancer* **53:** 65-74.
22. Stern RS, Nichols KT, Vakeva LH (1997) Malignant melanoma in patients treated for psoriasis with methoxsalen (psoralen) and ultraviolet A radiation (PUVA). *N Engl J Med* **336:** 1041-1045.

23. Jensen P, Hansen S, Moller B, *et al.* (1999) Skin cancer in kidney and heart transplant recipients and different long-term immunosuppressive therapy regimen. *J Am Acad Dermatol* **40:** 177-186.

24. Dei Tos AP, Maestro R, Doglioni C, *et al.* (1994) Ultraviolet-induced p53 mutations in atypical fibroxanthoma. *Am J Pathol* **145:** 11-17.

25. Miller RW, Rabkin CS (1999) Merkel cell carcinoma and melanoma: etiological similarities and differences. *Cancer Epidemiol Biomarkers Prev* **8:** 153-158.

26. Hardell L, Axelson O (1998) Environmental and occupational aspects on the etiology of non-Hodgkin's lymphoma. *Oncol Res* **10:** 1-5.

27. Garland FC, Garland CF, Gorham ED, Young JF (1990) Geographic variation in breast cancer mortality in the United States: a hypothesis involving exposure to solar radiation. *Prev Med* **19:** 614-622.

28. Kopelavich L (1983) Skin fibroblasts from humans predisposed to colon cancer are not abnormally sensitive to DNA damaging agents. *Cell Biol Int Rep* **7:** 369-375.

29. Little JB, Nove J, Weichselbaum RR (1980) Abnormal sensitivity of diploid skin fibroblasts from a family with gardner's syndrome to the lethal effects of X-irradiation, ultraviolet light, and mitomycin-C. *Mutat Res* **70:** 241-250.

30. Hanchette CL, Schwartz GG (1992) Geographic patterns of prostate cancer mortality. Evidence for a protective effect of ultraviolet radiation. *Cancer* **70:** 2861-2869.

31. Bioko S, ed. (1998) *Clinics in Dermatology,* Vol. 16.

32. Weinstock MA (1999) Do sunscreens increase or decrease melanoma risk: an epidemiologic evaluation. *J Invest Dermatol Suppl* **4:** 97-100.

33. Swerdlow AJ, Weinstock MA (1998) Do tanning lamps cause melanoma? An epidemiological assessment. *J Am Acad Dermatol* **38:** 89-98.

34. Whited JD, Grichnik JM (1998) Does this patient have a mole or melanoma? *JAMA* **279:** 696-701.

35. Weinstock MA, Goldstein MG, Dubé CE, Rhodes AR, Sober AJ (1998) Clinical diagnosis of moles vs melanoma. *JAMA* **280:** 881-882.

36. Weinstock MA, Goldstein MG, Dubé CE, Rhodes AR, Sober AJ (1996) Basic skin cancer triage for teaching melanoma detection. *J Am Acad Dermatol* **34:** 1063-1066.

37. Rampen FHJ (1998) Point: mass population skin cancer screening is not worthwhile. *J Cut Med Surg* **2:** 128-129.

38. Weinstock MA (1998) Counterpoint: mass population skin cancer screening can be worthwhile. *J Cut Med Surg* **2:** 129-132.

39. Berwick M, Begg CB, Fine JA, *et al.* (1996) Screening for cutaneous melanoma by skin self-examination. *J Natl Cancer Inst* **88:** 17-23.

Chapter 12

Radiation

John D. Boice, Jr., Sc.D. and John B. Little, M.D.
International Epidemiology Institute, Rockville, MD and Department of Cancer Cell Biology, Harvard School of Public Health, Boston, MA.

INTRODUCTION

Just over 100 years ago in 1895, Roentgen discovered the X-ray and revolutionized the practice of medicine. Over 50 years ago in 1945, World War II was brought to an end after the atomic bombs were dropped on Hiroshima and Nagasaki. The first commercial nuclear power plant began operating in 1957 and now nearly 20 percent of the electricity produced each year in the United States is from nuclear energy. In some countries, such as France, over 70 percent of the electrical power is from nuclear sources. Over the course of the century, radiation became pervasive in our world, sometimes with deleterious consequences. The Chernobyl nuclear reactor accident, for example, occurred in 1986 and spewed radioactivity throughout Europe and Asia. The beneficial uses of radiation have also become widespread, most notably in the treatment of cancer and the diagnosis of disease.

We live in a sea of low-level invisible radiation. Odorless and colorless, ionizing radiations continually bombard our bodies throughout life, and it is the release of ionizing energy within cells that can cause cancer. We know much about radiation risks. Comprehensive epidemiologic studies have been conducted of the Japanese atomic bomb survivors, patients given radiotherapy for benign and malignant conditions, workers occupationally exposed, populations living in areas of enhanced environmental radiation, and others (Table 12.1). Both the United Nations and the National Academy

G.A. Colditz et al. (eds.), Cancer Prevention: The Causes and Prevention of Cancer - Volume I, 123–136.
© 2000 *Kluwer Academic Publishers.*

of Sciences periodically publish authoritative volumes on the effects of radiation [1, 2]. No other environmental carcinogen, with the possible exception of tobacco, has been as extensively studied, yet there remains a public mystique about radiation that tends to exaggerate the actual hazard. While radiation is a human carcinogen, it is a relatively weak one, in part because it is such an effective cell killer. For example, nearly 100,000 women treated with radiation for cervical cancer were required to detect a significant doubling of the risk of leukemia [3], yet fewer than 1000 women with ovarian cancer were sufficient to identify a nearly 100-fold increase in leukemia risk due to chemotherapy [4].

Table 12.1 Epidemiologic studies with semiquantitative estimates of radiation doses to specific organs and cancer risks [1, 5-7]

Type of Exposure	Study
Atomic Bomb	Japanese bomb survivors
	Marshall Islanders
Radiotherapy for Malignant Disease	Cervical cancer
	Childhood cancer
	Breast cancer
	Endometrial cancer
	Hodgkin's disease
	Bone marrow transplant
Radiotherapy for Benign Disease	Ankylosing spondylitis
	Benign gynecologic disease
	Peptic ulcer
	Breast disease
	Tinea capitis
	Thymus enlargement
	Tonsil enlargement
	Hemangioma
	Bone disease, radium-224
	Hyperthyroidism, iodine-131
Diagnostic Procedures	Tuberculosis, fluoroscopic X-rays
	Thorotrast, thorium-232
	Thyroid, iodine-131
	Prenatal X-rays
Occupation	Radium dial painters, radium-226
	Underground miners
	Radiologists, technologists
	Nuclear Workers

The average *per capita* dose from all sources of radiation is about 3.4 mSv (millisieverts) per year of which natural sources (radon, cosmic rays, uranium, potassium-40) contribute 2.9 mSv/yr, or about **88** percent of the total. The remaining 12 percent are derived primarily from medical exposures (0.5 mSv per year). Based on linear extrapolation from high dose data (500-2000 mSv) it can be inferred that only a small fraction, about one to three percent of all cancers might be attributable to radiation arising largely from natural sources, in contrast to the 30 percent attributable to tobacco use. Lowering the risk of radiogenic cancer within the population can come mainly by exposure avoidance, such as reducing environments with high radon levels, minimizing unnecessary medical exposures, and improving medical applications by reducing the amount of radiation necessary to produce clinically informative images.

1.   RADIATION AS A CAUSE OF CANCER

Conclusive evidence that radiation can cause cancer comes from the studies of Japanese atomic bomb survivors, pioneering radiologists, and patient populations.   While the single most important study is of the survivors of the atomic bombs, there are well over 100 studies of patient populations linking radiation to cancer which confirm and extend our knowledge of radiation effects.   The major unanswered questions revolve around the magnitude of the risk at low levels of exposure, the ameliorating effect of spreading exposure over time, and the lifetime risk following exposures in childhood.   The following sections will touch on topics of current scientific and public health interest: Should I be concerned about breathing radon in my home?   Are X-ray mammographs dangerous?   Does genetic makeup affect my radiation risk?   Is living near a nuclear installation or power plant a cancer risk factor?   Can my radiation exposure affect the health of future children I might have?   Have studies of radiation exposures in the former Soviet Union provided new insights into radiation effects?   Since we know so much about radiation, why are there lingering controversies?

2.   SOME GENERAL PRINCIPLES

The amount of radiation needed to double the risk of cancer is quite large and of the order of 2000 mSv -- nearly 1000 times the annual exposure received from natural background sources. Risks at low levels are difficult to measure but can be estimated by extrapolation from high doses and applying principles from radiation biology. Some types of radiation are more effective in causing cancer than other types, in particular alpha particles (which are emitted during the decay of radon and radon progenies) and neutrons (which can be experienced during high altitude air travel). Children and females appear somewhat more sensitive to the carcinogenic effects of radiation than adults and males. Spreading the exposure to X-rays or gamma rays over time is seen to diminish considerably the carcinogenic effect in studies of animals, but the evidence from human studies is less conclusive. Leukemia can occur in excess within about two years after exposure but risk appears to return to near normal levels after 20 to 30 years have past. Other cancers, on the other hand, may take ten years or more before excesses can be detected and risk appears to remain high throughout the remainder of life. Age at exposure can modify the effectiveness of radiation to cause cancer; for example, radiogenic thyroid cancer is not apparent among adults exposed after age 20 and radiogenic breast cancer is not seen among women exposed past menopause. The major radiation-induced cancers are leukemia, female breast cancer, thyroid cancer following exposures in childhood, and lung cancer. Although many cancers have been linked to radiation exposure in human studies, many have not -- most notably chronic lymphocytic leukemia, adult T-cell leukemia, Hodgkin's disease, and cancer of the cervix, testis, prostate and pancreas.

3. RADON

Based on studies of underground miners exposed to high radon levels, it is estimated that approximately ten percent of all lung cancer deaths (or 15,400 to 21,800 per year) might be attributable to indoor radon [2]. Because the entire population, over 260 million citizens, breathes in radon with every breath, even a small risk can translate into large numbers of estimated deaths. Since most population exposure to radon is from very low levels, remediation of all homes above 4 pCi/L (picocuries per liter) -- the level at which the U.S. Environmental Protection Agencies recommends intervention -- would reduce the attributable risk by only one third or from ten percent to about six to eight percent. The main uncertainties in such estimates, however, are whether results from underground miner studies can be generalized to aboveground residential circumstances and whether extrapolation from high doses to very low doses is valid. Miners are exposed to silica dust, arsenic, diesel fumes, blasting smoke and other lung irritants or carcinogens that conceivably could exacerbate the effects of radon. Many miners were heavy cigarette smokers and convincing evidence suggests that radon and tobacco smoke interact to cause more lung cancers than expected from the sum of their individual effects.

Indoor radon studies have not provided a clear answer to whether levels in the home are hazardous, primarily because the risk is very small and is difficult to detect in the presence of other more powerful carcinogens such as tobacco smoke. Comprehensive studies in Sweden and England have suggested elevated risks while equally rigorous investigations in China, Canada and Missouri find no evidence of excess risk. A study of incident lung cancer among nonsmoking women in Missouri concluded that less than two percent of all lung cancers could be attributable to radon levels greater than 4 pCi/L, which was less than the risk attributable to passive smoking (6.1 percent) and other factors [8]. Because the lung cancer risk associated with exposures of 4 pCi/L is very low – of the order of a 10 to 30 percent relative increase – a single study is not powerful enough to detect convincingly a risk of this magnitude. Thus it is noteworthy that a recent meta-analysis of eight studies of indoor radon found a slight but significant elevation in lung cancer risk that was consistent with that estimated from studies of underground miners [9]. The graphical display of this analysis (Figure 12.1) indicates how difficult it is for epidemiology to detect convincingly radiation risks at very low levels, and how reliance on high dose studies is important. Recent evaluations of the miner data support their use in estimating risks from indoor radon and in forming the basis for public policy [2].

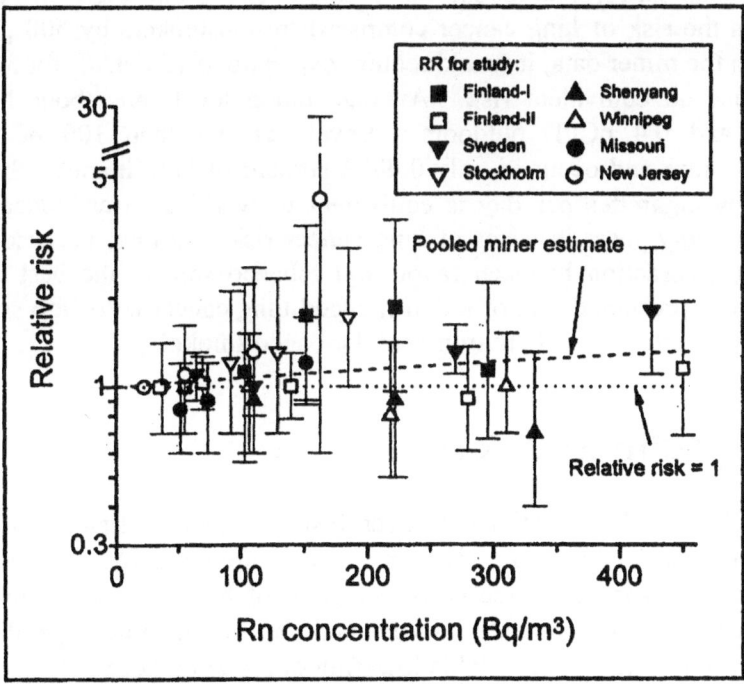

Figure 12.1 The risk of lung cancer associated with indoor levels of radon in eight studies contrasted with the level extrapolated from studies of underground miners [9]. 37 Bq/m³ is the same as 1 pCi/L. Thus 150 Bq/m³ would be about 4

pCi/L -- the action level recommended by the U.S. Environmental Protection
Agency for home remediation.

Some "ecological" studies have contrasted county-wide measures of
radon levels with county lung cancer deaths and find no evidence for an
association and even suggest a threshold below which the risk is negligible.
The problems associated with these geographical correlation studies include
the inability to control for smoking or for migration and the absence of any
knowledge of radon exposures to individuals who died in these counties [2].
To illustrate the problem of migration in the U.S., descriptive
epidemiologists like to remark how interesting it is that people in Florida are
born Hispanic but then die Jewish. Even if the county estimates of radon
were accurate for individuals, which is unlikely, the peripatetic nature of the
U.S. populace negates any meaning that could be ascribed to the
correlations. While the level of risk associated with indoor radon remains
uncertain, ecological surveys, because of their inherent limitations, should
not be used to conclude that there is no risk.

In terms of risk comparisons, tobacco use is a much more important
cause of lung cancer than radon. For example, one to nine cigarettes per day
increases the risk of lung cancer compared to nonsmokers by 500 percent.
Based on the miner data, it would require exposure to 120 pCi/L for 30 years
to produce an equivalent risk. Average radon levels are about 1 pCi/L
indoors and 0.4 pCi/L outdoors. Levels greater than 100 pCi/L are
extremely rare and occur in only 0.0002 percent of U.S. homes. Smoking
just a few cigarettes per day is equivalent to working in an underground
mine for many years in terms of lung cancer risk. Further, because of the
enhanced interaction between radon and tobacco smoke, the best way to
reduce your presumed risk of radon-induced lung cancer is to stop smoking
and/or reduce the level of environmental tobacco smoke.

4.   MEDICAL X-RAYS

In 1977, the U.S. National Cancer Institute held its first "consensus"
conference, and the topic chosen was mammography screening of
asymptomatic women for the early detection of breast cancer. Since that
time, there have been notable improvements in the imaging capabilities of
the X-ray units and an appreciable lowering of radiation dose to breast tissue
– by a factor of more than ten. The controversy today is not whether the
radiation exposures are hazardous, but whether young women, under the age
of 50, benefit from the mammographic examinations. A reduction in breast
cancer mortality of 30 percent has been convincingly demonstrated in

randomized trials of women over age 50 who received screening examinations that included mammographic X-rays. The benefit for younger women is less clear, but apparently lower. The possible hazard from mammographic X-rays is very low and should not be a factor in individual decisions to undergo this procedure. The same is true for most diagnostic X-ray procedures.

Nearly all studies of women exposed to radiation find that risk of induced breast cancer decreases appreciably with age at the time of exposure, and most studies fail to find a significant increase when exposures occur past the menopausal age [1, 10-12]. Despite recent claims that medical radiation is responsible for up to 75 percent of all breast cancers in the United States [13], a more reasonable estimate is that less than one percent of all breast cancers might be attributed to medical uses of radiation. For an individual woman, her lifetime risk might increase from 9.09 to perhaps 9.18 percent [14, 15]. It seems likely this small presumed risk is more than offset by the benefit of the diagnostic procedure. Nonetheless, unnecessary radiation exposures should be avoided and continued vigilance is required to ensure that the benefits associated with specific procedures outweigh the future risks.

The first reports that prenatal X-ray exposures were associated with an increased risk of leukemia and solid cancers during childhood were published in the 1950s [1, 5]. Evidence for a causal association comes almost entirely from case-control studies, whereas practically all cohort or prospective studies, including the atomic bomb survivors exposed *in utero*, find no association. Most of the case-control studies of medical exposure to diagnostic X-rays during pregnancy are consistent with a 40 to 50 percent increased risk of childhood cancer. Such studies are important because of the possibility that the developing fetus might be at higher radiation risk than children exposed after birth, and because there are few studies that provide direct evidence of radiation risks at relatively low levels. The association between prenatal X-ray and childhood cancer is not in doubt, but the causal nature of the association continues to be debated [1, 16, 17]. One peculiar observation in the case-control studies is the similarity in the excess relative risk estimates for each type of cancer — all are increased by 40 to 50 percent, whether the cancer is leukemia, lymphoma, Wilm's tumor, neuroblastoma or brain cancer. Such similarity suggests a possible underlying bias that has not been identified. Nonetheless, the medical profession has acted prudently, and pelvimetry X-rays have been replaced in large part by ultrasound procedures, which produce images from sound waves and do not involve ionizing radiation.

5.   NUCLEAR POWER PLANTS, CHERNOBYL, AND RUSSIAN EXPOSURES

Comprehensive surveys in several countries, including the United States, have failed to confirm increases in cancer risk associated with living in neighborhoods close to nuclear power plants or installations reported in the U.K. [1, 5]. This would be as expected if radiation releases during normal operations were as low as those reported, that is, much lower than natural background exposures [18]. The reactor accident at Chernobyl, however, was a major disaster. Radiation contaminated the environment surrounding the plant, and hundreds of thousands of workers came to cleanup the radioactive debris. The accident resulted from serious mistakes made by the operators; the release of radioactive was massive because of the absence of a containment vessel, a common safety feature in the West. The radiation released during the accident at Three Mile Island, for example, was very small.

It is yet too early to expect to see much increase in solid cancer rates within exposed Chernobyl populations because of the relatively long latency needed for radiation-induced cancer to be detected. While the latent period for leukemia is shorter, there have been no convincing reports of increases in childhood or adult leukemia among any exposed group suggesting that the radiation doses might not be sufficient to detect excesses [1, 19]. The only radiation effect to date appears to be a remarkable increase in childhood thyroid cancer [20]. A precise association with radioactive I-131 remains uncertain, however, because other radionuclides of iodine may have contributed to the thyroid dose, endemic goiter may have contributed to risk, convincing dose-response relationships have not been reported, and the increase occurs much earlier than expected based on current understanding of radiogenic thyroid cancer. It is also likely that increased surveillance contributed to detecting and reporting thyroid tumors [21].

Recently, it was disclosed that high levels of radioactive waste were dumped into the Techa river in the southern Urals from the Mayak nuclear facility in the former Soviet Union. Many villages downstream were eventually evacuated but only after the population ingested or inhaled large amounts of radioactive substances [22]. In the haste to develop a nuclear capability, radiation workers at the Mayak reactor plant also received large cumulative exposures [23]. Ongoing studies of workers at Russian nuclear installations and of surrounding populations in the southern Urals of Russia have the potential to contribute new information on the effects of chronic exposures to low levels of radiation that accumulate to large doses over time.

6.   RADIOACTIVE I-131

Radioactive iodine is used in medicine to treat and diagnose disease; it is released during nuclear reactor operations; and it is a component of radioactive fallout from weapons testing [1, 5, 6]. With the possible exception of thyroid cancer following exposures in childhood, there is little evidence that radioactive iodine, and I-131 in particular, is a potent carcinogen. This is probably because the thyroid absorbs most of the radioactive iodines ingested or injected – and the adult thyroid gland appears relatively immune to the carcinogenic effects of radiation – and other organs receive much lower doses. I-131 also has an eight day half life, which means that the radiation released during decay is protracted over time which might allow repair of radiation damage more readily than if the dose were received all at once. Very large studies of primarily adult populations given I-131 in medical settings have failed to find consistent increases in any cancer, including leukemia and thyroid cancer, despite substantial exposures [24, 25]. Studies of populations around Chernobyl, however, indicate an increase in thyroid cancer, but no other malignancy, among children exposed to radioactive iodines. Given the widespread use of I-131 in medicine, primarily among adults, the medical studies are reassuring in indicating that the adverse late effects appear very small in comparison with the medical benefit from improved diagnosis and treatment of thyroid disease.

7.   GENETIC PREDISPOSITION

Except in rare instances, it is not known whether an individual's genetic profile places him or her at unusually high (or low) risk of developing radiogenic cancers [26, 27]. One exception is heritable germline retinoblastoma, a rare childhood cancer of the eye. An affected child inherits a defective gene in one allele of the RB tumor suppressor gene, and then acquires a new mutation in the opposite allele. Such individuals are at high risk of developing osteosarcoma which is further enhanced following high dose radiotherapy [28]. Ataxia telangiectasia (AT) is another rare disorder associated with a high incidence of cancers of hematopoietic origin. Nonaffected gene carriers (heterozygotes), perhaps one percent of the population, may be at increased risk for breast cancer, but extreme sensitivity to the carcinogenic effects of ionizing radiation seems unlikely [27, 29] – an important question relative to the use of X-ray mammography in the >40 age group. Radiation and genetic susceptibility is an area of active research and could modify our understanding of radiation risk and mechanism. At the current time, however, small doses of radiation appear to contribute negligibly to the risk of cancer among individuals with familial cancer disorders (*i.e.,* persons with an inherent predisposition to cancer), whereas cancer risks seem important at high doses received during radiotherapy [28].

8.   GENETICS EFFECTS

There have been a number of reports out of England that radiation exposure to fathers might increase the risk of leukemia in their children [1, 5]. Subsequent research around the world did not confirm the initial reports which were based on small numbers of cancers [30]. While there is convincing evidence in fruit flies and mice that radiation exposure to the parent can be detrimental to future generations, no genetic effects in man have been demonstrated. Most notably, the comprehensive studies of the children of the survivors of the atomic bombings in Hiroshima and Nagasaki find no evidence for increases in childhood cancer, mortality, untoward pregnancies (defined as congenital malformations, stillbirths, and neonatal deaths), chromosome changes, sex ratio (male to female ratio), or blood protein changes [31]. These and other data from studies of the offspring of survivors of childhood cancer treated with radiation suggest that the human germinal cells may be relatively insensitive to the mutagenic effects of radiation that can be transmitted to offspring and lead to detrimental consequences in future generations.

9.   SOME CONTROVERSY REMAINS

Radiation protection guidelines exist to minimize exposures for occupational groups and the general population. The linear relationship to estimate risks at low levels is used by radiation protection committees to provide an appropriate standard of protection without unduly limiting the beneficial practices giving rise to radiation exposure [7]. The recommendations of these committees, however, are not universally accepted. Some contend that because cells efficiently repair damage to DNA that low doses might be beneficial by stimulating cellular repair systems so that subsequent exposures are more effectively repaired [32]. Others have argued that the linear response is not conservative and might underestimate radiation risk [33]. There appears little evidence for low doses of radiation to have beneficial effects based on animal or analytic epidemiologic data [1], and the relevance of the cellular response to afford protection against the mutagenic effects of low-level radiation is highly uncertain [7]. The weight of knowledge from comprehensive epidemiologic investigations on radiation and cancer risk is substantive [1] so that arguments that risks are greatly underestimated have become less tenable. It seems illogical that low doses of radiation would produce more cancers than high doses, especially when risks at high doses are not very large to begin with. There are several areas of molecular biology research, however, that suggest that exposures at low levels may not be free of risk, even though these risks cannot be measured by epidemiologic methods [34]. Genomic instability, for example, is a cellular response to radiation in which mutation or chromosome changes are not seen until many cell divisions have occurred [35]. The bystander effect is a phenomenon where radiation damage in some cells can lead indirectly to damage in neighboring cells that were not irradiated [36]. Radiation biology appears on the threshold of providing renewed understanding of the risks posed by low level exposures.

CONCLUSION

Radiation can cause cancer but the level of risk is much lower than perceived by the general public [37]. Most people exposed to radiation do not develop cancer. Even among the 100,000 Japanese atomic bomb survivors, only 400 to 500 cancer deaths (about one percent) of the over 40,000 deaths from all causes could be attributed to radiation. Reducing high levels of radon makes sense and unnecessary X-rays should be avoided. Radiogenic equipment improvements in medicine, such as mammography units, have reduced patient exposures without diminishing clinical usefulness. On the other hand, some radiation control measures are extremely costly and reduce risk only slightly [38, 39]. Understanding radiation risks and comparing them with other hazards of life should help society and individuals make informed decisions about medical and technological uses (see Summary Points and Recommendations).

SUMMARY POINTS

- Radiation can cause most types of cancer, most notably myelogenous leukemia and cancers of the breast, thyroid, and lung.
- Some cancers such as the sarcomas and cancers of the bone and rectum appear to develop only after very large, therapeutic exposures.
- A few cancers have not been linked convincingly to radiation, for example, chronic lymphocytic leukemia, non-Hodgkin's lymphoma,

Hodgkin's disease, and cancer of the cervix, testis, prostate, and pancreas.
- Based on extrapolation from data on people exposed to high doses, it is estimated that one to three percent of all cancers might be due to all forms of radiation (primarily from natural sources) and that 10 percent of lung cancer might result from indoor radon.

RECOMMENDATIONS

- Exposure to high levels of radiation in the past (*e.g.*, radiotherapy for enlarged tonsils)should be brought to the attention of your health care provider.
- Because of the enhanced interaction between radon and tobacco smoke, the best way to reduce presumed risk of radon-induced lung cancer is to stop smoking.
- Diagnostic procedure with possible radiation risk should not be refused because of clinical symptoms of a serious disease (the future risk is very low and the immediate benefit may be great).
- Most people will not develop radiation-related cancer because of radiation exposures in the past.

SUGGESTED FURTHER READING

1. United Nations Scientific Committee on the Effects of Atomic Radiation (UNSCEAR) (1994) *Sources and Effects of Ionizing Radiation. Publ E.94.IX.II.* New York, NY (USA): United Nations.
2. Boice JD Jr, Land CE, Preston D (1996) Ionizing radiation. In: Schottenfeld D, Fraumeni JF Jr, eds. *Cancer Epidemiology and Prevention.* New York, NY (USA): Oxford University Press, pp. 319-354.

REFERENCES

1. United Nations Scientific Committee on the Effects of Atomic Radiation (UNSCEAR) (1994) *Sources and Effects of Ionizing Radiation. Publ E.94.IX.11.* New York, NY (USA): United Nations.
2. National Research Council Committee on the Biological Effects of Ionizing Radiation (1999) *Health Effects of Exposure to Radon (BEIR VI).* Washington, DC: National Academy Press, pp. 500.

3. Boice JD Jr, Blettner M, Kleinerman RA, *et al.* (1987) Radiation dose and leukemia risk in patients treated for cancer of the cervix. *J Natl Cancer Inst* **79:** 1295-1311.

4. Greene MH, Boice JD Jr, Greer BE, *et al.* (1982) Acute nonlymphocytic leukemia after therapy with alkylating agents for ovarian cancer: a study of 5 randomized clinical trials. *N Engl J Med* **307:** 1416-1421.

5. Boice JD Jr, Land CE, Preston D (1996) Ionizing radiation. In: Schottenfeld D, Fraumeni JF Jr, eds. *Cancer Epidemiology and Prevention.* New York, NY (USA): Oxford University Press, pp. 319-354.

6. Boice JD Jr, ed. (1997) *Implications of New Data on Radiation Cancer Risk.* Bethesda, MD (USA): National Council on Radiation Protection and Measurements, pp. 315.

7. Upton AC (1999) The linear-nonthreshold dose-response model: a critical reappraisal. *NCRP Proc* **1:** 9-31.

8. Alavanja MCR, Brownson RC, Benichou J, *et al.* (1995) Attributable risk of lung cancer in lifetime nonsmokers and long-term ex-smokers (Missouri, United States). *Cancer Causes Control* **6:** 209-216.

9. Lubin JH, Boice JD Jr (1997) Lung cancer risk from residential radon: meta-analysis of eight epidemiologic studies. *J Natl Cancer Inst* **89:** 49-57.

10. Boice JD Jr, Preston D, Davis FG, *et al.* (1991) Frequent chest X-ray fluoroscopy and breast cancer incidence among tuberculosis patients in Massachusetts. *Radiat Res* **125:** 214-222.

11. Boice JD Jr, Harvey E, Blettner M, *et al.* (1992) Cancer in the contralateral breast after radiotherapy for breast cancer. *N Engl J Med* **326:** 781-785.

12. Thompson D, Mabuchi K, Ron E, *et al.* (1994) Cancer incidence in atomic bomb survivors. Part II: solid tumors, 1958-87. *Radiat Res* **137:** S17-S67.

13. Skolnick AA (1995) Claim that medical *X-rays* caused most U.S. breast cancers found incredible. *JAMA* **274:** 367-368.

14. Heath CW Jr (1995) Preventing breast cancer: the story of a major proven, preventable cause of this disease (Book Review). *JAMA* **274:** 657.

15. Evans JS, Wennberg JE, McNeil BJ (1986) The influence of diagnostic radiography on the incidence of breast cancer and leukemia. *N Engl J Med* **315:** 810-815.

16. Doll R, Wakeford R (1997) Risk of childhood cancer from fetal irradiation. *Br J Radiol* **70:** 130-139.

17. Boice JD Jr, Miller RW (1999) Childhood and adult cancer after intrauterine exposure to ionizing radiation. *Teratology* **59:** 227-233.

18. Jablon S, Hrubec Z, Boice JD Jr (1991) Cancer in populations living near nuclear facilities. A survey of mortality nationwide and incidence in two states. *JAMA* **265:** 1403-1408.

19. Rahu M, Tekkel M, Veidebaum T, *et al.* (1997) The Estonian study of Chernobyl cleanup workers: III. Incidence of cancer and mortality. *Radiat Res* **147:** 653-657.

20. Astakhova LN, Anspaugh LR, Beebe GW, *et al.* (1998) Chernobyl-related thyroid cancer in children of Belarus: a case-control study. *Radiat Res* **150:** 349-356.

21. Ron E, Lubin JH, Shore RE, *et al.* (1995) Thyroid cancer after exposure to external radiation: a pooled analysis of seven studies. *Radiat Res* **141:** 259-277.

22. Kossenko MM, Degteva MO, Vyushkova OV, *et al.* (1997) Issues in the comparison of risk estimates for the population in the Techa River region and atomic bomb survivors. *Radiat Res* **148:** 54-63.

23. Koshurnikova NA, Shilnikova NS, Okatenko PV, *et al.* (1997) The risk of cancer among nuclear workers at the 'Mayak' production association: preliminary results of an

epidemiological study. In: Boice JD Jr, ed. *Implications of New Data on Radiation Cancer Risk. NCRP Proc* **18:** 113-122.

24. Hall P, Mattsson A, Boice JD Jr (1996) Thyroid cancer following diagnostic administration of iodine-131. *Radiat Res* **145:** 86-92.

25. Ron E, Doody MM, Becker DV, *et al.* (1998) Cancer mortality following treatment for hyperthyroidism. *JAMA* **280:** 347-355.

26. Little JB (1993) Cellular, molecular, and carcinogenic effects of radiation. *Hematol Oncol Clin N Am* **7:** 337-352.

27. International Commission on Radiological Protection (ICRP) (1999) ICRP Publication 79. Genetic susceptibility to cancer. *Annals ICRP* **28:** 1-157.

28. Wong FL, Boice JD Jr, Abramson DH, *et al.* (1997) Cancer incidence after retinoblastoma: radiation dose and sarcoma risk. *JAMA* **278:** 1262-1267.

29. Lavin M (1998) Role of the ataxia-telangiectasia gene (ATM) in breast cancer. A-T heterozygotes seem to have an increased risk but its size is unknown. *Br Med J* **317:** 486-487.

30. Doll R, Evans HJ, Darby SC (1994) Paternal exposure not to blame. *Nature* **367:** 678-80.

31. Neel JV, Schull WJ, eds. (1991) *The Children of Atomic Bomb Survivors.* Washington, DC: National Academy Press, pp. 518.

32. Pollycove M (1998) Nonlinearity of radiation health effects. *Environ Health Perspect* **106**(Suppl 1): 363-368.

33. Nussbaum RH (1998) The linear no-threshold dose-effect relation: is it relevant to radiation protection regulation? *Med Phys* **25:** 291-299.

34. Fry RJ, Grosovsky A, Hanawalt PC, *et al.* (1998) The Impact of Biology on Risk Assessment -- workshop of the National Research Council's Board on Radiation Effects Research. July 21-22, 1997, National Academy of Sciences, Washington, DC. *Radiat Res* **150:** 695-705.

35. Little JB, Nagasawa H, Pfenning T, *et al.* (1997) Radiation-induced genetic instability: delayed mutagenic and cytogenetic effects of X-rays and alpha particles. *Radiat Res* **148:** 299-307.

36. Azzam EI, de Toledo SM, Gooding T, *et al.* (1998) Intercellular communication is involved in the bystander regulation of gene expression in human cells exposed to very low influences of alpha particles. *Radiat Res* **150:** 497-504.

37. Upton AC (1982) The biological effects of low-level ionizing radiation. *Sci Am* **246:** 41-49.

38. Tengs TO, Adams ME, Pliskin JS, *et al.* (1995) Five-hundred life-saving interventions and their cost effectiveness. *Risk Analysis* **15:** 369-90.

39. Clarke R. Control of low-level radiation exposure: time for a change? *J Radiol Prot* **19:** 107-115.

Chapter 13

Prescription Drugs

Alexander M. Walker, M.D., Dr.P.H.
Department of Epidemiology, Harvard School of Public Health, Boston, MA

INTRODUCTION

In 1887, Hutchinson reported that arsenic, which at that time was used for the treatment of syphilis, could cause skin cancer [1]. Since then there has been a recurrent fear that prescribed drugs might sometimes cause cancer as an unintended and disastrous side effect.

There is a rich literature of drugs that have been suspected of being carcinogenic, and have been exonerated, and there are a few drugs that are no longer in use that turned out to be carcinogenic. Neither of these is the focus of the current chapter but interested readers can find these reviewed elsewhere [2, 3].

For the vast majority of drugs in current use, there has never been any hint of a carcinogenic effect. Of the drugs that have been associated with cancer, many have been shown to increase the risks of some cancers, while decreasing others. Only in a few cases have the magnitude of these risks and benefits been as large as the risks posed by the diseases that the drugs are intended to treat. Cancer risk is therefore usually a secondary consideration in evaluating the global contribution of individual drugs, even those for which an association with cancer is clear.

The drugs that cause or prevent cancers fall into three main categories. The first includes drugs used in cancer therapy; these agents have been found to increase the risk of leukemia in particular. The second are immunosuppressive agents, used to get the body to accept transplanted organs, and used to arrest some uncommon diseases in which the immune system turns on the body's own tissues. Since one of the functions of the immune system appears to be the removal of aberrant, precancerous, and

G.A. Colditz et al. (eds.), Cancer Prevention: The Causes and Prevention of Cancer - Volume I, 137–143.
© 2000 *Kluwer Academic Publishers.*

cancerous cells, immunosuppression also raises the risk of cancer
occurrence. The third includes hormones and hormone antagonists. Many
of the body's internal regulatory mechanisms are under hormonal control,
and changing these with a drug appears to increase the risk for some cancers
and to decrease the risk of others.

Anyone concerned with drug carcinogenesis also has to contend with the
problem of mistaken attribution. Drugs by their nature generally are given to
people who already have an illness, and it sometimes emerges that the illness
itself is related to cancer. Until the dimensions of the relations between the
treated illness and cancer become clear, the drugs used to treat the illness
may sometimes stand wrongly accused, in a sort of medical guilt by
association.

1.   CANCER CHEMOTHERAPY

Several generations of cancer chemotherapeutic drugs were designed as
selective poisons that attack dividing cells, and which therefore are toxic to
rapidly growing cancers. One aspect of cellular metabolism that is uniquely
activated during cell division is the creation of new genetic material (DNA),
and an important class of anticancer agents consists of chemicals that attach
themselves to DNA in a manner that makes replication difficult and error
prone. Impaired replication may kill a rapidly growing cancer cell line, but
it may also lead slower growing cells to reproduce with mutations that
eventually lead to neoplasia. Chlorambucil, cyclophosphamide, melphalen,
myleran, thiotepa, and methyl-CCNU are all recognized as causing
leukemia, and cyclophosphamide and chlorpromazine both cause bladder
cancer [3-5]. Although these drugs are still available, most of them are
dropping out of current treatment regimens, replaced by more specific
agents.

2.   IMMUNOSUPPRESSANTS

The immune system recognizes a transplanted organ as an alien tissue
that needs to be attacked in much the same way that it recognizes a bacterial
invader. The steps in this process include the proliferation of cells that send
out signals in response to the presence of the foreign tissue, cells that mark
the tissues for destruction, and cells that actually carry out the attack on
foreign cells. The immune system has evolved a host of regulatory
mechanisms to ensure that attacks are proportionate and narrowly directed.

Immunosuppressant drugs are either naturally occurring substances that have been discovered to affect specific aspects of immune function or chemicals that been tailored to achieve precise effects. Each of the major immunosuppressants for which there has been adequate experience has also had the side effect of increasing the risk of some cancers, notably cancers of the skin and lips, and lymphomas [6-8]. The post-transplant lymphoproliferative disorders, which include the post-transplant lymphomas, are universally associated with Epstein Barr virus (EBV) infections, which in turn has been identified as the causative agent of a variety of other cancers [9]. Patients with end-stage renal disease, who comprise by far the largest group of transplant candidates, also have elevated rates for all the hematopoietic cancers, and it may be that some portion of the disease ascribed to immunosuppressants is related to changes that stem from chronic renal failure [10].

Post-transplant lymphomas appear to follow distinct time courses, according to the immunosuppressive regimens involved. Azathioprine-related lymphomas occur most commonly several years after transplant, whereas those associated with cyclosporine appear within the first year [11]. OKT3-induced tumors may arise within a few weeks [12].

3.   HORMONES

Women's menstrual patterns and childbearing are related to the incidence of several cancers. The connection is mediated by female hormones, particularly estrogens and progestins. With the realization that women's own hormones may affect the risk of cancer, there has been a major effort at research on the link between medically administered hormones and the incidence of cancer.

In brief, estrogen replacement therapy appears to slightly increase the risk of breast cancer and to decrease the risk of colon cancer. Contemporary estrogen replacement therapy is almost always given in combination with a progestational agent; together these result in a slight increase in risk for endometrial cancer. If the progestin is omitted, the risk is substantial. The addition of progestin appears to increase risk of breast cancer above that of estrogen alone. The issue has become increasingly complex with the introduction of selective estrogen receptor modulators, or SERMS, drugs like tamoxifen and raloxifene, which mimic some of the effects of natural estrogens, while inhibiting others. While both of these drugs appear to reduce the risk of breast cancer, and tamoxifen is approved in many countries for use as a chemopreventine agent, the overall story on risks and benefits for SERMs is still being played out. New SERMs are coming into use each year.

One unambiguous carcinogenic effect of an estrogenic drug involves an agent no longer used today, diethylstilbestrol (DES), but is an illustration of the complex and indirect ways in which hormonal agents can lead to cancer. From the late 1940s for over a decade, DES was used to prevent spontaneous abortion in women with history of pregnancy loss. The appearance of a cluster of the exceedingly rare disease adenocarcinoma of the vagina in young women in the early 1970s led to the detection of prenatal DES as the common exposure and undoubted initial cause [13]. Further research in DES-exposed sons and daughters revealed that the drug functioned as subtle teratogen of the genitourinary tract [14]. The cancers were in the end believed to be secondary to a misplacement of endocervical tissue into the vagina, followed by exposure at menarche to a microbial and chemical environment to which the cells were poorly suited.

4.   FALSE ATTRIBUTION

Cancers sometimes result from the same noxious stimuli that cause other systemic diseases, or they may be a consequence of the diseases themselves. Slow growing cancers may cause symptoms that are treated as if they were the primary disease, the cancer going unrecognized at first. The result of both of these phenomena is that cancer rates can be elevated in many groups of people with apparently benign diseases. For example, the incidence of pancreatic cancer is elevated in persons with diabetes, renal cancer is more common in persons with hypertension. Associations like these can give rise to the false impression that agents used to treat the condition are causative of the higher cancer rates in treated people. The only way to disentangle these associations is to compare individuals receiving different kinds of therapies for the same conditions carefully and to inquire as to whether the time course of the proposed drug-cancer relation fits with what is known about the biology of the cancer.

Almost all initial reports of commonly used drugs causing cancer have turned out to be wrong. Sometimes the false alarm rises when researchers are inattentive to alternate explanations for their findings. In other cases, spurious associations appear by chance, when many drugs or many cancers are studied simultaneously. Although they deserve open-minded follow-up, such initial results should be treated with considerable skepticism, particularly when they involve useful medications. Past examples of putative drug-cancer relations that have not been confirmed, usually after painstaking   and   time-consuming   research,   include   reserpine   (an antihypertensive) and breast cancer, cimetidine (which lowers gastric acidity) and gastric cancer, metronidazole (an antifungal) and cancer at multiple sites, and the artificial sweetener saccharin and bladder cancer [15-18]. A long-believed association between renal cancer and both phenacetin (an analgesic no longer on the market) and acetaminophen (a very widely used over-the-counter analgesic that is metabolized to phenacetin) now seems largely resolved, with a conclusion of no detectable harm [19].

One spectacular recent instance of false attribution has been the debate on calcium-channel blockers (CCBs). CCBs are used widely as antihypertensives, they also improve the symptoms of angina pectoris. Because the calcium channel is important for intercellular communication for many mammalian functions, researchers had posited the possibility of a variety of secondary effects of these drugs, and an initial small cohort study appeared to support the contention that they raised the risk for cancer generally [20]. The study gave rise to widespread concern, which abated only after more than half a dozen further studies failed to replicate the finding [21-27].

SUMMARY POINTS

- The great majority of first reports of commonly used drugs causing cancer have turned out to be wrong. Although they deserve open-minded follow-up, such initial results should be treated with considerable skepticism, particularly when they involve useful medications.
- Currently used drugs that affect cancer risk are found among immunosuppressive agents, anticancer drugs, and hormone replacements.
- The magnitude of the cancer risk or protection associated with contemporary medicines is very much smaller than the direct benefits of therapy.

SUGGESTED FURTHER READING

1. Stolley PD, Zahm SH (1995) Nonhormonal drugs and cancer. *Environ Health Perspect* **103**(Suppl 8): 191-196
2. IARC (1990) Pharmaceutical Drugs. In: *IARC Monographs on the Evaluation of the Carcinogenic Risk of Chemicals to Humans*, Vol. 50. Lyon: IARC.

REFERENCES

1. Hutchinson J (1887) Arsenic cancer. *Brit Med J* **2**: 1280-1.
2. Stolley PD, Zahm SH (1995) Nonhormonal drugs and cancer. *Environ Health Perspect* **103**(Suppl 8): 191-196
3. IARC (1990) Pharmaceutical Drugs. In: *IARC Monographs on the Evaluation of the Carcinogenic Risk of Chemicals to Humans*, Vol. 50. Lyon: IARC.
4. Boivin JF, Hutchinson J (1984) Second cancers after treatment for Hodgkin's disease: a review. In: Boice JD Jr, Fraumeni JF Jr, eds. *Radiation Carcinogenesis: Epidemiology and Biological Significance. Progress in Cancer Research and Therapy*, Vol. 26. New York, NY (USA): Raven Press, pp. 181-98.
5. Fisher B, Rockett H, Fisher ER, Wickerham DK, Redmond C, Brown A (1985) Leukemia in breast cancer patients following adjuvant chemotherapy or postoperative radiation: the NSABP experience. *J Clin Oncol* **3**: 1640-58.
6. Penn I (1993) Incidence and treatment of neoplasia after transplantation. *J Heart Lung Transplant* **12**: S328-S3236
7. Holm LE (1990) Cancer occurring after radiotherapy and chemotherapy. *Int J Radiation Oncol Biol Phys* **19**: 1303-8.
8. Cockburn ITR, Krupp P (1989) The risk of neoplasms in patients treated with cyclosporine A. *J Autoimmunol* **2**: 723-31.
9. Boubenider S, Hiesse C, Goupy C, *et al.* (1997) Incidence and consequences of post-transplantation lymphoproliferative disorders. *J Nephrol* **10**: 136-145.
10. Maisonneuve P, Agodoa L, Gellert R, *et al.* (1999) Cancer in patients on dialysis for end-stage renal disease: an international collaborative study. *Lancet* **354**: 93-99.
11. Penn I (1996) Cancers in cyclosporine-treated vs azathioprine treated patients. *Transplant Proc* **28**: 876-878.
12. Swinnen LJ, Costanzo-Nordin MR, Fisher SG, *et al.* (1990) Increased incidence of lymphoproliferative disorder after immunosuppression with the monoclonal antibody OKT3 in cardiac-transplant patients. *N Engl J Med* **323**: 1723-1728.
13. Herbst AL, Ulfelder H, Poskanzer DC (1971) Adenocarcinoma of the vagina. Association of maternal stilbestrol therapy with tumor appearance in young women. *N Engl J Med* **284**: 878-81.
14. Herbst AL, Scully RE, Robboy SJ (1979) Prenatal diethylstilbestrol exposure and human genital tract abnormalities. *Natl Cancer Inst Monogr* **51**: 25-35.
15. Labarthe DR, O'Fallon WM (1979) Methodologic variation in case-control studies of reserpine and breast cancer. *J Chronic Dis* **32**: 95-104.
16. Johnson AG, Jick SS, Perera DR, Jick H (1996) Histamine-2 receptor antagonists and gastric cancer. *Epidemiology* **7**: 434-436.
17. Falagas ME, Walker AM, Jick H, *et al.* (1998) Late incidence of cancer after metronidazole use: a matched metronidazole user/nonuser study. *Clin Infect Dis* **26**: 384-8.
18. IARC (1999) Saccharin [81-07-2] and its salts. In: *IARC Monographs on the Evaluation of the Carcinogenic Risk of Chemicals to Humans*, Vol. 73: Lyon: IARC.
19. McCredie M, Pommer W, McLaughlin JK, *et al.* (1995) International renal-cell cancer study. II. Analgesics. *Int J Cancer* **60**: 345-359.
20. Pahor M, Guralink JM, Ferrucci L, *et al.* (1996) Calcium-channel blockers and incidence of cancer in aged populations. *Lancet* **348**: 493-497
21. Olsen JH, Toft Sorensen HT, Friis S, *et al.* (1997) Cancer risk in users of calcium channel blockers. *Hypertension* **29**: 1091-1094.

22. Jonas M, Goldbourt U, Boyko V, *et al.* (1998) Nifedipine and cancer mortality: ten-year follow-up of 2607 patients after acute myocardial infarction. *Cardiovasc Drugs Ther* **12:** 177-181.

23. Hole DJ, Gillis CR, McCallum IR, McInnes GT, MacKinnon PL, Meredith PA, Murray LS, Robertson JWK, Lever AF (1998) Cancer risk of hypertensive patients taking calcium antagonists. *J Hypertens* **16:** 119-124.

24. Vaughan TL, Farrow DC, Hansten PD, *et al.* (1998) Risk of esophageal and gastric adenocarcinomas in relation to use of calcium channel blockers, asthma drugs, and other medications that promote gastroesophageal reflux. *Cancer Epidemiol Biomarkers Prev* **7:** 749-756.

25. Trenkwalder P, Hendricks P, Hense H-W (1998) Treatment with calcium antagonists does not increase the risk of fatal or non-fatal cancer in an elderly mid-European population: results from STEPHY II. *J Hypertens* **16:** 1113-1116.

26. Rosenberg L, Rao SR, Palmer JR, *et al.* (1998) Calcium channel blockers and the risk of cancer. *JAMA* **279:** 1000-10004.

27. Michels KB, Rosner BA, Walker AM, *et al.* (1998) Calcium channel blockers, cancer incidence, and cancer mortality in a cohort of U.S. women. *Cancer* **83:** 2003-2007.

Chapter 14

Electric and Magnetic Fields

Francine Laden, Sc.D.
Channing Laboratory, Department of Medicine, Brigham and Women's Hospital and Harvard Medical School, Boston, MA

INTRODUCTION

The carcinogenic effects of low frequency electric and magnetic fields have been the focus of a wide body of biological and epidemiological literature published during the last two decades. The seminal study by Wertheimer and Leeper (1979) suggested an elevated risk of leukemia and brain cancer among children exposed to residential power lines [1]. Subsequent residential and occupational studies have provided conflicting conclusions about the relationship of electric and magnetic fields with both childhood and adult cancers. Leukemias, brain tumors, and breast cancer are the cancers most frequently assessed; however, other cancers have been evaluated sporadically as well. Due to the ubiquitous nature of the exposure and the young ages of many of the potential victims, these studies have garnered considerable attention from policy makers, the popular press, and pseudoscientific books. In the scientific literature, many reviews and meta-analyses have been published. The U.S. Congress has commissioned two government agencies to develop summary documents and assess the potential risk to the public [2, 3]. Conclusions on whether there is a cause and effect relationship between electric and magnetic fields and cancer have varied. However, while the majority agrees that the carcinogenicity of electric and magnetic fields has not been established, weak associations of residential exposures with childhood leukemia and occupational exposures with adult leukemia have not definitively been ruled out.

G.A. Colditz et al. (eds.), Cancer Prevention: The Causes and Prevention of Cancer - Volume I, 145–159.
© 2000 *Kluwer Academic Publishers.*

The purpose of this chapter is to present the key findings from the epidemiological literature. An attempt has been made to give the reader a feel for the variation in results and the strengths of the associations. Because electric and magnetic fields are part of the ambient environment and in general experienced passively, exposure assessment has not been simple. Many different strategies have been developed and considerable discussion has focused on their strengths and limitations. Therefore, a basic introduction to these methods will be included in this chapter.

1.   SOURCES OF ELECTRIC AND MAGNETIC FIELDS

Alternating currents from electric power facilities and household appliances produce electric and magnetic fields in the extremely low-frequency range (60 Hz in the United States, 50 Hz in European countries). The intensity of the fields decreases rapidly with distance away from the source. Although, electric fields are shielded by common building materials and the electrically conducting nature of the body, magnetic fields are not blocked. Therefore, the etiologic component is believed to be the magnetic field, and exposure assessments have centered primarily on magnetic fields, measured in units of micro-Tesla (μT). Some occupational studies have also measured the electric field (in volts per meter [V/m]). Consistent with the majority of the epidemiological literature, the abbreviation EMF is used here in most cases to refer specifically to magnetic fields.

Power lines, the grounding system of the building, and electric appliances are the major source of residential exposure to EMF. There are two basic types of power lines: transmission lines and distribution lines. The high voltage transmission lines carry the electric power from the electrical generation facility to the substations. Transformers convert the high voltage power (>35 kV) to a lower voltage, 120 and 240 V, in a series of steps, and the distribution lines bring the power to the utility customers. Power delivery is dependent on voltage and current load. Electric fields are a function of voltage, and magnetic fields are proportional to the magnitude of the current. Because of their location, closer to the general population, commercial and residential power distribution systems are a more significant source of exposure to magnetic fields than transmission lines. Because the power is low voltage, the electric fields are small. Large magnetic fields are also associated with electric appliances. However, they are used intermittently and the magnitude of the field decreases quickly with distance. In a nationwide study of 996 randomly selected residences, the Electric Power Research Institute (EPRI) determined that the magnitude of the interior magnetic fields from all sources combined was 0.1 μT or less in approximately 72 percent of the homes. Magnetic fields exceeded 0.25 μT in 3.3 percent of the homes. In a survey of individual exposures in the general population, the distribution of 24-hour time weighted average (TWA) exposure was approximately lognormal with geometric mean of 0.09 μT and a geometric standard deviation of 2.2 [3].

Sources of occupational exposure range from those similar to those found in the residential environment (urban power lines and appliances in the office) to direct contact with the high voltage transmission lines. Most occupational epidemiological studies have focused on highly exposed individuals: employees in electrical jobs such as electricians, electric utility workers, and transportation engineers. The TWA magnetic fields and electric fields typically associated with "electrical occupations" range from approximately 0.5 to 4 μT and 0.1 to 2 kV/m, respectively [4]. See NIEHS (1998) [3] for a compilation of measurements from different occupational exposure assessments

2.   MEASUREMENT OF ELECTRIC AND MAGNETIC FIELDS IN EPIDEMIOLOGICAL STUDIES

Measurement of exposure to EMF during the etiologic time period in epidemiological studies has proved challenging. Because the cancers of interest are rare, the most practical and efficient study design has been the retrospective case-control study. Past exposures, experienced at a time when they might play a role in the cause of the disease, have to be recreated. In addition, the biological mechanism by which EMF might be carcinogenic, as well as the latency period of many of these cancers is unknown. (For a recent review of the biological data relating to the toxicity of EMF see NIEHS 1998 [3].) Therefore, researchers do not know when the relevant timing of exposure might be. Different studies include assessments of exposure for the residence occupied during the pre-natal period, at the time of diagnosis, at different times before diagnosis, and the residence lived in for the longest period of time. Thus, in some cases multiple residences need to be evaluated, often requiring permission from non-study participants who are currently residing in the houses previously lived in by the participants. Also, the exposure is ubiquitous and occurs in the ambient environment at very low levels. An unexposed population might not exist, and measurement error can be very influential.

Five methods for exposure assessment have been used in residential studies of EMF and cancer: wire codes, calculated levels (current and historical), direct measurements of magnetic fields, distance to the source, and reported use of appliances. Some epidemiological studies have utilized only one of these methods, while others have compared and contrasted the results from a combination of exposure metrics.

Wire codes were first developed for the Denver area by Wertheimer and Leeper in 1979 [1] and later modified [5, 6]. This classification scheme takes into account the type of power lines, the age of the lines, and the distance of the residence to the line. In the original study, houses were classified as either high current configuration (HCC) or low current configuration (LCC). The modified wire code consists of five levels, further dichotomizing the original two levels and adding a lowest exposure category, buried wire codes. The wire codes have been used with some alteration in subsequent studies performed in Denver and other locations. The strengths of this method are twofold. It is hypothesized to rank past exposures because it evaluates a stable entity of the residence, and it allows classification of exposure without requiring access to the homes. However, the codes are not necessarily generalizable to all geographic locations, and they are limited as a quantitative measure of magnetic fields. Wire codes rank homes reasonably well, but they only account for 15 to 20 percent of the variance in magnetic field measurements [2]. It has also been suggested that wire codes might be measuring some unknown exposure other than magnetic fields.

Theoretical calculations of magnetic fields utilize current and historical information from utility companies and derive a measure of average magnetic field exposure for each residence. The height of towers, distance between towers, distance between phases, ordering of phases, distance between the power line and the house, and average load on the power line during the relevant years are included in the equation. Cumulative exposure over time can also be assessed. This exposure metric was developed in Sweden where historical information is readily available [7]. It relies on a number of assumptions and requires reliable information from utility companies. However, unlike wire codes it supplies an estimate of the magnitude of the magnetic fields and uses established laws of physics [3].

Some studies have defined exposure by distance of the residence to power lines. In these studies subjects are divided into groups according to pre-selected cut-offs (*e.g.,* <100 and ≥100 meters from the source). Although distance is a significant component of magnetic field magnitude, this exposure metric is considered crude.

Two types of direct measurements of magnetic fields have been included in epidemiological studies: spot (short-term, 30 second) measurements and

24-hour measurements. The magnitude of the magnetic field is assessed using area monitors in various rooms of the house. The placement of the monitors and the number of measurements vary from study to study. Usually the subject's bedroom is measured, and sometimes other rooms in the house and near the front door are also included. Some studies obtain separate measurements under low-power use (when all appliances are turned off) and high-power use (all appliances are left on) conditions. These methods have the advantage of actually quantifying the potential magnetic fields experienced by an individual inside the home. However, there is uncertainty about the most appropriate location to place the monitors and how well fields measured in the present represent those experienced in the past. Furthermore, direct measurements require more effort from the study subjects than do surrogate assessments. This component of many studies suffers from low participation rates, compromising the usefulness of the data.

A few epidemiological studies have focused on the use of electric appliances. Electric blankets have been of particular interest because they provide a significant source of close body exposure for an extended period of time, approximately eight hours during the night. Overnight use of an electric blanket produced before 1990 (when they were reconfigured) was estimated to double an individual's average exposure to EMF [8]. Subjects have also been queried about their use of other appliances, particularly electric hair dryers, electric razors, bedside analog clocks, and black and white televisions. As mentioned previously, although the magnitude of magnetic fields from appliances can be high, most of them are used only intermittently. Also, reporting of past use is prone to recall bias.

Occupational studies usually use job title to define exposure. In many studies, the magnitude of exposure for each job is determined by enrolling a random sample of workers in a sub-study to wear personal monitors measuring EMF during a selected number of days and shifts. These measurements are combined with area monitoring and a time-weighted average (TWA) of exposure is calculated. Each job title is assigned a TWA and study subjects are grouped accordingly. Some studies obtain job titles at one point in time, while others evaluate the entire job history and incorporate duration at a given job into the exposure measurement.

None of these exposure metrics are ideal; each has its strengths and limitations. There is a good deal of opportunity for exposure misclassification. If this error is independent of disease status (nondifferential) then the relative risks for binary exposures are attenuated. This increases the difficulty of detecting a small real effect, and compromises assessment of dose response. Furthermore, because many strategies of exposure assessment, including different metrics, cutoffs and timing of exposure, have been used throughout the literature, comparison and summarization of results is difficult.

3.   EPIDEMIOLOGIC STUDIES OF ELECTRIC AND MAGNETIC FIELDS AND CANCER

Since 1979, when Wertheimer and Leeper published their study suggesting an association between childhood cancer and residence near power lines, numerous studies have been published assessing the association of EMF with childhood and adult cancers. Results have been inconsistent and interpretation varies depending on the author and the other experts who critique them. A few of the key studies and conclusions from recent comprehensive reviews are described briefly here.

3.1   Childhood leukemia

Using wire codes to define exposure, Wertheimer and Leeper [1] observed a three-fold increased risk of leukemia among children residing at the time of their death in high exposure homes. Like Wertheimer and Leeper, Savitz *et al.* conducted a study in the Denver area [6]. The odds ratio (OR) for high *vs.* low current homes occupied at the time of diagnosis, was 1.5 (95% confidence interval (CI) = 0.9-2.6). Seven cases lived in homes classified as very high, and the OR comparing them to children living in homes with the lowest classification, buried wire code, was 2.8 (95% CI = 0.9-8.0). Spot measurements for the same homes were also obtained. A nonstatistically significant two-fold increased risk was associated with homes with measured magnetic fields >0.2 µT under low power use conditions relative to less exposed homes. However, the association when all appliances were turned on, a more accurate reflection of normal living conditions, was lower and also not statistically significant (OR = 1.4; 95% CI = 0.6-3.5). In Los Angeles, London *et al.* observed a comparable effect estimate for wire codes (very high relative to very low and buried configuration combined) (OR = 1.7; 95% CI = 0.8-3.7). There was no association with spot measurements or 24-hour measurements [9].

In a landmark study of children living near high-voltage power lines in Sweden, a statistically significant increased risk was observed for homes with calculated magnetic fields ≥0.3 µT at the time of diagnosis compared to homes with fields ≤0.09 µT (OR = 3.8; 95% CI = 1.4-9.3). No elevated risk of leukemia was observed when exposure was defined by distance to the power lines or with spot measurements [7]. A study in Denmark also calculated historical fields and observed elevated but not statistically significant ORs for children in the highest group (≥0.4 µT) compared to the lowest (<0.1 µT) (OR = 6.0; 95% CI = 0.8-44.0) [10]. A cohort study in Finland did not observe an association of childhood leukemia with exposure to calculated magnetic fields, using incidence rates from the general population as the comparison [11].

Ever use, duration of use, and timing of use (prenatal and postnatal) of over 15 different appliances have been assessed. Elevated relative risks have been observed for prenatal exposure to electric blankets, postnatal use of hair dryers and black and white televisions, among others [12, 9]. However these exposure assessments are considered unreliable because of the high potential for recall bias, and the inadequacy of information on duration and intensity of use [3]. It has also been suggested that it is inadequate to define exposure one appliance at a time [13].

Overall, very modestly elevated relative risks were observed for surrogate measurements of EMF. Results from direct measurements of magnetic fields did not support these findings. Some researchers interpret the risks as suggestive and important. Others emphasize the low magnitude of the effect estimates, the wide non-significant 95% confidence intervals, and the inconsistency between the different exposure metrics. Common criticisms of these studies involve the small number of exposed cases, potential for selection bias, and misclassification of exposure. Participation rates, specifically for the direct measurements of magnetic fields were low, often less than 50 percent [6, 9]. Exposure was assessed many years after disease diagnosis, which itself is possibly years after the relevant etiologic period. Control selection by random digit dialing in many studies has also been criticized. It is possible that the controls are of a higher socioeconomic status than the cases and therefore less likely to live near high power lines, leading to artificially elevated relative risks. The risk assessment by the National Research Council included a detailed discussion of the possible selection, information, and confounding biases present in the studies [2].

A recent large multi-state case-control study of childhood acute lymphoblastic leukemia (ALL) was designed to address many of the limitations of the previous studies. Using Wertheimer and Leeper wire codes, they found no excess risk of ALL with very high current configurations at the main residence obtained within 24 months of diagnosis of the index case (OR: 0.9; 95% CI: 0.5-1.6). They calculated TWA exposures based on 24-hour measurements in the homes occupied for at least 70 percent of the children's lifetime. They found no significant excess risk with levels ≥0.2 µT and there was no evidence of a dose-response [14].

One of the most recent and comprehensive reviews was undertaken by the National Institute of Environmental Health Sciences (NIEHS), a division of the National Institutes of Health (NIH), and the Department of Energy (DOE), in response to congressional legislation [3]. The task of the working group consisting of experts in many disciplines, was to evaluate the quality of the research literature and the strength of the evidence. Their review included all of the studies discussed here, as well as many others. They concluded that overall, results from exposure assessments using wire codes and calculated historical fields, but not direct measurements, supported a modest association between EMF and the incidence of childhood leukemia [3]. The National Research Council, also commissioned by Congress, came to the same conclusion in their risk assessment. They determined that this weak association could not be explained by selection bias or uncontrolled confounding [2]. Again, the inconsistencies between and within the studies and the lack of a dose-response prevent a conclusive decision on the overall causative association of EMFs and leukemia. The fact that leukemia has not increased concurrently with the use of electric power has also been used as an argument to question the reliability of the observed associations.

3.2   Childhood brain tumors

In the 1979 Wertheimer and Leeper study, the unadjusted relative risk for brain tumors was 2.4 (95% CI = 1.2-5.0) for high current *vs.* low current exposure [1]. Savitz *et al.* observed similar results with wire codes; the OR for children living in high current homes was 2.0 (95% CI = 1.1-3.8) [6]. However, associations with spot measurements were essentially null. Two U.S. studies published in 1996 did not find evidence supporting an increased risk of brain tumors with wire codes and direct measurements [15] or wire codes and use of electric appliances [16]. The numbers of highly exposed cases in the three Nordic studies described earlier were small. Overall the results from calculated magnetic fields did not support an association with brain tumors [7, 10, 11]. The NIEHS working group determined that studies evaluating exposure with spot-measured magnetic fields, 24-hour measured magnetic fields and use of appliances had too few subjects and the results were too inconclusive to be useful in evaluating an association with childhood brain tumors [3]. In a review focused on this topic, Kheifets and colleagues concluded that there was no support for an association between EMF and childhood brain cancer [17].

3.3   Childhood lymphomas

Lymphoma cases were included in studies by Wertheimer and Leeper [1], Savitz *et al.* [6, 12], Olsen *et al.* [10], and Feychting and Ahlbom [7]. Modestly elevated but not statistically significant relative risks were observed in the former three studies. The number of cases in each of these studies was too small to draw any reliable inferences [3].

3.4   Adult leukemia

Risk of leukemia and other cancers in adults has been assessed for both occupational and residential exposures to EMF. Kheifets *et al.* published a meta-analysis in 1997 including 70 occupational studies representing 38 independent reports. For a broad group of electrical occupations, they calculated a pooled OR for leukemia of 1.2 (95% CI = 1.1-1.3). Associations for specific subtypes were also statistically significantly elevated: for acute myelogenous leukemia (AML) OR = 1.4 (95% CI = 1.2-1.7) and for chronic lymphocytic leukemia (CLL) OR: 1.6 (95% CI = 1.1-2.2) [18]. Based on the same studies and additional ones that were published after the meta-analysis was performed, NIEHS concluded that there was limited evidence to suggest a small association between occupational exposure to EMF and leukemia, specifically the subtype CLL [3]. This decision was supported by only half of the working group. The other half abstained or voted that there was "inadequate evidence".

Adult leukemias and residential exposures to EMF have been assessed by a number of researchers, including those who looked at childhood cancers. Wertheimer and Leeper did not observe an association of leukemia with wire codes among Denver area adults [19]. In Finland there was no association of calculated magnetic fields with all leukemias, but incidence of CLL was statistically significantly elevated with dichotomized cumulative exposures. For example, the standardized incidence ratio for ≥ 0.2 μT-years relative to <0.2 μT-years, at least ten years before diagnosis, was 2.8 (95% CI = 1.1-7.4) [20]. Li *et al.* grouped calculated exposures to magnetic fields in the year of diagnosis into three categories (<0.1, 0.1-0.2, >0.2 μT) in Taiwan. The ORs increased slightly with exposure, and the comparison of the highest category with the lowest was of borderline statistical significance (OR = 1.4; 95% CI = 1.0-1.9) [21]. Studies of electric appliance use either did not support an association with leukemia risk, or their design and exposure assessment were too limited to provide useful information [3]. Feychting *et al.* in a case-control study of Swedish adults attempted to account for both residential and occupational exposures at the same time. After excluding residentially unexposed subjects who were exposed at work, the OR for calculated magnetic fields ≥ 0.2 μT at the home was 1.3 (95% CI = 0.8-2.2) for all leukemias [22]. Although some elevated relative risks have been observed for leukemia in general and some specific subtypes, the weight of the evidence does not support an association of residential magnetic fields with leukemia in adults.

3.5   Adult brain tumors

As in residential childhood cancer studies, risk of brain tumors has also been extensively studied for adults. In a 1995 meta-analysis, Kheifets *et al.* identified 52 occupational studies of cancers of the central nervous system. Their pooled OR for "electrical occupations" was 1.2 (95% CI: 1.1-1.3) [23]. The previously described studies of adult leukemias and residential exposure to EMF also included assessments of brain tumors. Elevated relative risks were not observed in any of the studies. Although an elevated risk in electrical workers could not be ruled out, magnetic fields do not appear to be associated with brain tumors in adults [3].

3.6   Breast cancer

Breast cancer risk and EMF have been evaluated in occupational and residential studies. Evidence of an elevated risk of male breast cancer associated with presumed occupational EMF exposure based on job title has been observed in some studies but not in others (reviewed in Laden and Hunter [24]). Where an effect was present, measures of association ranged from 1.2 to 6.5. Because male breast cancer is a rare disease, these estimates were based on small numbers, sometimes as few as one to three cases, and were therefore unstable. Two case-control studies designed to examine occupational EMF exposure and breast cancer in women observed an approximately 40 percent increase in risk of mortality for women of all ages [25, 26]. Risk was higher among younger women than older women. Only the Coogan study accounted for potential confounding by known breast cancer risk factors [26].

Studies of residential exposure to EMF and breast cancer have focused either on residence near power lines or use of an electric blanket. Wertheimer and Leeper (1987) observed an almost threefold increase in premenopausal breast cancer associated with higher exposure as determined by distance to power lines [27]. Other studies have not reproduced these findings for breast cancer overall [24]. However, Feychting *et al.* did observe a nonstatistically significant increased risk at calculated magnetic field levels ≥ 0.1 μT (OR = 1.8; 95% CI = 0.7-4.3), but only when cases were restricted to women younger than 50 years of age at diagnosis [28]. Control for confounding in these studies was minimal and did not account for important known breast cancer risk factors.

The first case-control study of electric blanket use and female breast cancer was suggestive of a positive association with overnight use of the appliance during the ten years before diagnosis. Vena and colleagues observed a nonstatistically significant, approximately 40 percent increased risk among both pre- and postmenopausal women [29, 30]. A recent case-control study evaluating use of electric blankets, electric mattress pads and heated waterbeds did not observe an increased risk of breast cancer among women under the age of 45 (OR = 1.0; 95% CI = 0.9-1.2) [31].

There is the potential for a modest increased risk of both male and premenopausal female breast cancer among highly exposed electrical workers. However, these are rare diseases and because the exposure assessment has been based almost solely on job code the influence of chance cannot be ignored. There appears to be no risk of breast cancer to the general population from power lines and appliance use. Most of these studies were limited in their ability to control for confounding. There was no evidence of a dose-response effect, and increased risks, if observed, were only for the more rare breast cancers among premenopausal women.

3.7   Other cancers

Many of the studies described in this review included an analysis of total cancer, regardless of site. These results are not discussed here because they were dominated by leukemias and brain tumors. Elevated lung cancer rates were observed in one study and there have been reports of associations with malignant melanoma in occupational studies. There was no evidence of an association of occupational exposure to EMF and multiple myeloma, lymphoma, Hodgkin's disease, or non-Hodgkin's lymphoma. Testicular cancer was elevated in one occupational study, but there was no association reported in a study of electric blanket use [3]. A recent study looked at risk of prostate cancer and use of electric blankets and heated waterbeds. The OR was similar to that observed for breast cancer in the original electric blanket studies (OR = 1.4; 95% CI = 0.9-2.2) and there was no evidence of a dose-response effect [32]. No other studies to date have evaluated this endpoint. There is no evidence of an association of these other cancers with exposure to EMF.

CONCLUSIONS

The association of EMF and cancer has been studied extensively in the epidemiological literature, in both residential and occupational studies. A sampling of the results from across the literature is presented in this chapter, along with some recently published summary conclusions. In most studies where an effect was seen, the relative risks were less than 2.0, and the 95% confidence intervals were broad and not always statistically significant. Most of the elevated risks were observed with surrogate measurements, and were not supported by results from direct measurements even within the same studies. Also, there was little evidence of a linear dose-response effect. Researchers and reviewers have put varying emphasis on the inconsistency of the results between and within studies and on the importance of modestly elevated risks. Furthermore, some commentators point out that use of electric power has increased dramatically during the 20th century. They argue that if there is in fact an association with certain cancers then we would expect a much greater increase in the incidence of those diseases. Others counter that it cannot be assumed that population exposure to magnetic fields have increased proportionately to residential energy use [2], so they would not expect the incidence to be higher.

Assessments of exposure to magnetic fields and study design have often been criticized. Questions about what each exposure metric is actually measuring and its relationship to the actual exposure experienced by the study participants have ensued. The validity of direct measurements versus surrogate measurements has not been resolved. Also, if the exposures of the study participants are misclassified relative to each other, then the real relative risks might be greater than those observed. Furthermore, study design limitations, particularly the potential for bias in selection of the controls, have influenced interpretations of results. If the comparison population is not representative of the population the cases came from and have less opportunity for exposure, then the observed relative risks would actually be inflated. Finally, to date, a convincing biological mechanism for the carcinogenicity of magnetic fields has not been developed or supported in laboratory studies.

Because of these issues no strong consensus on this topic has been reached. Most experts agree that there is little evidence of an association between magnetic fields and most cancers. However, the possibility of a weak risk of childhood leukemia associated specifically with surrogate measurements of residential exposures and of adult chronic lymphocytic leukemia with occupational exposures has not been ruled out.

SUMMARY POINTS

- The major sources of electric and magnetic fields are from over-head power lines
- Both surrogate and direct measurements have been used to assess exposure to the electric and magnetic fields. Each metric has its own strengths and limitations, and exposure misclassification is a major issue in epidemiological studies.

- Many experts agree that there are suggestions of a modest association of surrogate measurements of residential exposures to EMF and childhood leukemia and of occupational exposures and adult chronic lymphocytic leukemia. However, results from across and even within epidemiological studies of EMF and cancer have been inconsistent and the biological mechanism is unknown.
- There is little evidence of an increased risk of other childhood and adult cancers.

RECOMMENDATIONS

- Due to the lack of a clear association between EMF and cancer, specific strategies and situations to avoid EMF exposure cannot be recommended at the present time.

SUGGESTED FURTHER READING

1. National Institute of Environmental Health Sciences (NIEHS), U.S. National Institutes of Health (1998) *Assessment of Health Effects from Exposure to Power-line Frequency Electric and Magnetic Fields: Working Group Report.* Research triangle Park, NC: NIH Publication No 98-3981.
2. National Research Council (NRC), Committee on the Possible Effect of Electromagnetic Fields on Biologic Systems (1997) *Possible Health Effects of Exposure to Residential Electric and Magnetic Fields.* Washington DC: National Academy Press.

REFERENCES

1. Wertheimer N, Leeper E (1979) Electrical wiring configurations and childhood cancer. *Am J Epidemiol* **109:** 273-284.
2. National Research Council (NRC), Committee on the Possible Effect of Electromagnetic Fields on Biologic Systems (1997) *Possible Health Effects of Exposure to Residential Electric and Magnetic fields.* Washington DC: National Academy Press.
3. National Institute of Environmental Health Sciences (NIEHS), U.S. National Institutes of Health (1998) *Assessment of Health Effects from Exposure to Power-line Frequency Electric and Magnetic Fields: Working Group Report.* Research Triangle Park, NC (USA): NIH Publication No 98-3981.
4. Moulder JE (1998) Power-frequency fields and cancer. *Crit Rev Biomed Eng* **26:** 1-116.

5. Wertheimer N, Leeper E (1982) Adult cancer related to electrical wires near the home. *Int J Epidemiol* **11:** 345-355.
6. Savitz DA, Wachtel H, Barnes FA, *et al.* (1998) Case-control study of childhood cancer and exposure to 60 Hz magnetic fields. *Am J Epidemiol* **128:** 21-38.
7. Feychting M, Ahlbom A (1993) Magnetic fields and cancer in children residing near Swedish high voltage power lines. *Am J Epidemiol* **138:** 467-481.
8. Florig HK, Hoburg JF (1990) Power-frequency magnetic fields from electric blankets. *Health Phys* **58:** 493-502.
9. London SJ, Thomas DC, Bowman JD, *et al.* (1991) Exposure to residential electric and magnetic fields and risk of childhood leukemia. *Am J Epidemiol* **134:** 923-937.
10. Olsen JH, Nielsen A, Schulgen G (1993) Residence near high voltage facilities and risk of cancer in children. *Br Med J* **307:** 891-895.
11. Verkasalo PK, Pukkala E, Hongisto MY, *et al.* (1993) Risk of cancer in Finnish children living close to power lines. *Br Med J* **307:** 895-898.
12. Savitz DA, John EM, Kleckner RC (1990) Magnetic field exposure from electric appliances and childhood cancer. *Am J Epidemiol* **131:** 763-773.
13. Poole C (1996) Invited commentary: evolution of epidemiologic evidence on magnetic fields and childhood cancers. *Am J Epidemiol* **143:** 129-131.
14. Linet MS, Hatch EE, Kleinerman RA, *et al.* (1997) Residential exposure to magnetic fields and acute lymphoblastic leukemia in children. *N Engl J Med* **337:** 1-7.
15. Preston-Martin S, Navidi W, Thomas D, *et al.* (1996) Los Angeles study of residential magnetic fields and childhood brain tumors. *Am J Epidemiol* **143:** 105-119.
16. Gurney JG, Mueller BA, Davis S, *et al.* (1996) Childhood brain tumor occurrence in relation to residential power line configuration, electric heating sources, and electric appliance use. *Am J Epidemiol* **143:** 120-128.
17. Kheifets LI, Sussman SS, Preston-Martin S (1999) Childhood brain tumors and residential electromagnetic fields (EMF). *Rev Environ Contam Toxicol* **159:** 111-129.
18. Kheifets LI, Afifi AA, Buffler PA, *et al.* (1997) Occupational electric and magnetic field exposure and leukemia: a meta-analysis. *J Occup Environ Med* **39:** 1074-1091.
19. Wertheimer N, Leeper E (1986) Possible effects of electric blankets and heated waterbeds on fetal development. *Bioelectromagnetics* **7:** 13-22.
20. Verkasalo PK (1996) Magnetic fields and leukemia – risk for adults living close to power lines. *Scan J Work Environ Health* **22**(Suppl 2): 1-56.
21. Li C-Y, Theriault G, Lin RS (1997) Residential exposure to 60-Hertz magnetic fields and adult cancers in Taiwan. *Epidemiology* **8:** 25-30.
22. Feychting M, Forssen U, Floderus B (1997) Occupational and residential magnetic fields exposure and leukemia and central nervous system tumors. *Epidemiology* **8:** 384-389.
23. Kheifets LI, Afifi AA, Buffler PA, *et al.* (1995) Occupational electric and magnetic field exposure and brain cancer: a meta-analysis. *J Occup Environ Med* **37:** 1327-1341.
24. Laden F, Hunter DJ (1998) Environmental risk factors and female breast cancer. *Annu Rev Public Health* **19:** 101-123.
25. Loomis DP, Savitz DA, Ananth CV (1994) Breast cancer mortality among female electrical workers in the United States. *J Natl Cancer Inst* **86:** 921-925.
26. Coogan PF, Clapp RW, Newcomb PA, *et al.* (1996) Occupational exposure to 60-hertz magnetic fields and risk of breast cancer in women. *Epidemiology* **7:** 459-464.
27. Wertheimer N, Leeper E (1987) Magnetic field exposure related to cancer subtypes. *Ann NY Acad Sci* **502:** 43-54.
28. Feychting M, Forssen U, Rutqvist LE, *et al.* (1998) Magnetic fields and breast cancer in Swedish adults residing near high-voltage power lines. *Epidemiology* **9:** 392-397.

29. Vena JE, Graham S, Hellmann R, *et al.* (1991) Use of electric blankets and risk of postmenopausal breast cancer. *Am J Epidemiol* **134:** 180-185.
30. Vena JE, Freudenheim JL, Marshall JR, *et al.* (1994) Risk of premenopausal breast cancer and use of electric blankets. *Am J Epidemiol* **140:** 974-979.
31. Gammon MD, Schoenberg JB, Britton JA, *et al.* (1998) Electric blanket use and breast cancer risk among younger women. *Am J Epidemiol* **148:** 556-563.
32. Zhu K, Weiss NS, Stanford JL, *et al.* (1999) Prostate cancer in relation to the use of electric blanket or heated water bed. *Epidemiology* **10:** 83-85

Summary – Causes of Cancer

Walter C. Willett, M.D., David Hunter, M.B.B.S., Sc.D. and Graham A. Colditz, M.D., Dr.P.H.
Department of Nutrition, Harvard School of Public Health, Department of Epidemiology, Harvard School of Public Health, Channing Laboratory, Brigham and Women's Hospital, and Harvard Medical School, Boston, MA

CAUSES OF CANCER

The purpose of this volume is to summarize what we know, and don't know, about the causes of cancer risk in the developed world. In this summary, we will highlight the important factors that have been reviewed in the previous chapters and provide an estimate of the percentage of cancer that could be avoided by implementing what we know already. An overall conclusion is that cancer is to a substantial degree a preventable illness.

In Table 1, we provide an estimate of the percentage of cancer deaths that are accounted for by the various factors discussed in the volume. These are to be regarded as rough estimates because of imprecision in epidemiologic studies and the complex interactions that can exist among causative factors (for example, the greatly reduced hazard of radon exposure among persons who do not smoke). Although the numbers have varied somewhat as evidence has accumulated, the overall relative importance of these causal factors is similar to summaries developed by other researchers over the last two decades.

G.A. Colditz et al. (eds.), Cancer Prevention: The Causes and Prevention of Cancer - Volume I, 161–171.
© 2000 *Kluwer Academic Publishers.*

Table 2. Causes of cancer in developed countries
**Estimated percentage of total cancer deaths
attributable to specific causes**

Casual Risk Factor	Percentage
Tobacco	30%
Adult diet/obesity	25%
Sedentary lifestyle	10%
Occupational factors	5%
Family history of cancer	5%
Viruses/other biologic agents	5%
Perinatal factors/growth	5%
Reproductive factors	5%
Alcohol	3%
Socioeconomic status	*
Environmental pollution	2%
Ionizing/ultraviolet radiation	2%
Prescription drugs/medical procedures	2%
Salt/other food additives/contaminants	1%

*An important underlying factor operating through other specified causes

1.   TOBACCO

With a barrage of new research findings constantly assaulting the public, it is easy to lose sight of the fact that stemming the epidemic of tobacco smoking is our most effective means for preventing cancer. An estimated 30 percent of all U.S. cancer deaths can be attributed to tobacco use.

Over the past decade, scientific studies have shown that the involuntary exposure of nonsmokers to smoke from other people's tobacco products - environmental tobacco smoke - poses a health risk for nonsmokers, including increased risks of lung cancer and other diseases. In 1993, the U.S. Environmental Protection Agency designated tobacco smoke as a Group A carcinogen, for which there is no known safe level of exposure.

2.   DIET AND OBESITY

An estimated 25 percent of all cancers in developed countries can be attributable to diet in adult life, including its effect on obesity. Evidence to date indicates that cancer risk can be reduced by taking the following steps:

- Staying lean throughout adult life. The common phenomena of gaining weight (more than five to ten pounds) during midlife is particularly important to avoid. This can to be achieved by incorporating regular exercise into daily life, and by avoiding excessive caloric intake, whether from carbohydrates or fats. Overweight increases the risk of endometrial cancer, postmenopausal breast cancer, and cancers of the colon, and kidney.
- Consuming a minimum of five or more servings of fruits and vegetables per day. The evidence of benefit is strongest for cancers of the lung, stomach, esophagus, and larynx, and reductions in cancers of the breast, colon, and prostate may exist. Although vitamin supplements are not an adequate substitute for fruits and vegetables, evidence does exist that taking a multiple vitamin containing folic acid can reduce risk of colon cancer, possibly because supplements contain a substantial amount of folic acid in a form that is readily absorbed.
- Reducing consumption of red meat to once a week or less.
- Wherever possible, use vegetable oils instead of animal fats. Olive oil appears to be a good choice for general use.

The above dietary suggestions will almost certainly have beneficial effects for reducing cardiovascular disease as well as cancer. Notably absent from the dietary suggestions for reducing cancer risk is advice to consume diets high in fiber. Despite strong belief in the notion that this would reduce risk of colon cancer, the evidence that whole grain cereal products have such an effect was always weak and recent data have also failed to support such a relationship. However, evidence is now strong that consuming grain products in a whole grain, high fiber form (as opposed to refined starches) is important for reducing risks of coronary heart disease and diabetes. Thus, as part of overall advice for a healthy diet, breads, pasta, and cereals should be consumed in whole grain form with attention to the calories that they contribute.

3.   SEDENTARY LIFESTYLE

Most adults need to engage in regular physical activity for successful weight control. This becomes increasingly important as we age because of the tendency for our bodies to require fewer calories as the years pass. Independent of assisting in weight control, regular physical activity can reduce the incidence of colon cancer and may help reduce cancers of the breast and prostate.

Regular physical activity during childhood and adolescence may prevent excessive weight gain and delay onset of menstruation (early age at menarche is a major risk factor for breast cancer).

4.   OCCUPATIONAL FACTORS

Control of occupational carcinogens in the U.S. and other industrialized countries represents an important but insufficiently recognized triumph for primary cancer prevention. Collectively, occupational factors are thought to cause about five percent of all fatal cancers, mostly in the lung, bladder, and bone marrow, and this percentage will decline because exposures have already been dramatically reduced.

Continuing progress in reducing cancers due to occupational causes can also be expected in developed countries because of technological advances and a continuing shift away from industrial employment. The public must continue to insist that governmental regulations be enforced to minimize occupational exposure to carcinogens.

5.   FAMILY HISTORY OF CANCER

Certain individuals have susceptibility to cancer due to inherited mutations in genes running in families. Fortunately, the occurrence of such mutations is not common, resulting in about five percent of all fatal cancers. Preventive measures that can be taken include genetic counseling, through which couples may decide not to have children, and more frequent screening among those at high risk, or surgery to remove the organs at risk.

Cancer incidence is also influenced by inherited polymorphisms in genes that affect the absorption, transport, metabolic activation, or detoxification of dietary and environmental carcinogens. Genetic susceptibility due to these variation in the rates of these processes could play an interactive role with environmental factors in the majority of cancer cases.

6.   VIRUSES AND OTHER BIOLOGIC AGENTS

Infectious agents, overlooked as causes of human cancer only 30 years ago, are now considered to be a factor in five percent or more of all fatal cancers in the developed countries. Among the more significant infectious agents are human papilloma viruses (HPV) types 16 and 18, which are implicated in cancer of the uterine cervix, and hepatitis B virus (HBV), which is implicated in liver carcinoma.

Hepatitis B and C viruses are responsible for a minority of cases of liver carcinoma in the U.S. The proportion of such cases is likely to decrease following the availability of anti-HBV vaccine, improved screening of blood and blood products, and more frequent use of disposable syringes and needles by injection drug users. Measures directed against HIV transmission, coupled with declining mortality from cervical cancer due to effective Pap screening programs, suggest that human papilloma virus-related cancer mortality is also likely to decline.

7.   PERINATAL GROWTH FACTORS

Excess energy intake early in life may be responsible for the positive association between height and the risk of breast cancer, colon, and possibly other cancers. Evidence is also emerging that larger birth weight is associated positively with some cancer types, notably breast cancer and possibly prostate cancer. However, benefits of higher birth weight exist for cardiovascular disease. Thus, attempts to modify perinatal factors for cancer prevention would be premature.

8.   REPRODUCTIVE FACTORS

Among physiologic processes, reproductive factors are the most closely linked to human cancer. Early age at menarche, late age at first birth, and late age at menopause tend to increase the risk for breast cancer, while parity is associated inversely with cancers of the endometrium and ovaries.

Several other associations have been noted, but they have not been established conclusively, are of marginal importance, or are thought to be surrogates for other recognized causal factors. For example, having multiple sexual partners, an established risk factor for cancer of the cervix, reflects likelihood of exposure to sexually transmitted viruses that are carcinogenic.

9.   ALCOHOL

The use of alcoholic beverages interacts with tobacco smoking in the causation of cancers of the upper respiratory and gastrointestinal tracts. Moreover, alcohol alone is implicated in cirrhosis-mediated liver cancer and also may cause a proportion of cancer of the breast and the large bowel. The combination of low folic acid intake and regular alcohol consumption may be especially hazardous. In contrast, moderate alcohol consumption does reduce risk of coronary heart disease.

Because the epidemiologic findings here are complicated, the advice to minimize cancer risk is also complex. Most importantly, heavy alcohol consumption should be avoided. Current guidelines define moderate drinking as two or fewer drinks per day for men and no more than one drink per day for women. Women in particular should be cautious about their level of consumption because evidence is strong that alcohol increases breast cancer incidence moderately. Indeed, women who are at high risk for breast cancer (*e.g.*, because of family history) should be particularly cautious about drinking alcohol and should ensure that their folic acid intake is adequate.

10.   SOCIOECONOMIC STATUS

Cancers of the lung, stomach, and uterine cervix, and possibly other cancers as well, are particularly common among poor and underprivileged population groups. Poverty may be thought of as an important underlying cause for these cancers, since it is associated with increased exposure to tobacco smoke, alcoholism, poor nutrition, and certain infectious agents.

11.   ENVIRONMENTAL POLLUTION

The search for carcinogenic agents from environmental pollution has been an active area of investigation, yet few causal links have been firmly established. Investigations have focused on water fluoridation, chlorinated water by-products, metabolites of organochlorine pesticides (*e.g.*, DDT), and residential proximity to hazardous waste sites or contaminated wells.

Ecologic studies have indicated higher mortality from lung cancer in urban areas with high air pollution levels than in rural areas. On the other hand, epidemiologic studies have not documented an increased risk of lung cancer among nonsmokers living in urban rather than in rural areas but do suggest higher risks for urban smokers compared with rural smokers.

12. IONIZING AND ULTRAVIOLET (UV) RADIATION

The ultraviolet (UV) part of the sunlight spectrum is responsible for over 90 percent of skin cancers, including skin melanomas. Both prolonged sun exposure and a history of severe sunburns have been implicated in skin cancer. Experience in Australia and other countries demonstrates that both higher public awareness of the cancer risk associated with prolonged sun exposure and greater use of sunscreens can be achieved, both resulting in reduced UV exposure.

Ionizing radiation is unquestionably carcinogenic, but the risk of cancer following exposure to low levels of radiation is generally overestimated. Even among Japanese atomic bomb survivors, only one percent have died from radiation-related cancers.

Extremely low-frequency magnetic fields have been intensively studied. The collective evidence suggests that if a risk exists at all, it is small. Radio-frequency-range electromagnetic radiation, as used in cellular telephones, is being studied currently for possible brain carcinogenicity, but at present there is no empirical evidence to substantiate this claim.

13. PRESCRIPTION DRUGS AND MEDICAL PROCEDURES

Several medical products and procedures can cause cancer, but when they are administered to patients suffering from serious disease, they result in exceedingly favorable benefit-to-risk ratios. The problem is more complicated when pharmaceutical agents or procedures are applied to healthy persons for preventive purposes, since the potential benefit is smaller.

Radiotherapy can cause cancer. It is also conceivable that medical diagnostic radiation is responsible for some cancer cases, although this has been documented only for intrauterine exposures in relation to childhood leukemia. It is now generally recognized that mammography conveys a negligible risk but a substantial benefit.

Several pharmaceutical agents are human carcinogens (at different sites): cancer chemotherapeutic and immunosuppressive drugs (bone marrow); tamoxifen (endometrium); anabolic steroids (liver); and phenacetin analgesics (kidney, pelvis). The use of estrogen and progesterone therapy after menopause represents a dilemma for many women because important benefits exist for osteoporosis and coronary heart disease, whereas risk of breast cancer increases with duration of continued use (for women currently using hormone replacements with ten years or more of use, the risk of breast cancer can increase 1.5 to two-fold compared to nonusers). Modified estrogenic compounds (SERMs) that may provide similar benefits and even reduce breast cancer risk are now entering the market; their long term effects will require continued monitoring. Other drugs with established carcinogenicity are not used anymore (*e.g.*, DES).

Oral contraceptives, above and beyond their social benefits, prevent many more cancers of the ovary and endometrium than they cause in the liver, while their effect in causing breast cancer appears to be minimal.

14.   SALT AND OTHER FOOD ADDITIVES AND CONTAMINANTS

As noted above, reduction of salt intake could reduce stomach cancer risk. No other food additive or contaminant has been linked conclusively to cancer.

15.   THE POTENTIAL FOR CANCER REDUCTION

As suggested by Table 1, the potential for reducing death (as well as incidence) due to cancer is large. Some of the causes of cancer, although well known, are not directly amenable to prevention, for example, inherited gene mutations. Other causes are theoretically modifiable, but doing so would have other adverse consequences. For example, promoting teen pregnancies and high parity would reduce breast cancer incidence, but would have severe social and environmental impacts. Fortunately, the dominant causes of cancer, specifically tobacco use, unhealthy diets and overweight, and sedentary lifestyle, are potentially avoidable. If the whole population of a developed country would stop smoking, exercise regularly, avoid midlife weight gains, and consume a healthy diet and avoid excessive alcohol consumption, then cancer mortality rates could be reduced by approximately two thirds. Moreover, besides reducing cancer risk, avoidance of these causes can have major benefits for cardiovascular disease and positive environmental impacts. For example, walking or bicycling for transportation will reduce risks of cancer, heart disease, diabetes, other consequences of obesity, and at the same time reduce air pollution and traffic congestion.

The adoption of known healthy dietary and lifestyle behaviors will reduce different cancers to a variable degree. Although the large majority of cancers of the lung and colon would be avoided, the impact on cancers of the breast and prostate would be more modest. Most likely, realistically obtainable lifestyle and reproductive behaviors will not be adequate to eliminate the majority of these cancers. Fortunately research during the last several years has begun to elucidate the relationships between circulating hormone levels and risks of these important cancers, and at that same time pharmacologic agents are being developed that should be able to modify risk. Thus, in the future, it is likely that we will be able to identify persons at increased risks of breast or prostate cancer by measuring their hormone levels, as we currently do for cholesterol in determining risk of heart disease, and then combining lifestyle and pharmacologic means to reduce risk.

Although it is unrealistic to expect that all persons will adopt the full set of healthy diet and lifestyle behaviors needed to reduce cancer mortality by two-thirds, individuals can act on this information to reduce their personal risk. Indeed, many already have and we have observed a decline in lung cancer rates in men. For our population as a whole, we believe that cancer mortality can realistically be reduced substantially, perhaps by as much as one-third, by addressing these causes of cancer. Progress is likely to be incremental, however, and not the result of major breakthroughs. Ultimately, the prevention of cancer will depend on changes in individual lifestyles, development and implementation of government regulations, societal change, and further research.

Widespread recognition that cancer can be prevented would represent a major shift in how the public thinks about this disease. Avoiding or stopping tobacco use is broadly known to lower cancer risk, but beyond that, cancer is commonly viewed as a mystery whose cause eludes our intellectual grasp and therefore our ability to prevent it. Instead, the public's focus has largely been on cancer treatment. This is due, in part, to rhetoric about finding a 'cure for cancer.' This focus also results from the fact that the diagnosis of cancer in a friend or family member is a landmark event whose successful treatment is celebrated, while the results of effective prevention cannot be individually recognized and therefore goes unnoticed. While the search for better treatment of cancer is important, the most effective strategy for reducing cancer mortality will require at least an equal emphasis on prevention.

Unfortunately, public interest in cancer prevention has been largely directed to potential environmental carcinogens, especially chemicals, electromagnetic fields, and other products of our technological age. Recent years have seen increases in rates of some type of cancer, which the public thinks can be attributed to environmental pollution or occupational exposures. Continued vigilance on these fronts is necessary, of course, but in fact these appear to be far less important sources of cancer risk than most people assume.

CONCLUSION

Preventing cancer deaths in the U.S. will not be easy, given the scope of individual and societal change that must occur. But change is possible. Studies of migrant populations show that they tend to adopt the cancer pattern of the host country within a period of time that varies from less than 20 years (*e.g.*, cancer of the large bowel) to a few generations (*e.g.*, cancer of the breast). Cancer rates are malleable, and with the proper commitment of resources, and with time, we believe that the United States can realistically reduce cancer rates by as much as one-third.

SUGGESTIONS

- Reduced exposure to tobacco smoke, including environmental tobacco smoke, is the first priority.
- The following dietary practice changes are likely to contribute substantially to the primary prevention of cancer:
- Consumption of at least five servings of vegetables and fruits per day.
- Reduced consumption of red meat, refined carbohydrates, and salt;
- Replacement of animal fat, with plant oils (*e.g.*, olive oil) as added fats.
- Reduction of excess energy intake in early life, avoidance of obesity in adult life, and increased physical activity throughout life are also desirable;
- Alcoholic beverages should be consumed only in moderation, especially by smokers (because of the interactive effects of tobacco and alcohol) and by women (because alcohol intake may be involved in the etiology of breast cancer).
- Avoidance of exposure to ultraviolet radiation, prudent use of potentially carcinogenic medical products and procedures, strict control of occupational exposures, sound environmental policies with strict enforcement, and continuous scrutiny of food additives and contaminants can also contribute to cancer prevention, but only to a small degree compared with reduced smoking, dietary changes, reduced obesity, and greater physical activity.

2

PREVENTION OF HUMAN CANCER

Chapter 15

Prevention of Tobacco Use

Nancy A. Rigotti, M.D.
Tobacco Research and Treatment Program, Massachusetts General Hospital and Harvard Medical School

INTRODUCTION

Tobacco is the leading preventable cause of death in the United States. Although tobacco - related disease takes its toll among adults, tobacco use begins early in life. Nearly 90 percent of smokers smoke their first cigarette by the age of 18, and half of smokers try their first cigarette by the age of 14 years [1, 2]. Former Food and Drug Administration Commissioner Dr. David Kessler has called tobacco use - and the nicotine dependence which sustains it - a "pediatric disease" [3]. Because tobacco use starts early in life, tobacco prevention efforts must focus on children and adolescents.

1.   PATTERNS OF TOBACCO INITIATION AND USE

Tobacco use is common among youths. Each day, an estimated 6000 U.S. children and adolescents try cigarettes and 3000 start to smoke regularly [4]. According to the Youth Risk Behavior Survey (YRBS), in 1997, 70 percent of high school students in grades 9 to 12 had ever tried a cigarette, 36 percent had smoked within the past month, and 17 percent smoked cigarettes frequently (on at least 20 of the past 30 days) [5]. In contrast to adult smoking prevalence, which has declined since the 1960s, adolescent smoking prevalence did not change during the 1980s and has

G.A. Colditz et al. (eds.), Cancer Prevention: The Causes and Prevention of Cancer - Volume I, 175–192.
© 2000 *Kluwer Academic Publishers.*

increased since 1991 (Figure 1) [1, 2, 6]. Between 1991 and 1997, the last year for which data are available, cigarette smoking among high school students rose by 32 percent, from 27.5 percent to 36.4 percent [5]. These teenagers are carrying their smoking into young adulthood. Among college students, smoking prevalence increased by 28 percent between 1993 and 1997 [7]. Only 10 percent of these smokers began to smoke while in college, but 25 percent of them started smoking regularly during college.

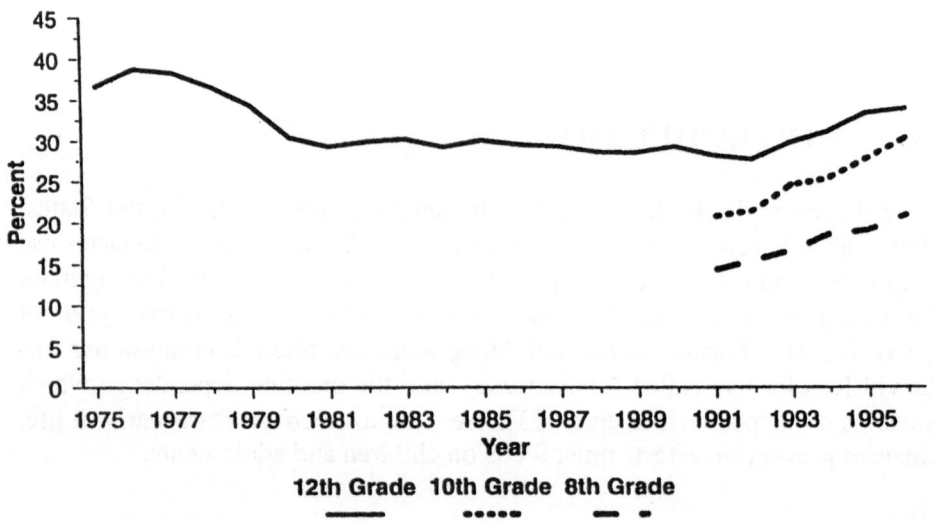

Source: Institute for Social Research,
University of Michigan, Monitoring the Future Project
*Smoking 1 or more cigarettes during the previous 30 days

Figure 15.1 Trends in Cigarette Smoking Anytime in the Past *30 Days by Grade in School -- United States, 1975-1996

Young people's tobacco use is not limited to cigarettes. In the 1997 YRBS, 42.7 percent of high school students reported having used any tobacco product in the past 30 days; this included 36.4 percent who had smoked cigarettes, 22.0 percent who had smoked cigars, and 9.3 percent who had used smokeless tobacco (Figure 2) [5]. There was little gender difference in cigarette use (37.7 percent of males *vs.* 34.7 percent of females), but males were far more likely than females to use smokeless tobacco (15.8 percent *vs.* 1.5 percent), or cigars (31.2 percent *vs.* 10.8 percent). In contrast, there are marked ethnic differences in tobacco use by teens [6]. Whites and Native Americans have the highest rate of tobacco use, while African-Americans have the lowest. Use rates among Hispanics are intermediate. In the 1997 YRBS survey, the prevalence of current smoking (*e.g.,* smoking within the past 30 days) was 40 percent among white high school students, 34 percent among Hispanics and 23 percent among African-Americans [5]. Considerable research has been done to try to understand the markedly lower rates of tobacco use among African-Americans in hopes of learning lessons applicable to other sociodemographic groups. There is no evidence that the finding represents error in measurement. Qualitative research suggests that tobacco has very different roles in the subcultures of white and African American youth and that this may explain the differences in prevalence [1, 6].

Like other drug dependence syndromes, nicotine dependence is characterized by a compulsive pattern of use that persists in spite of an individual's desire or unsuccessful effort to cut down on use. Nicotine-dependent individuals develop tolerance to the adverse effects of nicotine and withdrawal symptoms if they stop drug use abruptly [2]. Current models of the natural history of nicotine dependence postulate a gradual process requiring several years between the first use of tobacco and established nicotine dependence [1, 2]. Not all youths who try a cigarette progress to nicotine dependence, which is thought to require regular daily smoking. According to cross-sectional surveys, of the 70 percent of young people who try a cigarette, 36 percent report that they have ever smoked daily [8]. There are few prospective data examining the development of nicotine dependence and some suggestions that nicotine dependence may precede the establishment of regular daily smoking. Prospective observational studies designed to better define the development of nicotine dependence are underway.

Regardless of how quickly nicotine dependence develops, surveys of adolescent smokers indicate that most are nicotine dependent [2]. When adolescents try to stop smoking, they report withdrawal symptoms that are similar to those reported by adult smokers [1]. According to the 1997 YRBS, 73 percent of daily smokers have tried unsuccessfully to quit [8]. In another study, 74 percent of daily cigarette smokers aged 10 to 22 reported that one reason they used tobacco was that it was hard to quit [9]. Despite these data, adolescents underestimate their risk of becoming dependent on nicotine. In high school, only five to ten percent of daily smokers think that they will definitely be smoking in five years, but longitudinal data show that 75 percent of them are still smoking five years later [10].

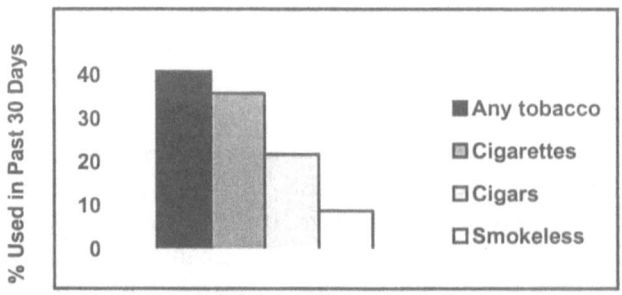

MMWR April 2, 1999

Figure 15.2 Tobacco use by high school students. 1997 Youth Risk Behavior Survey

2. RISK FACTORS FOR SMOKING INITIATION

Factors operating at the environmental, family, peer, and individual levels have been associated with smoking initiation [1]. Pro-smoking messages, which portray cigarettes as symbols of independence, rebellion, and adulthood, permeate the environment [2]. This symbolism has appeal for children and adolescents who are eager to try out adult behavior as part of the process of establishing independence. Messages also communicate the misinformation that smoking is a common, safe, attractive, and relaxing habit [2]. These messages are delivered by tobacco advertising in newspapers and magazines and by tobacco promotional activities such as the sponsorship of sporting events and entertainment, in-store displays, and distribution of items with tobacco company logos. Smoking in movies and on TV by role models such as actors, musicians, models, and sports celebrities also conveys the message that smoking is desirable and normative. Furthermore, tobacco products are readily available to youths who seek them. Cigarettes are relatively inexpensive and youths report little difficulty obtaining tobacco products, despite laws in all 50 states that prohibit tobacco sales to minors. These factors presumably explain why 70 percent of teens try a cigarette at least once.

However, only about half of the adolescents who try cigarettes continue to experiment with cigarettes, implying that forces at the family, peer group, and individual levels must also contribute to the initiation of tobacco use. Studies have repeatedly shown that youths whose parents, siblings, and peers smoke are at higher risk of becoming smokers than are youths surrounded by nonsmokers. Other studies indicate that families in which there is less overt parental disapproval of tobacco use are more likely to produce smokers[1]. Behavioral factors associated with tobacco use include poor academic achievement and less involvement in school, fewer skills to resist peer influences, and fewer problem-solving skills. Tobacco use during adolescence is associated with an array of other behaviors that put individuals at risk, including using alcohol and other drugs, carrying weapons, being involved in fights, and engaging in high-risk sexual behavior [1]. Psychological risk factors for tobacco use include low self-image, low self-esteem, and depressive symptoms. Females with concerns about weight, especially white females, are at greater risk of smoking. Individuals who manifest conduct problems in childhood or adolescence are at higher risk of becoming smokers. A relationship between attention-deficit hyperactivity disorder (ADHD) and smoking has also been observed, although it is not clear whether ADHD is a risk factor for smoking in the absence of conduct disorders [11]. In short, many of the characteristics that are associated with early tobacco use put these youths at risk of other behavioral and health problems. Furthermore, tobacco is generally the first drug used by youths who progress to other drug use [1].

Genetic factors may also contribute to the risk of becoming nicotine dependent [2]. Factors that affect nicotine uptake or metabolism might make some youths more vulnerable to becoming addicted when they try tobacco or make it more difficult for some smokers to stop. Twin studies indicate that approximately 50 percent of smoking is heritable. The mechanisms by which genetic factors may influence smoking behavior are unknown. Potential genes and mechanisms are under active investigation, including those coding for nicotine and dopamine receptors in the brain. Another candidate, the CYP2A6 gene, codes for an enzyme that metabolizes nicotine to cotinine. Individuals carrying the variant allele metabolize nicotine more slowly and have higher blood nicotine levels after smoking a cigarette. They may have more severe adverse physical effects following initial tobacco use, which might discourage repetitive use and protect these individuals from developing nicotine dependence. Consistent with this hypothesis, one study found a lower prevalence of smoking among individuals with the variant CYP2A6 allele, compared with those with the wild type [12].

3. HEALTH CONSEQUENCES

The long-term health impact of the cigarette smoking that children are now starting is substantial. Of all U.S. children under the age of 18 in 1995, the CDC estimated that 16 million will smoke regularly and 5 million will die prematurely of a tobacco-related disease [13]. The risk of developing a tobacco-related disease is related to the duration and intensity of an individual's tobacco exposure. Smokers who begin before age 15 are more likely to develop strong nicotine dependence, to have more difficulty stopping smoking, and to continue to smoke through adulthood [1, 14]. Greater nicotine dependence leads to greater duration and intensity of exposure to tobacco, and hence greater risk of disease. In the short term, a rise in tobacco use by teens and young adults, who are in their reproductive years, has the potential to increase tobacco related pregnancy complications (*e.g.,* infants with low birth weight) and children's exposure to environmental tobacco smoke. In the long term is the risk that future decades will see a stalling or even a reversal of the declines in adult tobacco prevalence that have accounted for decreases in deaths due to tobacco-related diseases.

4.   PREVENTION OF TOBACCO USE

The ultimate goal of a tobacco prevention program is to prevent any new tobacco use, but given the fact that the majority of youths try at least one cigarette, this cannot be the only measure of success (Table 1). An alternate goal of prevention programs is to prevent the development of nicotine dependence among youth by blocking the transition from experimentation with tobacco to regular tobacco use. This would still reduce adult smoking prevalence and the consequent health harms. Even just delaying the onset of tobacco use without preventing it could conceivably reduce the ultimate harms of tobacco, because early tobacco onset is associated with greater risk of adverse health consequences, stronger nicotine dependence, and a lower likelihood of cessation [14]. Finally, promoting smoking cessation by nicotine-addicted youths would contribute to reducing teen and ultimately adult tobacco use. Though cessation does not prevent tobacco use *per se*, it does serve public health goals by reducing the proportion of adults who smoke and are at risk of tobacco related disease. To achieve any of these goals, a tobacco prevention program can focus on altering individual behavior directly or on changing the environment in which young people make decisions about whether to start smoking (Table 15.2). Ultimately, a comprehensive program that targets both individuals and the environment is likely to be most effective.

Table 15.1 Potential goals of tobacco prevention.

- Prevent all tobacco use (*e.g.,* stop experimentation with tobacco)
- Block the transition from experimentation to nicotine dependence
- Delay the onset of tobacco use
- Promote smoking cessation

---

5. TOBACCO PREVENTION EFFORTS THAT TARGET INDIVIDUALS

5.1 School-based Programs

Most tobacco-prevention efforts that target individuals are school-based programs designed to discourage young people from starting to use tobacco [1, 2]. This is because outside of the home, schools are the major environment of children and adolescents. Schools provide the opportunity to communicate nonsmoking norms, teach children to resist environmental pressures to try tobacco, and educate children about the hazards and addictiveness of tobacco. Several decades of research have demonstrated that the most effective programs train young people to resist peer influences to try tobacco and teach general problem-solving or social skills, especially assertiveness. They also educate young people about the health harms and addictiveness of tobacco products, but programs providing information alone without skills training are generally ineffective. In controlled studies, these programs have produced significant reductions in youth smoking prevalence that lasts for several years after the program ends. More intense programs, involving as many as 30 sessions delivered over several years, are more effective than less intense programs. School-based programs are more effective if combined with community-wide mass media campaigns that target adolescents or community-wide tobacco education or smoking cessation programs that involve parents and other adults [1]. Unfortunately, school-based tobacco prevention programs demonstrated to be effective in research settings have not been widely adopted by schools nationwide [2].

The Centers for Disease Control and the National Cancer Institute have developed guidelines for school-based programs based on experimentally-validated programs [15, 16]. Both recommend that school programs include information about the short- and long-term negative physiologic consequences of tobacco use, make students aware that smoking is not the norm for adolescents, and teach students the skills to recognize and resist the social influences that encourage smoking. Programs are most important for grades 6 to 9, but to remain effective, booster sessions should continue through high school. Programs are most effective if they start in elementary school. The National Cancer Institute recommends a minimum of five sessions over two years in middle school, followed by annual booster sessions through high school. Effective programs require careful teacher training and the support of parents and families. Tobacco prevention programs in schools should be accompanied by no-smoking policies in schools and support for smoking cessation by students and staff who use tobacco.

5.2   Counseling by Health Care Providers

Children's and adolescents' contact with the health care system provide another opportunity for tobacco use prevention at the individual level. Visits for preventive care are recommended regularly throughout childhood and adolescence. These provide the setting for addressing tobacco use at all ages. Formal recommendations for the content and delivery of adolescent preventive visits have been made by numerous organizations. These include the American Medical Association's Guidelines for Adolescent Preventive Services (GAPS), the Maternal and Child Health Bureau's Bright Futures, the U.S. Preventive Services Task Force's Guide to Clinical Preventive Services, and the American Academy of Pediatrics [17]. All recommend that physicians screen and counsel children and teens about tobacco use. Specific guidelines for addressing tobacco use by adolescents have been developed or endorsed by the National Cancer Institute, the American Academy of Pediatrics, the American Academy of Family Physicians, and the Agency for Health Care Policy and Research [17, 18]. Despite a clear consensus from these organizations, data indicate that physicians' practices fall far short of these recommendations [17, 19, 20]

Unlike school-based tobacco prevention programs, whose efficacy has been established, no available evidence demonstrates the efficacy of tobacco use prevention in the health care setting, largely because the topic has not been studied [17, 21]. Even less attention has been paid to smoking cessation among adolescents [21]. The little evidence that exists indicates that recruiting and retaining adolescents into formal smoking cessation programs is difficult and those programs have low success rates [1]. A number of tobacco prevention and treatment studies targeting youth have recently been funded and better information should be forthcoming. Until more is known about what tobacco prevention or cessation approaches work for youths, expert panels have concluded that it is appropriate to adapt what is known to be effective for adults to the developmental level of children [21, 22]

A substantial body of research indicates that office-based counseling for smoking cessation is effective in adults. This evidence was reviewed by the Agency for Health Care Policy and Research (AHCPR) and used to develop formal smoking cessation guidelines for primary care practice [22]. The Agency concluded that both behavioral counseling and nicotine replacement therapy were effective treatment methods and that combining the two produced the best success. No evidence for efficacy was found for hypnosis, acupuncture, or other smoking cessation methods. Brief physician advice to quit smoking delivered to all adult smokers seen in medical practice increased cessation rates, but adding brief (<3 minutes) counseling was more effective. The Food and Drug Administration has approved several drugs for use to aid smoking cessation; these include nicotine replacement therapies (gum, skin patch, nasal spray, and inhaler) and the antidepressant bupropion (Zyban or Wellbutrin SR). None of these products is approved for use by children under the age of 18 [23]. The nicotine skin patch has been tested in teenagers and found to be safe but not effective in a single published trial [24]. Bupropion is being tested in teens as an aid for smoking cessation and as a tool to prevent smoking initiation among youths with attention-deficit hyperactivity disorder.

The AHCPR consensus panel concluded that physicians should provide pediatric and adolescent patients (and their parents) with a strong message to abstain from tobacco use at every visit[22]. The National Cancer Institute and the American Academy of Pediatrics developed a pediatric smoking intervention model based on the NCI's adult model [18]. This algorithm includes 5 steps: (1) anticipate the risk of tobacco use or exposure in all pediatric and adolescent patients; (2) ask about exposure to tobacco and tobacco use at each visit; (3) advise all children not to use tobacco products and all tobacco users to stop; (4) assist children to resist tobacco use and assist smokers to quit; and (5) arrange follow-up visits as needed (Table 15.3).

Table 15.2 Components of comprehensive tobacco prevention

Efforts Targeting Individuals	School-based programs
	Counseling by health care providers
Public Health Efforts	Increase tobacco excise taxes to raise price of tobacco products
	Restrict or ban tobacco advertising and promotion
	Fund mass media counter-advertising campaigns
	Restrict smoking in public places, work places, restaurants, and schools
	Reduce youth access to tobacco products

6. PUBLIC HEALTH AND PUBLIC POLICY FOR TOBACCO PREVENTION

Public health efforts to prevent tobacco use aims to remove or counter the environmental influences that promote smoking. Most public health efforts focus on reducing the demand for tobacco products by young people, but recently efforts have also attempted to reduce the supply of tobacco products to youth. Public policies that have been proposed to prevent smoking initiation include increasing the price of tobacco products by raising tobacco excise taxes, reducing or eliminating tobacco advertising and promotion, conducting counter-advertising campaigns (*e.g.,* using marketing techniques to discourage smoking), mandating school-based tobacco prevention programs, stopping the sale of tobacco products to minors, and adopting policies that prohibit smoking in schools, public places, restaurants, and work sites [1, 2] (Table 15.2). Varying levels of evidence support the efficacy of these individual policies for discouraging tobacco use.

Table 15.3 Smoking counseling model for pediatric practice

ANTICIPATE	the risk of use or exposure in all patients
ASK	about exposure to tobacco and tobacco use at each visit
ADVISE	all children not to use tobacco products and all tobacco users to stop
ASSIST	children to resist tobacco use and assist smokers to quit
ARRANGE	follow-up visits as needed

6.1   Increasing the Price of Tobacco Products

The strongest case can be made for increasing the price of tobacco [1, 2]. Multiple econometric studies demonstrate that increasing the price of tobacco products reduces the demand for cigarettes by both adults and teens, as measured by *per capita* tobacco consumption and smoking prevalence. In part because younger smokers are less nicotine-addicted than adult smokers, the effect of a price increase on youth demand for cigarettes is two to three times greater than the effect on adult demand. A ten percent increase in price of tobacco products will reduce adult smoking prevalence by one to two percent but reduce youth smoking prevalence by as much as seven percent. Overall, the ten percent increase in price produces a three to four percent decline in adult tobacco consumption and a larger decline in adolescent tobacco consumption [25].

6.2   Restricting Tobacco Advertising and Promotion

Definitive evidence that reducing tobacco advertising and promotion reduces youth smoking is difficult to obtain because there have been few opportunities to test this hypothesis in the U.S. However, a strong circumstantial case can be made that tobacco industry advertising and promotional activity encourages adolescents to smoke, and there is evidence from other countries (Canada, New Zealand, Finland, and Norway) that tobacco advertising bans or restrictions reduce tobacco consumption [1, 2, 26]. Tobacco manufacturers themselves attributed the large increase in tobacco use that occurred in the first half of the 20th century to the effectiveness of their advertising and promotional campaigns. A long-term decline in adolescent smoking and overall *per capita* cigarette consumption began in 1973, shortly after 1971 when the U.S. banned tobacco advertising on radio and television. Tobacco industry leaders responded to this trend by focusing on the youth market. The best-funded effort was the Joe Camel campaign, launched in 1987. This cartoon character was shown to be attractive to young children and was followed by an increase in adolescent smoking prevalence beginning in 1991 [2]. Additional research has been shown that the brand preferences of teenage smokers are linked much more closely to tobacco industry advertising expenditures than are adult brand choices. Longitudinal studies of nonsmoking adolescents have found that having a favorite cigarette advertisement or a tobacco industry promotional item is associated with progression toward becoming a smoker.

6.3   Counter-Advertising Campaigns

Counter-advertising campaigns use marketing techniques to educate youths and adults about the harms of tobacco use and persuade youths not to start smoking. They provide an alternative to advertising restriction as a method to reduce the power of tobacco industry marketing efforts. Evidence to support this approach derives from a natural experiment in the U.S., where *per capita* tobacco consumption dropped for the three years when anti-tobacco messages were mandated and broadcast widely on radio and TV (1968-70) [2]. This extensive counter-advertising campaign ended in 1971 when Congress banned tobacco advertising in all broadcast media. More recently, several states have funded large-scale counter-advertising campaigns that were funded by increases in state tobacco excise taxes (California and Massachusetts) or by funds provided by the tobacco industry to settle litigation (Florida). In Florida, small but significant declines in tobacco use by students in public middle schools and high schools were observed following one year of an aggressive, well-funded counter-advertising campaign aimed at and created in part by teenagers [27]. The pure effect of counter-advertising campaigns in other states is more difficult to assess because price increases and other policies were implemented simultaneously.

6.4   Implementing Smoke-free Policies

Laws and policies that prohibit smoking in public places, work places, and restaurants have been adopted to protect nonsmokers from the hazards of involuntary tobacco smoke exposure. In practice, these policies reduce smokers' daily tobacco consumption and may encourage cessation. These policies may also discourage youth smoking by reducing the visibility and perceived prevalence of tobacco use and by altering social norms about the acceptability of smoking. Currently no data are available to test the hypothesis [2].

6.5   Reducing Youth Access to Tobacco

Young people report having little difficulty obtaining tobacco from commercial sources (stores and vending machines), despite laws in all 50 states prohibit tobacco sales to minors [28]. Youths also obtain tobacco from noncommercial sources such as older friends and relatives. It has been proposed that enforcing existing tobacco sales restrictions could discourage youth smoking by reducing the supply of cigarettes to youth. Efforts to educate tobacco retailers not to sell tobacco to minors has had limited success, but active enforcement of tobacco sales laws, with fines for violators, has reduced the proportion of stores that sell tobacco to minors. However, there is conflicting evidence about the effect of supply reduction strategies on the prevalence of smoking by youths [29, 30]. It is likely to be difficult to stop the supply of tobacco to youth, since cigarettes are available through noncommercial sources and because tobacco retailers have economic incentives to sell tobacco to minors. However, supply reduction is likely to be a useful component of comprehensive efforts to prevent tobacco use, along with efforts to reduce young people's demand for tobacco products.

6.6   Comprehensive State Tobacco Control Programs

The policies described above have been combined into several large-scale efforts aimed at preventing and treating tobacco use. Comprehensive statewide tobacco control programs were funded in California (1988) and Massachusetts (1992) by increases in state tobacco excise taxes. Preventing tobacco initiation was a major focus of both programs, which combined mass media counter-advertising programs, school-based tobacco prevention programs, expanded access to smoking cessation programs, promotion of no-smoking policies, and enforcement of tobacco sales restrictions with tobacco price increases. *Per capita* tobacco consumption and adult smoking prevalence declined more rapidly in California and Massachusetts than in the other 48 states after the implementation of these comprehensive programs [31, 32]. The programs have had less effect on youth smoking rates, showing at best a slowing of the rise in adolescent smoking prevalence as compared to a more rapid rise in these rates observed in the rest of the U.S.

Arizona and Oregon have also implemented comprehensive tobacco control programs funded by increases in state tobacco excise taxes.

Similar comprehensive tobacco control programs have been promoted for all states, using funds generated by the settlement of lawsuits filed by 46 state attorneys general against the tobacco industry [33]. These lawsuits, which sought to recover the costs of treating tobacco-related disease among Medicaid recipients, were settled out-of-court in late 1998. The multi-state settlement stipulated that the tobacco industry would pay each participating state substantial monetary damages over several decades. These funds could support comprehensive tobacco control programs in each state that could substantially reduce tobacco initiation among youth as well as support cessation efforts by adult smokers. However, as of early 2000, little of this revenue will be used for tobacco control.

6.7   Tobacco Product Regulation

In 1996, the U.S. Food and Drug Administration asserted the right to regulate nicotine as a drug [3, 34]. Subsequently, the agency issued regulations aimed at reducing the appeal and availability of tobacco to youth. The provisions established 18 as the minimum age of tobacco purchase nationwide and banned vending machines in most locations (except those where children are not permitted). Tobacco advertising and promotion were also restricted. Tobacco promotional items and tobacco-industry sponsorship of sporting and entertainment events were banned, and restrictions were placed on the content of advertising in magazines with significant youth readership. The FDA also mandated that the tobacco industry fund a counter-advertising campaign aimed toward youth. Full implementation of the FDA regulations have been delayed pending the outcome of a legal challenge from the tobacco industry. The U.S. Supreme Court will decide the case in the 1999/2000 term.

CONCLUSION

Effective tobacco prevention will require a comprehensive effort to counter the multiple risk factors for tobacco initiation that operate at the environmental, family, peer, and individual levels. Efforts will need to target both individual behavior and the environmental context in which it occurs. A number of tobacco prevention approaches have been proposed. The evidence supporting individual strategies varies. Best substantiated are school-based tobacco prevention programs and increases in the price of tobacco products. Evidence also supports the efficacy of mass media counter-advertising campaigns, restrictions on tobacco advertising and promotion, efforts to reduce youth access to tobacco products, and comprehensive state tobacco control programs that combine all of these elements. The efficacy of tobacco prevention or cessation counseling in pediatric and adolescent medicine practice has received little study, but expert panels recommend that physicians routinely counsel children and adolescents about tobacco use prevention, adapting approaches shown to be effective in adult medicine practice. While further research is needed to define optimal prevention strategies, we also need to disseminate measures already shown to be effective at reducing youth smoking, ideally in comprehensive tobacco control programs.

Recently, new opportunities to fund comprehensive tobacco prevention programs have arisen from the settlement of litigation against the tobacco industry. Whether these funds will be used for tobacco control remains to be determined. Also in doubt, pending the outcome of a lawsuit filed by the tobacco industry, is the fate of the landmark regulations on tobacco products issued the U.S. Food and Drug Administration in 1996. The current environment holds great opportunity but also great uncertainty regarding future tobacco prevention efforts.

SUMMARY POINTS

- Because tobacco use starts early in life, tobacco prevention efforts must focus on children and adolescents, in whom tobacco use is rising.
- Tobacco prevention efforts can attempt to stop all tobacco use, but given the ubiquity of experimentation among youth, it may be more realistic to try to block the transition from experimental to regular, nicotine-dependent use. Tobacco cessation by youths, while not prevention, *per se*, will also have the effect of preventing the health harms of tobacco use.
- Multiple risk factors operating at environmental, family, peer, and individual (behavioral, psychosocial, and genetic) levels have been associated with smoking initiation. A comprehensive program that targets both individual and environmental risk factors is likely to be most effective for tobacco prevention.
- Most tobacco-prevention efforts that target individuals are based in schools. Programs demonstrated to be effective in research settings have not been widely adopted. Evidence-based guidelines for school-based tobacco prevention programs have been developed by the Centers for Disease Control.

- Counseling by health care providers is widely recommended, but not widely practiced. The efficacy of counseling for tobacco prevention in the pediatric settings has not been studied and little is known about effective tobacco cessation programs for youths. Until more is known, expert panels recommend adapting what is known to be effective for adults to the developmental level of children and adolescents. The National Cancer Institute has developed a model program for pediatric practice.
- Public policies that have been proposed to prevent smoking initiation include increasing tobacco excise taxes in order to raise the price of tobacco products, reducing or eliminating tobacco advertising and promotion, funding mass media counter-advertising campaigns, stopping the sale of tobacco products to minors, and adopting policies that prohibit smoking in schools, public places, restaurants, and work sites.
- Comprehensive tobacco control programs which combine these individual components have been implemented in several states. Preliminary results indicate that they reduce *per capita* consumption and adult tobacco use, although the effect on youth tobacco use is less dramatic. The U.S. Food and Drug Administration has also proposed regulations on tobacco products designed to reduce youth smoking. The recent multi-state settlement of litigation against the tobacco industry provides a new opportunity to fund comprehensive statewide tobacco control programs.

RECOMMENDATIONS

- The following public policies could contribute to reductions in youth tobacco use and should be undertaken or expanded:
  - Substantial increases in federal and state tobacco excise taxes
  - Widespread dissemination of effective school-based tobacco education programs, ideally offered each year (K-12), but especially in grades 6 through 9.
  - Well-funded mass media counter-advertising campaigns to counter the appeal of tobacco to youths.
  - Restrictions on tobacco advertising and bans on tobacco promotional activities.
  - Expansion of no-smoking policies in public places, work places, restaurants, and schools.
  - Efforts to reduce young people's access to tobacco by actively enforcing laws that ban tobacco sales to minors.

- Comprehensive tobacco control programs that combine the elements listed above should be implemented by all states or by the federal government. Funds generated by the settlement of tobacco industry litigation should be used by each state to support these programs, as well as to support expanded tobacco cessation services.
- The Food and Drug Administration's authority to regulate nicotine as a drug should be upheld and its 1996 recommendations implemented.
- Further research should identify effective tobacco prevention and cessation counseling approaches for use in pediatric and adolescent medicine practice. In the meantime, physicians caring for children and teens should adopt current recommendations of professional organizations to address smoking routinely at all visits.

SUGGESTED FURTHER READING

1. U.S. Department of Health and Human Services (1994) *Preventing Tobacco Use Among Young People: A Report of the Surgeon General.* Atlanta, GA: Public Health Service, Centers for Disease Control and Prevention, Office on Smoking and Health.
2. Institute of Medicine (1994) *Growing Up Tobacco Free: Preventing Nicotine Addiction in Children and Youths.* In: Lynch BS, Bonnie BJ, eds. Washington, DC: National Academy Press.
3. *Addicted to Nicotine: A National Research Forum.* Sponsored by the National Institute on Drug Abuse, NIH, and the Robert Wood Johnson Foundation. Bethesda, MD, July 27-28, 1998. [Conference papers to be published as a supplement to *Nicotine and Tobacco Research* (in press)].
4. (1998) Tobacco cessation and youth. *Prev Med* **27**(Suppl): A1-A63

REFERENCES

1. U.S. Department of Health and Human Services (1994) Preventing Tobacco Use Among Young People: *A Report of the Surgeon General.* Atlanta, GA (USA): Public Health Service, Centers for Disease Control and Prevention, Office on Smoking and Health.
2. Institute of Medicine (1994) *Growing Up Tobacco Free: Preventing Nicotine Addiction in Children and Youths.* In: Lynch BS, Bonnie BJ, eds. Washington, DC: National Academy Press.
3. Kessler DA, Witt AM, Barnett PS, *et al.* (1996) The Food and Drug Administration's regulation of tobacco products. *N Engl J Med* **335**: 988-994.
4. Centers for Disease Control (1998) Incidence of initiation of cigarette smoking - United States, 1965-1996. *MMWR Morb Mortal Wkly Rep* **47**: 837-840.

5. Centers for Disease Control (1998) Tobacco use among high school students-United States, 1997. *MMWR Morbid Mortal Wkly Rep* **47**: 224-233.
6. Giovino GA (1999) Epidemiology of tobacco use among U.S. adolescents. *Nicotine Tobacco Res* **1**: S31-S40.
7. Wechsler H, Rigotti NA, Gledhill-Hoyt J, *et al.* (1998) Increased levels of cigarette use among college students. *JAMA* **280**: 1673-1678.
8. Centers for Disease Control (1998) Selected cigarette smoking initiation and quitting behaviors among high school students – United States, 1997. *MMWR Morb Mortal Wkly Rep* **47**: 386-389.
9. Centers for Disease Control (1994) Reasons for tobacco use and symptoms of nicotine withdrawal among adolescent and young adult tobacco users-United States, 1993. *MMWR Morb Mortal Wkly Rep* **43**: 745-750.
10. National Institute on Drug Abuse (1993) *National Survey Results on Drug Use from Monitoring the Future Study, 1975-1992.* Rockville, MD (USA): U.S. Department of Health and Human Services, Public Health Service, DHHS publication no. (NIH)93-3597.
11. McMahon RJ (1998) Child and adolescent psychopathology as risk factors for tobacco use. *Addicted to Nicotine: A National Research Forum.* Bethesda, MD: Sponsored by the National Institute on Drug Abuse, NIH, and the Robert Wood Johnson Foundation., July 27-28 *Nicotine and Tobacco Research* (In press).
12. Pianezza ML, Sellers EM, Tyndale R (1998) Nicotine metabolism defect reduces smoking. *Nature* **393**: 750.
13. Centers for Disease Control (1996) Projected smoking-related deaths among youth-United States. *MMWR Morb Mortal Wkly Rep* **45**: 971-974.
14. Breslau N, Peterson EL (1996) Smoking cessation in young adults: age at initiation of cigarette smoking and other suspected influences. *Am J Public Health* **86**: 214-20.
15. Centers for Disease Control and Prevention (1994) Guidelines for school health programs to prevent tobacco use and addiction. *MMWR Morb Mortal Wkly Rep* **43**(No. RR-2): 1-15.
16. Glynn TJ (1990) *School Programs to Prevent Smoking: The National Cancer Institute Guide to Strategies that Succeed.* U.S. Department of Health and Human Services, Public Health Service, National Institutes of Health, NIH Publication No. 90-500.
17. Hedberg VA, Klein JD, Andresen E (1998) Health counseling in adolescent preventive visits: effectiveness, current practices, and quality measurement. *J Adolesc Health* **23**: 344-353.
18. Epps R, Manley M (1991) A physician's guide to preventing tobacco use during childhood and adolescence. *Pediatrics* **88**: 140-144.
19. Thorndike AN, Ferris TG, Stafford RS, *et al.* (1999) Do physicians address smoking with adolescents? Results of the National Ambulatory Medical Care survey. *J Natl Cancer Inst* (In press).
20. Centers for Disease Control (1995) Health care provider advice on tobacco use to persons aged 10-22 years-United States, 1993. *MMWR Morb Mortal Wkly Rep* **44**: 826-837.
21. Schubiner H, Herrold A, Hurt R (1998) Tobacco cessation and youth: the feasibility of brief office interventions for adolescents. *Prev Med* **27**: A47-A54.
22. (1996) The Agency for Health Care Policy and Research Smoking Cessation Clinical Practice Guideline. *JAMA* **275**: 1270-1280.
23. Hughes JR, Goldstein MG, Hurt RD, *et al.* (1999) Recent advances in the pharmacotherapy of smoking. *JAMA* **281**: 72-76.
24. Smith TA, House RRF, Croghan TT, *et al.* (1996) Nicotine patch therapy in adolescent smokers. *Pediatrics* **98**: 659-667.

25. Chaloupka FJ (1998) Economics. In: *Addicted to Nicotine: A National Research Forum*. Bethesda, MD: Sponsored by the National Institute on Drug Abuse, NIH, and the Robert Wood Johnson Foundation. July 27-28. *Nicotine and Tobacco Research* (In press).

26. Pierce JP (1998) Advertising and promotion. In: *Addicted to Nicotine: A National Research Forum*. Bethesda, MD: Sponsored by the National Institute on Drug Abuse, NIH, and the Robert Wood Johnson Foundation. July 27-28. *Nicotine and Tobacco Research* (In press).

27. Centers for Disease Control (1999) Tobacco use among middle and high school students-Florida, 1998 and 1999. *MMWR Morb Mortal Wkly Rep* **48**: 248-53.

28. Forster JL, Wolfson M (1998) Youth access to tobacco: policies and politics. *Annu Rev Public Health* **19**: 203-235.

29. Rigotti NA, DiFranza JR, Chang YC, *et al.* (1997) The effect of enforcing tobacco sales laws on adolescents' access to tobacco and smoking behavior. *N Engl J Med* **337**: 1044-1051.

30. Forster JL, Murray DM, Wolfson M, *et al.* (1998) The effects of community policies to reduce youth access to tobacco. *Am J Public Health* **88**: 1193-1198.

31. Centers for Disease Control (1996) Cigarette smoking before and after an excise tax increase and an antismoking campaign – Massachusetts, 1990-96. *MMWR Morb Mortal Wkly Rep* **45**: 966-970.

32. Pierce JP, Gilpin EA, Emery SL, *et al.* (1998) Has the California tobacco control program reduced smoking? *JAMA* **280**: 893-899.

33. Bloch M, Daynard R, Roemer R (1998) A year of living dangerously: the tobacco control community meets the global settlement. *Public Health* **113**: 488-497.

34. (1996) FDA regulations restricting the sale and distribution of cigarettes and smokeless tobacco to protect children and adolescents (executive summary). *Tob Control* **5**: 236-246.

Chapter 16

Cessation from Tobacco Use

Jennifer B. McClure, Ph.D., Susan J. Curry, Ph.D. and David W. Wetter, Ph.D.
Center for Health Studies, Group Health Cooperative of Puget Sound, Seattle, WA

INTRODUCTION

Tobacco use is the most preventable cause of death and illness in the United States [1]. It is responsible for one out of every five deaths, or more than 400,000 people per year [2]. There are essentially three ways to reduce the morbidity and mortality attributable to tobacco: prevent initiation of its use, promote cessation, and limit exposure to the dangerous toxins and carcinogens in tobacco. Since 1964 when the first Surgeon General's report linking smoking and disease was released, there has been increasing attention focused on each of these goals, particularly smoking cessation. Effective behavioral and pharmacological treatments for smoking have been developed. Tobacco cessation efforts have also broadened to include community and population-based interventions. As a result, smoking prevalence in the United States has declined from 41 percent in 1966 to 25 percent in 1995 [3, 4].

The following chapter reviews effective smoking cessation treatments and discusses several public health strategies that have been employed to promote smoking cessation at the federal, state, and local levels. Although effective interventions exist, the development and systematic implementation of more efficacious treatments and community-wide interventions are needed to further reduce tobacco use in the U.S.

G.A. Colditz et al. (eds.), Cancer Prevention: The Causes and Prevention of Cancer - Volume I, 193–204.
© 2000 *Kluwer Academic Publishers.*

1.   SMOKING CESSATION TREATMENT

Smoking cessation treatment is typically delivered by healthcare professionals (*e.g.,* physicians, nurses, psychologists, and pharmacists) or specially trained smoking cessation counselors. Although a variety of providers may offer this assistance, research does not show any single provider type is more effective than another. The important factors for treatment success are content and intensity [5]. The most efficacious interventions are those that involve behavioral counseling and pharmacotherapy, and there is some evidence that the combination of these components produces the highest long-term abstinence rates. Furthermore, there is a strong dose-response relation between treatment intensity and long-term abstinence. In general, treatments, which involve four to seven contacts of at least 20 minutes duration spread over several weeks, are ideal. However, even brief interventions ($\leq$3 minutes) can increase cessation rates and should be offered when more intensive interventions are not feasible [5].

1.1   Behavioral Intervention

Behavioral counseling can be delivered in a variety of formats, from intensive programs that meet regularly prior to and following the quit date for up to several months to brief quit advice combined with self-help materials. Behavioral interventions can be delivered individually or in a group format. They can be administered in person, over the phone, or by computer. The active ingredients of behavioral interventions are problem solving/skills training and supportive encouragement. Behavioral programs that include these components are more effective in helping people achieve long-term abstinence than those that do not [5]. Problem solving includes coping skills training, relapse prevention, and stress management. Smokers are taught how to anticipate smoking triggers, manage cravings and urges without smoking, and manage stress and other negative emotions without smoking. Programs should also provide supportive encouragement for any quit attempts – successful or not. Because smoking cessation typically involves multiple serious attempts to quit, providing this type of support can help motivate smokers to remain engaged in the cessation process.

1.2   Pharmacotherapy

Although behavioral interventions are effective, long-term abstinence rates increase when counseling is combined with pharmacotherapy. Presently there are two types of medication approved by the Food and Drug Administration (FDA) for smoking cessation: nicotine replacement products (nicotine replacement therapy [NRT]; *i.e.,* patch, gum, inhaler, and nasal spray) and bupropion (Zyban). Each is an effective smoking cessation aid and has been found to approximately double quit rates compared to placebo in well-controlled clinical trials [6].

1.2.1 Nicotine Replacement Therapy

The nicotine gum and nicotine patch were the first NRT products approved by the FDA and are the only pharmacotherapies that are available over-the-counter (OTC). The nicotine patch is available in a variety of dosing regimens and is typically worn 24 hours a day for six to eight weeks. The gum comes in two doses, 2 mg and 4 mg. Smokers are instructed to "chew" one to two pieces of gum every hour to alleviate withdrawal and to use the gum for up to three months. Of the two, the nicotine patch is recommended for routine clinical use because it requires less training, yields greater compliance, and is easier to use than the gum [5].

Two new forms of NRT were recently approved for prescription administration, the nicotine inhaler and the nicotine nasal spray. Unlike the patch and gum, the nasal spray and inhaler were designed to provide immediate relief from withdrawal symptoms and cravings. The nicotine inhaler consists of a small plastic rod containing a nicotine plug. When puffed, nicotine vapor is inhaled and absorbed bucally. The inhaler can be used 6 to 16 times a day for three to six months. The nicotine nasal spray resembles standard OTC nasal sprays. Smokers are advised to use one to two doses per hour for three to six months. The side-effect profile for both of these products is similar and includes nasal and throat irritation, rhinitis, sneezing, coughing, and watery eyes, but tolerance commonly occurs after the first week of use. Both the inhaler and nasal spray increase abstinence rates compared to placebo [7-12] (Table 16.1).

1.2.2 Bupropion

Bupropion (Zyban) is the only non-nicotine medication currently approved as a smoking cessation aid. Recommended dosage is 300 mg per day for seven to twelve weeks. Few bupropion trials have been published, but short- and long-term abstinence rates are significantly increased with this medication [13-14] (Table 16.1). Overall, bupropion appears to be at least as effective as the nicotine patch.

Table 16.1 Abstinence rates for the nicotine inhaler, nicotine nasal spray, and bupropion

	% Abstinent at 6 Months[a]		% Abstinent at 12 Months[a]	
	Active	Placebo	Active	Placebo
Nasal Spray				
Blondal *et al.*, 1997	29	18	25	17
Schneider *et al.*, 1994	25	10	18	8
Hjalmarson *et al.*, 1994	35	15	28	18
Inhaler				
Schneider *et al.*, 1996	17	9	13	8
Leischow *et al.*, 1996	21	6	11	5
Tonnesen *et al.*, 1993	17	8	15	5
Bupropion				
Jorenby *et al.*, 1999[b,c]	34.8	18.8	30.3	15.6
Hurt *et al.*, 1997[b,c]	26.9	15.7	23.1	12.4

[a]Continuous abstinence rates unless noted otherwise.
[b]300 mg daily dose
[c]Point prevalence abstinence.

1.2.3 Experimental Pharmacological Treatments

New ways to maximize the effectiveness of pharmacologic cessation aids are constantly under investigation. One area of promise is combination pharmacotherapies. Combined patch and nicotine nasal spray use results in greater abstinence than use of either alone [15]. Similar results have been reported for combined patch and bupropion use [13]. To date, however, there are no treatment guidelines pertaining to combination pharmacotherapy.

1.2.4 Pharmacotherapy and Counseling.

Though NRT and bupropion are effective cessation aids, it is important to note that pharmacotherapy alone is not a substitute for advising and assisting smokers to quit smoking. When used without adjuvant behavioral therapy, such as when obtained OTC, abstinence rates decline substantially [6]. Even when obtained by prescription, the effectiveness of these drugs may vary depending on the provision of concomitant behavioral treatment. Efficacy can also be limited by improper usage of these medications or premature discontinuation due to side-effects. Thus, it is important when prescribing pharmacotherapies or when instructing patients to purchase them OTC those smokers are fully informed of their potential side-effects, dosing regimens, and proper administration procedures.

1.3   Role of Healthcare Providers

Healthcare providers play a critical role in tobacco cessation, particularly physicians and their medical staff. As many as 70 percent of smokers see a primary care physician each year [16]. Thus, medical professionals have the opportunity to intervene with the majority of smokers. Intervention can include providing brief quit advice, self-help materials, pharmacotherapy, and/or appropriate treatment referrals. Because physicians have tremendous access to smokers, even minimal efforts such as brief quit advice can have an enormous public health impact when systematically implemented. Clinicians can also intervene with individuals who are not ready to make a quit attempt and help motivate them to do so. This is important since the majority of smokers are not ready to quit at any given time.

1.4   Smoking Cessation Clinical Practice Guidelines

To guide clinicians' treatment efforts, the Agency for Health Care Policy and Research (AHCPR) released the first evidence-based clinical practice guideline for smoking cessation in 1996 [5]. The guideline lays out a treatment model for physicians and other healthcare providers to assist patients in quitting smoking. Recommendations are based on a comprehensive review of the literature and meta-analyses of randomized, controlled trials. The basic treatment recommendations can be summarized as follows:
- Smokers should be systematically identified at every clinical contact.
- All smokers should be urged to quit smoking and offered assistance appropriate to their readiness to quit (*e.g.*, either motivational or cessation focused).
- Brief counseling (≤3 minutes) can increase abstinence and should be offered to every patient, although more intensive treatments consisting of multiple contacts lasting at least 20 minutes each, over several weeks are optimal.
- Treatment should include NRT (except under special circumstances), social support, and skills training/problem-solving.

At the time the AHCPR guideline was released, the only pharmacotherapies available were the nicotine patch and gum. Given the relative effectiveness and safety of the newer medications (nicotine inhaler, nicotine nasal spray, bupropion), these should also be used when treating smoking. It is anticipated that more specific recommendations regarding these drugs will be included in future clinical treatment guidelines.

In the AHCPR model, primary care professionals serve as the front-line for proactive treatment of tobacco use. That is, all tobacco users are identified and offered an intervention at every clinical contact. The level of the intervention is tailored to each patient's readiness to quit smoking. Those not interested in quitting receive feedback intended to increase their motivation for quitting. Those ready to quit are offered problem-focused assistance ranging from a treatment referral to planning a quit date and discussing strategies for quitting. The intensity of this assistance can vary depending on the clinician's time and expertise. This type of proactive, systematic intervention is critical to reducing the public health burden of smoking in this country, but the model's effectiveness is dependent on a number of factors. Practice-wide methods are needed for consistently identifying all smokers during their medical contacts (*e.g.,* use of chart stickers or adding tobacco use status to vital sign measures) and all medical staff should be trained in identifying and counseling smokers. Take-home materials such as self-help brochures and referral information for community smoking cessation programs need to be routinely available. And finally, insurance reimbursement should be provided for smoking-cessation treatment. There is evidence that full-coverage for smoking cessation treatments increases their reach into the population of smokers without significant declines in effectiveness. The net result is a potential two-fold increase in the impact of smoking cessation programs with full coverage [17].

2.   COMMUNITY AND POPULATION-BASED INTERVENTIONS

Over the last few decades the concept of tobacco cessation has expanded from individual-level treatments to include more broadly focused community and population-based interventions. These initiatives have been implemented by federal, state, and local governments, as well as by public and private agencies. Such large-scale interventions produce smaller absolute abstinence rates than effective individual treatments, but have greater reach and can significantly impact tobacco use among the general population. Community and population-based interventions promote cessation through a variety of means, such as providing self-help treatment materials to smokers, educating the public about the health risks of smoking, discouraging tobacco use *via* economic barriers, and constraining access and use of tobacco products. A comprehensive discussion of community and population-based interventions is beyond the scope of this chapter, but several examples are presented.

2.1   Self-Help Materials

Self-help interventions represent a bridge between clinical and public health treatment approaches. They are appealing to smokers who are often reluctant to seek treatment because they can be applied at the smoker's own pace and are low cost. Likewise, they appeal to providers because they contain intensive treatment information, can be disseminated to large segments of the population, and are cost-effective [18]. However, self-help materials are often criticized because, at best, one in five smokers will be abstinent one year after receiving a self-help program and only one in twenty will have sustained at least six months of continuous abstinence at that point [18]. Nevertheless, even a five percent abstinence rate can have a significant public health impact if the treatment materials are systematically disseminated on a community or population level. Thus, the challenge facing self-help programs is how to get the materials used by a large enough segment of the population to maximize the treatment impact (impact = participation [reach] x efficacy). Proactive dissemination to a targeted population, such as smokers in a health maintenance organization (HMO) is one way to enhance the reach of self-help programs. Centralized clinical information systems that routinely track smoking status could be used to provide motivational interventions and population-based self-help programs to smokers without requiring them to actively seek treatment.

2.2   Community-Based Interventions

Several large-scale community-wide interventions to reduce smoking have demonstrated mixed results. The Minnesota Heart Health project lasted for five years and targeted four communities. At the end of the intervention, no significant differences were found between the treatment and control communities in smoking [19]. The Community Intervention Trial for Smoking Cessation (COMMIT) used a multi-channel intervention targeting schools, worksites, physicians, and the general public in eleven matched-pair communities. Like the Minnesota Heart Health Project, no significant reduction in smoking was found among heavy smokers, but a modest reduction was seen among light-to-moderate smokers [20]. Another community intervention, the American Stop Smoking Intervention Study for Cancer Prevention (ASSIST) was recently completed. ASSIST was the first federally funded program to develop state-level infrastructures for tobacco control and was being conducted in seventeen states. Although the final results of this trial are not yet available, at mid-point review, smokers in the intervention states were consuming seven percent fewer cigarettes *per capita* than in the comparison states [21].

2.3   Taxation

Another strategy for reducing smoking at the community and population level is increased taxation.   Research clearly demonstrates that increasing tobacco taxes results in decreased tobacco usage, particularly among individuals who are sensitive to price increases such as younger age groups [22].   After federal excise taxes were doubled in 1983, cigarette purchases dropped nationwide by 12 percent [3].   Although most states levy some excise tax on cigarettes, three states have voted to significantly increase tobacco taxes and use the revenue to develop statewide tobacco intervention programs.   After implementation of these programs in Massachusetts and California, *per capita* cigarette consumption between 1992 and 1996 declined by 20 percent in Massachusetts and 16 percent in California, compared to six percent in the remaining U.S. states [23].   In 1996 Oregon passed an increased cigarette tax of $.68 per pack, ten percent of which is dedicated to the Tobacco Prevention and Education Program, a comprehensive community-based program modeled after those in California and Massachusetts. After institution of this tax, taxable *per capita* consumption of cigarettes declined 11.3 percent (from 1996 to 1998).   In comparison, nationwide *per capita* consumption between 1996 and 1997 declined by only one percent [24].   As a result of findings such as these, the National Cancer Policy Board has recognized increased tobacco taxation as the "single most direct and reliable method for reducing [tobacco] consumption" [22].

2.4   Tobacco Control Regulations

Tobacco control regulations have been implemented at the local, state and federal levels.   These regulatory restrictions limit the sales, advertisement, and public use of tobacco products.   Though they are primarily intended to discourage tobacco initiation among youths and limit nonsmokers' environmental exposure to passive smoke, they also promote a social norm of no-smoking and help motivate smokers to quit.

2.5   Public Stop Smoking Campaigns: The Great
         American Smoke Out

One of the most high-profile smoking cessation interventions is the Great American Smoke Out (GASO), sponsored by the American Cancer Society. For more than 20 years, the GASO has publicly encouraged smokers to quit smoking for one day each November. It is not clear how many people have quit smoking and maintained long-term abstinence as a result of the GASO, but it has been an effective catalyst for altering smoking behavior. In 1996, it was estimated that 26 percent of smokers either quit or cut-back their smoking in response to the GASO. NRT sales increased by 11 percent during the four-week promotional period and 30 percent during the week of the GASO [25].

3. AREAS FOR FUTURE WORK

Smoking prevalence in this country has declined significantly, but more needs to be done to address this issue. The majority of smokers, although interested in quitting "someday", are not ready to take action to quit and those who are ready are often reluctant to seek assistance. Thus, it is critical to develop better ways of motivating individuals to make a quit attempt and to make treatment more acceptable and accessible. This includes developing more, and more effective, population-based interventions that promote a non-smoking culture and promote cessation attempts. It is also essential that we increase the efficacy of individual treatments. Even with the best treatments as many as 70 to 80 percent of smokers will begin smoking again by one year, so further emphasis needs to be placed on preventing relapse.

CONCLUSION

Tobacco cessation is a national health priority. Research and public health initiatives over the past three decades have led to the development and implementation of a number of effective means of motivating smokers to quit and helping them to do so, but continued work is needed. In order to continue impacting the prevalence of smoking in the U.S., current treatments will need to be systematically implemented at the community and individual level. Furthermore, interventions will need to continue broadening their scope to emphasize motivational strategies, relapse prevention, and making effective treatments more accessible and acceptable to smokers.

SUMMARY POINTS

- Tobacco cessation is a public health priority.
- Healthcare providers should routinely advise and assist their patients to stop smoking.

- At present, the most effective smoking cessation treatments combine behavioral counseling and pharmacotherapy.
- Population- and community-based interventions can have a substantial public health impact on reducing tobacco use.
- Future research is needed emphasizing motivational interventions, relapse prevention, and how to make treatment more accessible and acceptable to smokers.

RECOMMENDATIONS

- Healthcare providers should identify and intervene with all smokers.
- Smokers should be offered behavioral and pharmacological treatments for cessation.
- Motivational interventions should be used to encourage behavior change among smokers not currently interested in quitting.
- Effective community level interventions should be systematically implemented on a nationwide basis.

SUGGESTED FURTHER READING

1. Fiore MC, Bailey WC, Cohen SJ, *et al.* (1996) *Smoking Cessation. Clinical Practice Guideline No. 18.* Rockville, MD (U.S.A): U.S. Department of Health and Human Services, Public Health Service, Agency for Health Care Policy and Research, AHCPR Pub. No. 96-0692.
2. U.S. Department of Health and Human Services (1990) *The Health Benefits of Smoking Cessation: A Report of the Surgeon General.* Atlanta, GA (U.S.A): U.S. Department of Health and Human Services, Public Health Service, Centers for Disease Control, Center for Chronic Disease Prevention and Health Promotion, Office of Smoking and Health, DHHS Pub. No. (CDC) 90-8416.
3. Hughes JR, Goldstein G, Hurt RD, Shiffman S (1999) Recent advances in the pharmacotherapy of smoking, *JAMA* **281:** 72-76.

REFERENCES

1. U.S. Department of Health and Human Services (1990) *The Health Benefits of Smoking Cessation: A Report of the Surgeon General.* Atlanta, GA (U.S.A): U.S. Department of Health and Human Services, Public Health Service, Centers for Disease Control, Center

for Chronic Disease Prevention and Health Promotion, Office of Smoking and Health, DHHS Pub. No. (CDC) 90-8416.

2. CDC (1993) Cigarette smoking-attributable mortality and years of potential life lost— United States, 1990. *MMWR Morb Mortal Wkly Rep* **42**: 645-649.

3. U.S. Department of Health and Human Services (1989) *Reducing the health Consequences of Smoking: 25 Years of Progress. A Report of the Surgeon General.* Rockville, MD (USA): U.S. Department of Health and Human Services, Public Health Service, Centers for Disease Control, Center for Chronic Disease Prevention and Health Promotion, Office of Smoking and Health, DHHS Pub. No. (CDC) 89-8411.

4. CDC (1997) Cigarette smoking among adults – United States, 1995. *MMWR Morb Mortal Wkly Rep* **46**: 1217-1220.

5. Fiore MC, Bailey WC, Cohen SJ, *et al.* (1996) *Smoking Cessation.* Clinical Practice Guideline No. 18. Rockville, MD (U.S.A): U.S. Department of Health and Human Services, Public Health Service, Agency for Health Care Policy and research, AHCPR Pub. No. 96-0692.

6. Hughes JR, Goldstein G, Hurt RD, *et al.* (1999) Recent advances in the pharmacotherapy of smoking, *JAMA* **281**: 72-76.

7. Blondal T, Franzon M, Westin A (1997) A double-blind randomized trial of nicotine nasal spray as an aid in smoking cessation. *Eur Respir J* **10**: 1585-1590.

8. Schneider NG, Olmstead R, Mody FV, *et al.* (1995) Efficacy of a nicotine nasal spray in smoking cessation: a placebo-controlled, double-blind trial. *Addiction* **90**: 1671-1682.

9. Hjalmarson A, Franzon M, Westin A, *et al.* (1994) Effect of nicotine nasal spray on smoking cessation. *Arch Intern Med* **154**: 2567-2572.

10. Schneider NG, Olmstead R, Nilsson F, *et al.* (1996) Efficacy of a nicotine inhaler in smoking cessation: a double-blind, placebo-controlled trial. *Addiction* **91**: 1293-1306.

11. Leischow SJ, Nilsson F, Franzon M, *et al.* (1996) Efficacy of the nicotine inhaler as an adjunct to smoking cessation. **20**: 364-371.

12. Tonnesen P, Norregaard J, Mikkelsen K, *et al.* (1993) A double-blind trial of a nicotine inhaler for smoking cessation. *JAMA* **269**: 1268-1271.

13. Jorenby DE, Leischow SJ, Nides MA, *et al.* (1999) A controlled trial of sustained-release bupropion, a nicotine patch, or both for smoking cessation. *N Engl J Med* **340**: 685-691.

14. Hurt RD, Sachs DPL, Glover ED, *et al.* (1997) A comparison of sustained-release bupropion and placebo for smoking cessation. *N Engl J Med* **337**: 1195-1202.

15. Blondal T, Gudmundsson LJ, Olafsdottir I, *et al.* (1999) Nicotine nasal spray with nicotine patch for smoking cessation: randomized trial with six year follow-up. *Br Med J* **318**: 285-288.

16. Ockene JK (1987) Smoking intervention: the expanding role of the physician. *Am J Public Health* **77**: 782-83.

17. Curry SJ, Grothaus LC, McAfee T, *et al.* (1998) Use and cost effectiveness of smoking-cessation services under four insurance plans in a health maintenance organization. *N Engl J Med* **339**: 673-679.

18. Curry, SJ (1993) Self-help interventions for smoking cessation. *J Consult Clin Psychol* **5**: 790-803.

19. Luepker RV, Murray DM, Jacobs DR, *et al.* (1994) Community education for cardiovascular disease prevention: risk factor changes in the Minnesota Heart Health Project. *Am J Public Health* **84**: 1383-1393.

20. The COMMIT Research Group (1995) Community Intervention Trial for Smoking Cessation (COMMIT): I. Cohort results from a four-year community intervention. *Am J Public Health* **85**: 183-92.

21. Manley, MW, Pierce, JP, Gilpin, EA, *et al.* (1997) Impact of the American Stop Smoking Intervention Study on cigarette consumption. *Tob Control* 6(Suppl 2): S12-16.
22. National Cancer Policy Board, Institute of Medicine and Commission on Life Sciences, National Research Council (1998) Raise Prices to Reduce Use. In: *Taking Action to Reduce Tobacco Use.* Washington, DC (USA): National Academy Press, pp. 4-6.
23. Centers for Disease Control (1996) Cigarette smoking before and after excise tax increase and an antismoking campaign – Massachusetts, 1990-1996. *MMWR Morb Mortal Wkly Rep* 45: 966-970.
24. Centers for Disease Control (1999) Decline in cigarette consumption following implementation of a comprehensive tobacco prevention and education program – Oregon, 1996-1998. *MMWR Morb Mortal Wkly Rep* 48: 140-143.
25. Centers for Disease Control (1997) Impact of promotion of the Great American Smokeout and availability of over-the-counter nicotine medications, 1996. *MMWR Morb Mortal Wkly Rep* 45: 961.

Chapter 17

Dietary Change Strategies

Karen Glanz, M.P.H., Ph.D.
Cancer Research Center of Hawaii, University of Hawaii, Honolulu, HI

INTRODUCTION

Nutrition plays an important role in the initiation, promotion and progression of cancer although the role of diet in cancer is complex and continues to be studied actively. Cancers are a diverse group of diseases, and their relationships with diet vary [1]. The most consistent findings for many cancers are protective effects of vegetables, and to a lesser extent fruits. High intakes of vegetables and fruits decrease the risks of lung, stomach, colon, esophagus and oral cavity cancers. Recent evidence also suggests protective effects for breast and prostate cancers. High fat intakes increase risk for prostate cancer, while high intakes of meat and/or saturated fat increase the risk of colon cancer. Obesity has been shown to be associated with breast and colorectal cancers; while it reflects a complex set of factors including nutrition, physical activity, and genetics, eating patterns appear to be major contributors. Alcohol, even in modest quantities, increases the risk of breast cancer, and high alcohol consumption increases risks of colon, liver, esophagus and oral cavity cancers. Much progress is being made in understanding the associations of diet with cancer, with a focus on identifying the components of fruits and vegetables that reduce risk.

Even as research into dietary causation of cancer continues, most professional and scientific organizations believe the evidence is sufficient to support official dietary guidance. Dietary guidelines for health promotion and cancer prevention recommend consumption of less animal fat; more fiber (20 to 30 g/day), fruits and vegetables ($\geq$5 servings/day); prevention of obesity; and avoidance of excess alcohol intake [1, 2]. This advice is quite similar to what is recommended for reducing the incidence of other serious chronic illnesses. In 1999, the leading voluntary and scientific organizations

205

G.A. Colditz et al. (eds.), Cancer Prevention: The Causes and Prevention of Cancer - Volume I, 205–217.
© 2000 *Kluwer Academic Publishers.*

in the United States agreed upon a set of Unified Dietary Guidelines. The guidelines suggest that healthy eating plans include: a variety of foods; five or more servings of fruits and vegetables each day; most foods from plant sources, six or more servings of bread, pasta, and cereal grains daily; limited high-fat foods, especially from animal sources; and minimal levels of simple sugars and sodium.

During the past decade, there has been positive movement in several dietary intake and risk factor markers, as well as in the context and environment of eating. Population trends in sentinel Healthy People 2000 diet indicators show decreases in percent of calories from fat (36 percent to 34 percent) and saturated fat (13 percent to 12 percent) [3]. Concern about dietary fat has increased dramatically, more processed foods bear nutrition labels, a greater proportion of restaurants offer low-fat and low-calorie selections, and more worksites offer nutrition education and weight management programs. Further, the food and restaurant industry has developed products that better meet national recommendations for healthful eating. On the other hand, considerable challenges remain. The prevalence of overweight has increased among teens (15 percent to 21 percent) and adults (26 percent to 34 percent) [3]. Intake of fruits, vegetables, grains, and dietary fiber remain well below recommendations.

Eating habits are influenced by many biological, social, psychological, and cultural factors, and achieving successful dietary change is a great challenge. Much research on strategies to promote eating patterns that may prevent or control some cancers has been conducted over the past two decades. This research has addressed efforts to control cancer and also to prevent and control other chronic diseases and risk factors, especially cardiovascular disease, diabetes, and obesity [4, 5].

The current state of knowledge about strategies for dietary change reflects the varying conditions under which nutrition intervention research has been conducted, from clinical trials to population-wide prevention campaigns. In general, clinical trials have shown large effects in small groups of select, motivated participants. Population-wide strategies have reached many people and achieved smaller effects for large groups [6]. Often, similar strategies have been delivered through different channels, for example communities, worksites, schools, and healthcare settings; and by various types of providers. This chapter provides an up-to-date summary of what is known about selected strategies and settings and should not be considered a comprehensive review of all research on dietary change.

1.   INDIVIDUAL AND COMMUNITY STRATEGIES

Nutrition interventions for the prevention and control of cancer and other chronic diseases are intended to encourage long-term adoption of healthful eating patterns in free-living populations. The major settings and channels for nutrition intervention to reduce chronic disease risk are: healthcare settings, schools, worksites, community social and religious organizations, and the consumer marketplace. Various settings and channels hold opportunities to reach different audiences.

Early research on promoting healthful dietary change focused mainly on information and skill enhancement through classes, and intensive small-group and individual nutrition counseling. These strategies were often found effective at improving knowledge and promoting short-term behavior changes, but they reached only the most motivated individuals. However, behavioral research on dietary change has become more rigorous in the past decade. Clear evidence exists from controlled clinical trials that intensive educational and behavioral interventions are effective in promoting sustained reductions in dietary fat intake among motivated subjects [7]. Interventions that include counseling, group education, and mediated strategies are effective in high-risk persons [8] (Table 17.1).

2.   STRATEGIES IN HEALTHCARE SETTINGS

Although the evidence is mixed, promising findings exist for nutritional risk reduction in medical settings. Despite consensus among health professionals that diet can promote health and reduce risks of chronic disease, actual counseling practices are much less common than recommended by authoritative groups. Some studies of group education and intensive nutrition counseling have found positive dietary changes achieved in healthcare settings. Also, primary care settings have been the venue for self-help programs [9] and personally tailored messages [10], described below.

Some large clinical trials of dietary change have been conducted in healthcare settings. These clinical trials have used behavioral science intervention models and systematically studied changes in eating patterns, maintenance of change, and correlates of change. The largest trials to date have been the Multiple Risk Factor Intervention Trial (MRFIT) (n=12,866 men aged 35 to 57) [11] and the Women's Health Trial (WHT) Vanguard Study and its extension (n=2064 women aged 45 to 69) [7]. Both MRFIT and WHT used multiple educational strategies including group education, individual behavioral counseling, periodic monitoring, feedback, and reinforcement. In MRFIT, family involvement (usually of wives) was also included. Both trials found significant changes in the intervention groups compared to control participants. In MRFIT, men in the experimental group achieved average cholesterol reductions of 7.5 percent and reductions in saturated fat intake from 13.9 percent to ten percent of calories [11]. The WHT Vanguard Study intervention group reported reductions in fat intake from 39.1 percent to 20.9 percent of calories, and concurrent reductions in weight and cholesterol [7]. In both studies, the greatest changes occurred in the first year and changes were maintained for several years.

These clinical trials of dietary change strategies show clearly that significant dietary change is possible in selected, highly motivated participants. Each of the studies used intensive, multi-component educational and behavioral strategies. The interventions were much more intensive and expensive than typical outpatient nutrition interventions. To better understand what strategies might be used to prevent cancer or improve health through diet in free-living populations, we need to look beyond clinical trials to clinical interventions studies and community-based interventions.

3. SELF-HELP, MINIMAL-CONTACT, AND TAILORED INTERVENTIONS

Accumulating data support the efficacy of *self-help and minimal-contact interventions*, including print guides, tailored messages, and supportive telephone counseling [9, 10, 12]. In a randomized trial, tailored materials providing feedback about fat reduction, fruit and vegetable intake, and intentions, attitudes, and self-efficacy expectations led to improved eating behaviors [12]. These strategies, as well as computerized and interactive interventions, hold great promise for expanding the reach of interventions aimed at individuals. These interventions may produce small effects relative to those achieved with more intensive behavioral interventions, but the net public health effects may be equal to or greater than those with small, highly selected audiences.

4. WORKSITE NUTRITION INTERVENTIONS

Worksite interventions using public health approaches attempt to change the health milieu at the worksite using several intervention techniques in concert. They use strategies such as employee involvement in planning, environmental changes, competitions, incentives, and self-help programs. Research suggests that the most effective worksite health promotion programs are those that use multiple strategies and aim to achieve multiple goals of awareness, information transmission, skill development, and supportive environments and policies [8]. The majority of published evaluations of worksite nutrition programs report on four types of interventions: group education, group education with individual counseling, cafeteria-based programs, and group education combined with cafeteria-based programs [8]. While most published evaluations report some positive outcomes, it is not always possible to clearly attribute those results to the interventions due to non-randomized designs or overly liberal analysis methods.

During the mid-1990s, there have been several new trials of worksite nutrition programs to reduce the risks of cardiovascular disease and cancer, and to lower employees' elevated cholesterol levels. The Working Well Trial (WWT) used multiple strategies including awareness activities, education, cafeteria changes, and participatory strategies to improve diet and reduce tobacco use. One hundred fourteen worksites were randomized to treatment or control conditions. After two years of intervention, there was a significant net decrease in energy from fat (-0.9 percent en fat), increase in fiber density (+0.13 g/1,000 kcal), increase in fruit and vegetable intake (+0.18 svgs/day) [13], and improvements in the healthy eating environment [14]. It is difficult to determine the specific effective and/or ineffective components of the WWT intervention because the evaluation was designed to compare a multi-method program with a control condition. The changes were modest but significant because of the large sample (114 worksites, more than 30,000 workers), and the practical significance of the dietary changes found in the WWT, while considered encouraging, remains a matter of debate.

The Next Step Trial tested interventions encouraging prevention and early detection practices in automotive-industry employees at increased colorectal risk. The nutrition intervention, provided at half of the 28 worksites who were randomly assigned to the experimental arm, included nutrition classes, self-help materials, and computer-generated personalized feedback. At one year, there were modest but significant intervention effects for fat (-0.9 percent), fiber (+-.5 g/1000 kcal), and fruits/vegetables (+0.2 servings/day), all p <.007. At two years, intervention effects were smaller and remained significant for fiber only. Intervention effects were larger in younger, active employees, and those who attended classes [15].

The Treatwell 5-A-Day study compared a minimal intervention control group, a worksite intervention, and a worksite-plus-family intervention for increasing fruit and vegetable intake, in 22 community health center worksites. The intervention used a community-organizing strategy and was structured to target multiple levels of influence. The control group showed no change, the worksite intervention group increased their fruit and vegetable intake by seven percent, and the worksite-plus-family group increased total fruit and vegetable intake by 19 percent; the group with the largest increases improved by about one-half serving per day [16].

The Seattle 5 A Day Worksite Program evaluated an intervention based on the stage of change model, and using 28 worksites randomly assigned to intervention or control arms. The intervention included an Employee Advisory Board, a study interventionist, materials targeting transition points between stages of change, and addressed both individual and worksite environments. There was a significant net intervention effect of 0.3 daily servings, favoring the intervention worksites [17].

It is difficult to draw definitive conclusions about the strategies that work best in promoting dietary change as part of worksite nutrition programs. We cautiously conclude that group education programs produced some dietary changes. Cafeteria programs appear to hold promise, as do computer-tailored messages and worksite interventions enhanced with family outreach. Comprehensive programs addressing both individual and environmental changes deserve particular further attention, and it would be useful for future multiple-strategy studies to use evaluation designs that would help determine the impact of various contributing strategies. More recent publications point to the promising strategies of family outreach, stage-based interventions, group programs for large groups of high-risk workers.

5.   SCHOOL-BASED NUTRITION EDUCATION

School-based instructional and food service programs, aiming at fat and sodium reduction and increasing complex carbohydrate intake, generally show positive but inconsistent results [18]. Programs focusing on younger children and involving parents have been most successful. Dietary behavior change can be enhanced by modifying institutional food service offerings, as demonstrated in the ongoing CATCH (Child and Adolescent Trial for Cardiovascular Health) trial and other studies [19]. An experiment using substantial price reductions in high school cafeterias found significant increases in fruit and vegetable purchase during the low-price periods, though most of the changes did not persist when regular pricing policies were reinstated [20].

Recently, results have been published from school-based interventions designed especially to increase fruit and vegetable consumption. The Gimme 5 high school program in Louisiana [21] and the 5-A-Day Power Plus elementary school program in Minnesota [22] were multi-component intervention trials affiliated with the 5 A Day for Better Health program. They both included behavioral curricula in classrooms, school food service changes, and parental involvement; and Gimme 5 also used an extensive media marketing campaign. Both studies found that the interventions increased fruit and vegetable intake in the children in the treatment schools compared to control schools. These new studies are encouraging, though it is not possible to ascertain which strategies contributed the most to the dietary improvements because of their control *vs.* multi-component program designs.

6.   INTERVENTIONS FOR DISADVANTAGED GROUPS

Nutrition education for maternal and child health has long focused on less educated, low income, and ethnically diverse populations, often through food assistance programs. In the past decade there has been increasing emphasis on developing and evaluating adult-oriented nutrition improvement programs for disadvantaged groups, principally because they may have poorer nutritional health status and limited access to or participation in programs offered through worksites, schools, healthcare settings. The Stanford Nutrition Action Program (SNAP) tested a classroom-based intervention to lower fat intake in an ethnically diverse population with low literacy skills who were enrolled in vocational training and GED classes in California. The six classes emphasized interactive learning and skill building, and used few written materials and food tasting demonstrations. Compared to a control group receiving a general nutrition curriculum, the SNAP class groups showed improvements in knowledge, attitudes, and fat density, although they did not differ in BMI or cholesterol levels [23].

The Maryland WIC 5-A-Day Promotion Program was a multifaceted intervention program for low-income women attending WIC (Women, Infants, Children nutrition program) sites. This program used peer educator nutrition sessions, print materials, and direct mail. Changes in fruit and vegetable consumption were significantly greater in treatment group participants, and were closely associated with the number of sessions attended [24]. The Black Churches United for Better Health Project tested a multi-component church-based intervention in rural North Carolina. The intervention included tailored bulletins, print materials, gardening, education sessions, cookbook and recipe tasting, lay health advisors, community coalitions, pastor support, grocer involvement, and church-initiated activities. After two years, the intervention group consumed 0.85 servings of fruits and vegetables more than the delayed intervention (control) group [25].

These new studies are encouraging, and provide clear evidence that well-designed and well-implemented, culturally sensitive interventions for low literacy and lower socioeconomic populations can be effective. The SNAP program used a fairly well circumscribed intervention package and thus can inform future intervention planning. The 5-A-Day studies are less easily interpreted because of their research designs testing delayed interventions *vs.* broad multi-component program designs.

Table 17.1 Examples of promising interventions for dietary change

Individual, Community and, Healthcare Interventions	•	Counseling, and intervention for individuals at increased cancer risk
	•	Behavioral interventions (group instruction and individual counseling) to reduce dietary fat intake and increase fruit and vegetable intake
	•	Minimal contact and self-help interventions to promote healthy eating
	•	Worksite programs that include family outreach
	•	School-based programs including classroom instruction and food service changes
Environmental, Regulatory, and Policy Strategies	•	Point-of-choice nutrition information programs (*e.g.*, grocery stores, restaurants)
	•	Federal nutrition information policy and strategies (*e.g.*, ingredient and nutrient labeling requirements)
	•	Increased access to health foods (*e.g.*, in cafeterias, growing more fresh fruits and vegetables)
	•	Nutrition services in health care (*e.g.*, reimbursement for nutrition counseling, more emphasis in medical education)
	•	Economic strategies (*e.g.*, food pricing policies, monetary incentives/disincentives for healthy eating through taxation)

7.   REGULATION, ENVIRONMENTAL, AND POLICY STRATEGIES

The environmental and organizational context plays an important role in shaping and maintaining individual change. Modification of cafeterias, dining facilities and vending services, along with other supportive policies and incentives are increasingly the focus of programs to encourage healthy eating patterns [26]. Nutrition policy and environmental interventions include provision of dietary guidance, and nutrition information and regulatory strategies (labeling, regulation of health claims, point-of-purchase information), increased access to healthy foods, nutrition services in schools, worksites, and health care settings, and economic strategies (*e.g.*, food pricing strategies, catering policies, reimbursement for nutrition counseling). One of the key features of these interventions is that they can reach all persons in a target group, and not just those who are at high-risk or more highly motivated. These strategies were included in several of the interventions described above, in schools, worksites, and churches (Table 17.1). However, virtually no data exist about the incremental effects of these interventions when combined with behaviorally-oriented nutrition education strategies and the use of media.

Food access strategies can increase the availability of nutritious foods in cafeterias and vending machines, use recipe modifications to improve the composition of foods that are already available, or establish policy guidelines for foods served at company functions (*i.e.,* catering policies). Point-of-choice programs provide nutrition information to individuals at the point of food selection or purchase, thereby increasing awareness and prompting people to select healthier foods [26]. Economic strategies can reduce the prices of healthier choices, or use other incentives. Incentive programs can be used to bolster participation on an organized worksite nutrition program or to draw attention to point-of-choice programs, awareness events, games, and competitions.

Few evaluations have reported the results of programs trying to modify the eating environment on the environment *per se,* and/or on social norms. Recent data from the Working Well Trial (WWT) intervention trial are encouraging. In 111 WWT workplaces, it was found that, at the time of follow-up surveys, the intervention sites showed improved access to healthy food, more nutrition information at work, and more favorable social norms regarding dietary choices [14].

CONCLUSION

Although the exact role of dietary factors and nutritional risk in cancer are still being studied, the evidence is sufficient to warrant concerted efforts to promote healthful dietary behavior. The potential public health benefit from improved eating patterns, coupled with the low risk of adopting the present guidelines for healthy eating, provides a strong foundation for efforts to understand and encourage good nutrition in the general population, inpatients, and in persons at high risk for cancer.

Clear evidence exists for the effectiveness of intensive educational and behavioral interventions in teaching and persuading motivated individuals and small groups to change their diets. Clearly, much experience has been gained in the 1980s and 1990s in conducting and evaluating the nutrition intervention strategies cited in this chapter. However, no single type of intervention has proven consistently successful, and there are many reports of ineffective or minimally effective interventions, as well. The most intensive strategies (*e.g.,* those used in clinical trials) have produced the greatest effects of dietary behavior and physiological risk factors. The cost per person reached is also greatest for the most intensive strategies. The largest effects of interventions have been in high-risk and highly motivated groups.

Nutrition interventions must be sensitive to audience and contextual factors. Food selection decisions are made for many reasons other than just nutrition: taste, cost, convenience, and cultural factors all play significant roles. The design and implementation of dietary change strategies must take these issues into consideration. The health promotion motto "know your audience" has a true and valuable meaning.

Further, change is incremental. Many people have practiced a lifetime of less than optimal nutrition behaviors. It is unreasonable to expect that significant and lasting changes will occur during the course of a program that lasts only a few months. Programs need to pull participants along the continuum of change, being sure to be just in front of those most ready to change with attractive, innovative offerings.

In population-focused programs, it appears to be of limited value to adopt a program solely oriented toward modifying individual choice (*e.g.,* teaching and persuading individuals to choose low-fat dairy products). A more productive strategy would also include environmental change efforts, *e.g.,* expanding the availability of more nutritious food choices. When this is done in conjunction with individual skill training, long-lasting and meaningful changes can be achieved.

Research methodology for research on dietary change has improved considerably in the past decade. As research methods have become more sophisticated, there is a need to continue to grapple with issues of design, measurement, and analysis. Even though study designs have improved markedly in the past few years, it is still usually difficult to determine which *strategies* within a program account for observed effects. Also, the reported effects are generally modest even where they are significant, and no single study can be taken as conclusive regarding a particular type of strategy. Recent diet change research has contributed to an understanding of determinants of behavior and change processes and needs to be paired with intervention research in future studies. A related focus of study should aim toward specifying the minimum necessary level of intervention to achieve a meaningful impact on dietary behavior. A rigorous evidence-based review of dietary change strategies to prevent cancer and other chronic diseases is now under way with support from the Agency for Health Care Policy Research and the National Cancer Institute, and the results will be available by the middle of the year 2000.

There is a need for further research on diffusion of effective intervention models, as few studies have addressed how best to disseminate tested interventions [27]. Dissemination of proven interventions has been uncoordinated, and this is another fertile area for future activity [28].

Finally, program designers should strive to be creative. Nutrition interventions should be as entertaining and engaging as the other activities they are competing with. People will want to participate if they can have fun with the nutrition programs. Emerging communication technologies are opening up new channels for engaging people's interest in better nutrition. E-mail support and motivation systems, "internet buddies," and interactive web-based approaches can be used creatively to promote healthful eating. The communication of nutrition information, now matter how important it is to good health, is secondary to attracting and retaining the interest and enthusiasm of the audience.

SUMMARY POINTS

- There is clear evidence that intensive educational and behavioral interventions are effective for teaching and persuading motivated persons and small groups to change their diets. However, no single type of intervention has proven consistently successful, and there are many reports of ineffective or minimally effective interventions, as well.
- The most intensive strategies (*e.g.,* those in clinical trials) have produced the greatest effects on dietary behavior and physiological risk factors. The cost per person reached is also the greatest for the most intensive strategies.
- Recently published research demonstrates that well-designed and implemented, culturally sensitive multi-component interventions for low literacy and lower socioeconomic populations can be effective.
- Policy interventions and changes in the food and nutrition environment have great potential to enhance the effects of individually focused interventions.

RECOMMENDATIONS

- Dietary change research should aim toward specifying the minimum necessary level of intervention to achieve to achieve a meaningful impact on dietary behavior.
- There is a need for continued advances in the areas of theory application, design, measurement, and analysis in dietary change research.
- Innovative communication technologies should be adapted and tested for their impact on cancer-preventive dietary change.

- Current and emerging knowledge, tools, and change technologies should be disseminated to professionals and the public.

SUGGESTED FURTHER READING

1. Glanz K (1997) Behavioral research contributions and needs in cancer prevention and control: dietary change. *Prev Med* **26**: S43-S55.
2. Sorensen G, Emmons K, Hunt MK, *et al.* (1998) Implications of the results of community intervention trials. *Annu Rev Public Health* **19**: 379-416.
3. Brunner E, White I, Thorogood M, *et al.* (1997) Can dietary interventions change diet and cardiovascular risk factors? A meta-analysis of randomized controlled trials. *Am J Public Health* **87**: 1415-1422.
4. Glanz K (1994) Reducing breast cancer risk through changes in diet and alcohol intake: from clinic to community. *Ann Behav Med* **16**: 334-346.
5. Glanz K, Sorensen G, Farmer A (1996) The impact of worksite nutrition and cholesterol intervention programs. *Am J Health Promot* **10**: 453-470.

REFERENCES

1. World Cancer Research Fund and American Institute for Cancer Research (1997) *Food, Nutrition and the Prevention of Cancer: A Global Perspective.* Washington, D.C.: World Cancer Research Fund/American Institute for Cancer Research.
2. Butrum R, Clifford CK, Lanza E (1988) NCI dietary guidelines: rationale. *Am J Clin Nutr* **48**: 888-895.
3. McGinnis JM, Lee PR (1995) Healthy people 2000 at mid decade. *JAMA* **273**: 1123-1129.
4. Thomas P, ed. (1991) *Improving America's Diet and Health: From Recommendations to Action.* Washington, D.C.: National Academy Press.
5. Glanz K (1997) Behavioral research contributions and needs in cancer prevention and control: dietary change. *Prev Med* **26**: S43-S55.
6. Glanz K (1994) Reducing breast cancer risk through changes in diet and alcohol intake: From clinic to community. *Ann Behav Med* **16**: 334-346.
7. Henderson MM, Kushi LH, Thompson DJ, *et al.* (1990) Feasibility of a randomized trial of a low-fat diet for the prevention of breast cancer: Dietary compliance in the Women's Health Trial Vanguard Study. *Prev Med* **19**: 115-133.
8. Glanz K, Sorensen G, Farmer A (1996) The impact of worksite nutrition and cholesterol intervention programs. *Am J Health Promot* **10**: 453-470.
9. Beresford SA, Curry SJ, Kristal AR, *et al.* (1997) A dietary intervention in primary care practice: The eating patterns study. *Am J Public Health* **87**: 610-616.
10. Campbell MK, DeVellis BM, Strecher VJ, *et al.* (1994) Improving dietary behavior: the effectiveness of tailored messages in primary care settings. *Am J Public Health.* **84**: 783-787.

11. Gorder DD, Dolecek TA, Coleman GG, *et al.* (1986) Dietary intake in the Multiple Risk Factor Intervention Trial (MRFIT): nutrient and food group changes over six years. *J Am Diet Assoc* **86:** 744-751.

12. Brug J, Glanz K, van Assema P, *et al.* (1998) The impact of computer-tailored feedback and iterative feedback on fat, fruit, and vegetable intake. *Health Educ Behav* **25:** 517-531.

13. Sorensen G, Thompson B, Glanz K, Feng A, *et al.* (1996) Work site-based cancer prevention: primary results from the Working Well Trials. *Am J Public Health* **86:** 939-47.

14. Biener L, Glanz K, McLerran D, *et al.* (1999) Impact of the Working Well Trial on the worksite smoking and nutrition environment. *Health Educ Behav* **16:** 478-494.

15. Tilley B, Glanz K, Kristal A, *et al.* (1999) Nutrition intervention for high-risk auto workers: results of the Next Step Trial. *Prev Med* **28:** 284-292.

16. Sorensen G, Stoddard A, Peterson K, *et al.* (1999) Lederman R. Increasing fruit and vegetable consumption through worksites and families in the Treatwell 5-A-Day study. *Am J Public Health* **89:** 54-60.

17. Beresford SA, Thompson B, Feng Z, *et al.* (1999) Seattle 5 A Day worksite program to increase fruit and vegetable consumption. Personal Communication/Manuscript, June.

18. Contento IR, Manning AD, Shannon B (1992) Research perspective on school-based nutrition education. *J Nutr Educ* **24:** 247-260.

19. Luepker RV, Perry CL, McKinlay SM, *et al.* (1996) Outcomes of a field trial to improve children's dietary patterns and physical activity: the Child and Adolescent Trial for Cardiovascular Health (CATCH). *JAMA* **275:** 768-776.

20. French S, Story M, Jeffery R, *et al.* (1997) Pricing strategy to promote fruit and vegetable purchase in high school cafeterias. *J Am Diet Assoc* **97:** 1008-1010.

21. Nicklas T, Johnson CC, Myers L, *et al.* (1998) Outcomes of a high school program to increase fruit and vegetable consumption: *Gimme 5* – A fresh nutrition concept for students. *J Sch Health* **68:** 248-253.

22. Perry CL, Bishop D, Taylor G, *et al.* (1998) Changing fruit and vegetable consumption among children: The 5-A-Day Power Plus Program in St. Paul, Minnesota. *Am J Public Health* **88:** 603-609.

23. Howard-Pitney B, Winkleby MA, Albright CL, *et al.* (1997) The Stanford Nutrition Action Program: a dietary fat intervention for low-literacy adults. *Am J Public Health* **87:** 1971-1976.

24. Havas S, Anliker J, Damron D, *et al.* (1998) Final results of the Maryland WIC 5-A-Day promotion program. *Am J Public Health* **88:** 1161-1167.

25. Campbell MK, Demark-Wahnefried W, Symons M, *et al.* (1999) Fruit and vegetable consumption and prevention of cancer: The Black Churches United for Better Health Project. *Am J Public Health* **89:** 1390-6

26. Glanz K, Lankenau B, Foerster S, *et al.* (1995) Environmental and policy approaches to cardiovascular disease prevention through nutrition: opportunities for state and local action. *Health Educ Q* **22:** 512-527.

27. Sorensen G, Emmons K, Hunt MK, *et al.* (1998) Implications of the results of community intervention trials. *Annu Rev Public Health* **19:** 379-416.

28. Brunner E, White I, Thorogood M, *et al.* (1997) Can dietary interventions change diet and cardiovascular risk factors? A meta-analysis of randomized controlled trials. *Am J Public Health* **87:** 1415-1422.

Chapter 18

Physical Activity and Cancer Prevention

Beverly Rockhill, Ph.D. and Graham A. Colditz, M.D., Dr.P.H.
Channing Laboratory, Department of Medicine, Brigham and Women's Hospital and Harvard Medical School, Boston, MA

INTRODUCTION

Physical activity has many health benefits. It reduces risk of premature mortality in general, as well as risk of cardiovascular diseases, hypertension, diabetes mellitus, osteoporosis, and colon cancer in particular [1]. It also improves mental health, and the health of muscles and bones [1]. Finally, physical activity is an important complement to dietary management for avoiding weight gain or losing weight.

The diseases linked to sedentariness are major causes of morbidity and mortality in industrialized societies, and thus the impact of sedentariness on public health is enormous. Together with detrimental dietary patterns, inactivity is ranked as the second leading contributing factor to premature mortality in the United States, after tobacco use [2]. Sedentary lifestyle has been linked to 23 percent of deaths from major chronic diseases [3]. This is a large percentage, yet it still does not address the burden of morbidity, loss of functional capacity and disability, suffering, and health care costs due to sedentariness [1].

In 1996, the first Surgeon General's report on physical activity and health was published [1]. This report grew out of an emerging consensus that physical activity need not be vigorous in intensity to have a beneficial effect on health. Because more than 60 percent of American adults are not regularly physically active (25 percent are not active at all), and because physical activity levels have declined dramatically even among children and adolescents (over one-third of children aged 10 to 17 years do not get enough physical activity to enhance their cardiorespiratory fitness) [1], the

G.A. Colditz et al. (eds.), Cancer Prevention: The Causes and Prevention of Cancer - Volume I, 219–233.
© 2000 *Kluwer Academic Publishers.*

message that significant health benefits are achievable with moderate amounts of physical activity is especially important.

In order to substantially reduce the public health burden of disease due to sedentariness, the population distribution of physical activity levels must be shifted upward. Because the large majority of morbidity and mortality due to low physical activity arises from the mass of the population with activity levels close to "average," a high-risk strategy that focuses only on the most inactive tail of the distribution, while improving the health of those in the inactive tail, will not have a large public health impact. In order to favorably shift the population distribution of physical activity, strategies that seek to influence the underlying social determinants of this distribution, rather than those that merely seek to persuade inactive individuals to become more active, are necessary.

The major barrier to population-wide shifts in physical activity is the age in which we live [1]. In the past, most activities of daily living involved significant expenditures of energy. In contrast, the overarching goal of modern technology has been to reduce this expenditure, seemingly to zero, through production of devices and services explicitly designed to obviate physical labor [1]. Today, many Americans engage in little or no physical activity in the course of their work, often spending eight hours or more per day sitting at a desk or standing at a counter. At the end of their workday, most people spend additional hours sitting and viewing television, playing video games, or using a computer terminal. Such devices have contributed substantially to the sedentariness of people's lives.

1. INDIVIDUAL-LEVEL INTERVENTIONS

The modifiable determinants of physical activity include individual, interpersonal, and environmental factors [1]. To date, physical inactivity has proved difficult to modify on a large scale by using individually-focused approaches to behavior change. Where effects have been demonstrated, they have often been small and relatively short-lived.

1.1 Children

Behavioral research on physical activity promotion in children is more limited than in adults. The most extensive research in children has been conducted in schools, primarily at the elementary grade level. The Know Your Body (KYB) program [4], which has been the focus of three school-based studies, included health screening, behaviorally-oriented health education curricula, and special interventions for students with one or more cardiovascular disease risk factors (*e.g.,* obesity, lack of physical exercise, cigarette smoking). In only one study [5], a randomized trial among African-American 4th through 6th graders, physical activity was reliably assessed. The intervention was not effective in increasing levels of physical activity; in both the intervention and control schools, physical activity levels of the students declined, by equivalent amounts, over the four-year follow-up period. The Stanford Adolescent Heart Health Program [6] was a classroom-based randomized cardiovascular disease risk reduction trial for 10th graders from four high schools. After receiving a 20-week risk reduction curriculum, which included information on physical activity, students from the intervention schools had significantly higher gains in knowledge about physical activity than students in the control schools, and among students not exercising regularly at baseline, those in the intervention schools had greater increases in activity than did those in the control schools. Nothing is known about the long-term effectiveness of this intervention. The Child and Adolescent Trial for Cardiovascular Health (CATCH) [7] was a multicenter-randomized trial to test the effectiveness of a cardiovascular health promotion program in 96 schools. A major component of CATCH was a physical education program, beginning in the third grade, for elementary school students. For two and a half years, intervention schools received a standardized physical activity intervention, including new curriculum, staff development, and consultations. In these intervention schools, participation in moderate/vigorous activity during physical education classes increased more than in the control schools, although no such treatment effect was observed in a family intervention component.

The summary of evidence on school-based interventions shows that such approaches generally have had positive short-term effects on increasing physical activity among elementary school students [1]. Little is known, however, about the long-term effects of such early interventions. Further, most physical activity engaged in by youth occurs outside of the school setting, so knowledge of the effects of school interventions on outside activity is critical. Little is also known about how best to increase physical activity among older students, or in settings other than school physical education classes. Finally, there is little research on how to prevent the rapid decline in physical activity that usually occurs in late childhood and adolescence, particularly among girls [1].

1.2   Adults

Interventions designed to increase physical activity among adults have been based in the health care setting, the workplace, and in the general community. Health care settings offer the opportunity to individually counsel persons about physical activity and other healthful behaviors. Only a few studies attempting to improve the physical activity counseling skills of primary care physicians have been reported in the literature; results suggest small but positive effects, with seven to ten percent of sedentary persons beginning a physical activity regimen on the advice of their provider [1]. Providers are often pressed for time during their brief appointments with patients, and many may not believe that physical activity is an important priority for discussion. Many may also lack effective counseling skills. Even if the barriers to effective provider counseling could be overcome, the strategy is limited in its potential population benefit by its restriction to individuals who regularly visit a health care provider.

Physical activity programs conducted at the worksite have the potential to reach a large percentage of the United States population [1, 8]. The proportion of worksites offering physical activity and fitness programs has grown in recent years, from 22 percent in 1985 to 42 percent in the early 1990s. In each worksite size category, the percentage with exercise programs in 1992 had already exceeded the year 2000 national objective for worksite health promotion listed in the Healthy People 2000 goals [9]. The limited research conducted on worksite physical activity programs shows that widespread employee involvement, coupled with managerial support, is critical to the success of worksite physical activity programs [1]. Approaches to increasing physical activity in the worksite can be both active (*e.g.*, offering on-site exercise classes and encouraging individuals to attend) and passive. Passive approaches are those that make it easier for an individual to choose to be more physically active. They include measures such as flexible-time policies allowing individuals who commute to work by bicycle or by foot to arrive and leave during non rush-hour times; providing secure bicycle racks and shower facilities for employees; and making workplace stairways safe, well-lit, and as easily accessible as elevators.

While it is very unlikely that the trends in workplace mechanization and job sedentariness will be reversed, worksites are an important venue in which to seek to increase physical activity levels, since many persons spend a large proportion of their waking time at their workplace. However, research on the long-term effectiveness of such programs is limited. Further, virtually all studies have been conducted in larger worksites with on-site physical activity facilities; it is not known what methods are best in smaller worksites where physical activity facilities are often not available, or in worksites where many employees are traveling for much of the working day (*e.g.*, repair services, transportation services).

Community-wide programs to prevent chronic disease have evolved from the concept that population-based, rather than individual-level, strategies are needed to achieve meaningful reductions in disease burden. Despite this theoretical foundation, however, such programs have tended to rely predominantly on individually-focused health education and on persuading individuals within communities to improve their behaviors, rather than on changing structural/environmental factors and relevant policies (see below) to set new social norms. Perhaps this should not be surprising; changing policies and social norms is often a very slow process, and community intervention trials have, by necessity dictated by funding limits, been relatively short-lived.

Three trials of community-based cardiovascular disease prevention have been conducted in the United States. These three trials (the Minnesota Heart Health Project [10], the Pawtucket Heart Health Program [11], and the Stanford Five-City Project [12]) used mass media, health professionals, and local organizations and institutions (such as schools and workplaces) to educate adults and children in the intervention communities about the benefits of healthy diet, physical education, management of hypertension, and weight control. The Minnesota investigators reported small but significant effects for physical activity in the first three years in a cross-sectional random-sample comparison of individuals in intervention and control communities; in a cohort of individuals followed over time in the two types of communities, little effect of intervention was found. In the Pawtucket program, individuals enrolled in a six week "Imagine Action" program reported being more active after the intervention compared to previous activity levels [13]. In the Stanford Five-City Project, overall the educational intervention had no significant impact on physical activity levels, knowledge, self-efficacy, or attitudes toward physical activity. The published literature on these three trials is large. On the whole, in each of the trials, effects of the interventions were disappointingly small and short-lived with regard to physical activity and many of the other outcome variables.

The underlying theme of the above-discussed behavioral interventions, even those based in worksites and communities, has been to educate individuals about the benefits of increased physical activity, thereby, in theory, encouraging individuals to become more active. However, as noted by Rose, it is difficult to convince seemingly healthy individuals to change their lives in order to reap the possible future benefit of better health. As he pointed out in his exposition of the prevention paradox [14], a preventive measure that brings large benefits to the population offers little to each participating individual. Given such a small expected payoff, it is especially difficult to induce individuals to act outside the conventional social norms that confront them everywhere. It is difficult to convince individuals to walk instead of driving to the grocery store when they must cross busy streets and trudge through long parking lots; to convince them to commute to work by foot or by bicycle if there are no safe pathways, if there are no workplace facilities for showering and changing, and if the external costs associated with automobiles are widely subsidized by society; and to convince them to walk up stairs, rather than take elevators, when stairways often require special keys and are usually poorly-lit and located at extreme ends of buildings.

In such a setting, policies that move beyond the realm of individual choice about individual risk and benefit are necessary to substantially reduce the population burden of disease.   To create lasting population-wide behavioral change, social structures, norms, and policies, in addition to individuals, must change. There are important environmental barriers, some of which were mentioned above, which strongly inhibit a meaningful population-wide transition from a sedentary to an active lifestyle.   The failure to eradicate such barriers likely explains the disappointing results of many intervention trials, including the community-based ones. For instance, although the intervention trials employed mass media to communicate their messages about healthy behavior choices, the Stanford group concluded that the average adult in one of their intervention communities was exposed to only 100 educational messages per year [15]. The total duration of these messages was estimated at about five hours per year, with one of these five hours coming from radio and television. In contrast, the average American adult is exposed annually to 35,000 television advertisements (many of which promote products and lifestyles that are not beneficial and even are detrimental to health), equalling 292 hours, or 12 days, of such exposure [15].   The study of changes in social norms show that such change is often slow, and full of conflict [16]. Intervention trials can accomplish only a small part of what a social movement brings to bear on an issue. An important strategy of many social movements is to seek to change the social environment and the laws/policies governing a population [16].

2.   ENVIRONMENTAL AND POLICY APPROACHES TO INCREASING PHYSICAL ACTIVITY

Environmental and policy approaches to increasing physical activity have the potential to influence large segments of the population simultaneously, and therefore can often be less costly (on a *per capita* basis) and more enduring than approaches that focus on convincing individuals to get more physical activity [8]. By incorporating promotion of physical activity into the mission and objectives of local and state health departments, and developing and maintaining an appropriately trained and staffed unit within the health department that focuses on physical activity, a foundation for strong environmental and policy actions to increase physical activity in the population can be built [8]. Such actions should ideally involve many groups, public and private, who have as part of their mission increasing physical activity in the population. For example, state and local health departments can actively collaborate with other public agencies, such as the departments of parks and recreation, education, and transportation, in order to develop consistent and unified plans to encourage increased physical activity [8]. Parks may charge lower, or no, fees to visitors who are on foot or on a bicycle; the education department might develop a curriculum about the health benefits of increased physical activity, and the environmental and aesthetic benefits associated with a decrease in automobile usage; and the transportation department might work in conjunction with community employers to develop and enforce incentives for non-automotive commuting. By collaborating actively with worksites to promote physical activity, health departments and transportation departments can help to institutionalize new social norms.

The transportation department can also work to build bike paths and walking paths in high-use areas in the local community. Here, the United States might take a lesson from its European counterparts (see sidebar): European countries generally locate bicycle/walking paths or lanes a safe distance from streets, whereas in the United States bicycle lanes are often located right on the street, often with few or no demarcating lines. Such a practice greatly reduces the safety and comfort of cyclists, and is a strong disincentive for many who contemplate using their bike for either recreation or commuting [8].

With regard to the construction of bicycling and walking paths, the Intermodal Surface Transportation Efficiency Act (ISTEA) provides federal funds for bicycle and pedestrian transportation projects [17]. Such projects can include the building of new cycling or pedestrian paths, modification of existing roadways for use by pedestrians and cyclists, and development or modification of commuting policies that reward walking and cycling. This Act gives authority to states to dispense funds for such projects, and each state is required to appoint a bicycle/pedestrian coordinator [17]. However, ISTEA does not *require* states to make any funding allocations for such bicycle/pedestrian purposes; thus, advocacy and other forms of public support from health departments, transportation departments, and local coalitions are necessary for its success [8].

Physical activity can also be fostered through public policies that enhance recreational space outdoors. Increased environmental awareness has led to zoning restrictions in many United States communities to protect open spaces for recreational use [8]. Such greenways are becoming particularly popular in urban areas both as means of connecting neighborhoods and of fostering alternative modes of transportation such as bicycling and walking [8]. Parks, open spaces, and greenways are more plentiful in affluent communities than in less affluent urban centers, while sedentariness, and its negative health consequences, are more prevalent among lower socioeconomic (SES) groups. Grassroots organizations in such urban areas can play a critical role in working with governmental agencies to help insure that recreational spaces, such as neighborhood parks and other recreational spaces, remain safe and well-maintained [8].

Two large sub-populations may be especially important to address in environmental and structural interventions to increase physical activity: young people and older adults [1]. Communities face a growing need to provide supportive, safe, healthy environments for children and adolescents. In addition to organized sports, all communities need to provide recreational programs and opportunities for their young people, because such programs may encourage a lifetime habit of physical activity. They may also produce other community benefits, as well. The Trust for Public Land reported that arrests among young people in one community decreased by 28% after the community instituted an academic and recreational support program for teenagers [18]. In another community, juvenile crime dropped 55% when community recreational facilities stayed open until 2 a.m. [18].

Communities will also need to meet the needs of a growing population of older adults, as the population in the United States continues to age. The health benefits of regular, moderate, physical activity among older adults are enormous. Various sites in the community, including schools, senior centers, and libraries, are increasingly serving as venues for physical activity programs for older adults. Also, in recent years, indoor shopping malls have become popular meeting sites for walking groups and clubs [1, 8]. State and local health departments can encourage using such settings as safe and appropriate places for physical activity.

Concerns about crime can be a major barrier to physical activity for both adults and young people. In a recent national survey of parents, 46% believed that their neighborhood was not very safe from for their children [19]. Minority parents were half as likely as white parents to report that their neighborhood was safe. Successful policy implementations may help to address such concerns [1]. Putting more police on a beat in a high-crime area may help residents feel safer when they go outside to a park, or to walk. As discussed above, opening schools for community recreation and malls for walking can provide safe venues for all community members to get more physical activity. Neighborhood watch groups, often formed to increase safety and reduce crime, can help promote increased physical activity among neighborhood residents. Such groups, as well as transportation and community planners, can help ensure that children can safely walk or bike to school, and that adults can walk or bike to work. Fear of traffic is one of the most frequently cited reasons for not bicycling (see below) [20, 21]. Adult pedestrians and bicyclists account for 14 percent of yearly traffic fatalities [20, 21]. In a survey of adults who had ridden a bicycle in the preceding year, 53 percent said they would commute to work by bicycle if safe, separate, designated bike paths existed. Forty-seven percent said they would do so if their employer offered financial or other incentives. More than half the respondents indicated they would walk, or walk more, to work, if there were safe pathways protected from automobiles and if crime were not a consideration [20].

> Bicycling boom in Germany (summarized from: Pucher, J (1997) Bicycling boom in Germany: a revival engineered by public policy. *Transportation Quarterly* **51**: 31-46)

CONCLUSION

Few studies have assessed the effects of environmental and policy intervention approaches to increase physical activity [8]. The history of tobacco control efforts in this country is informative, however, and several conclusions can be drawn from this history. First, to bring about notable change in ingrained behaviors, and to have the change diffuse through the population, time is needed to ignite and build a social movement at non-governmental levels [16]. Such a social movement results from many local-based programs and initiatives. Potential efforts within communities to increase physical activity within the schools and workplaces include: (1) offering incentives for physically-active commuting; (2) opening schools and malls and other venues for community activity programs; (3) increasing safety (with regard to both crime and traffic) for walkers, bicyclists, and others engaged in outdoor activity; and (4) educating individuals about the health benefits of physical activity. These are all fundamental components of a social movement to shift the distribution of physical activity upward in the population.

A second lesson from the tobacco control effort is that once a social movement is strong enough to induce government leaders and policymakers to bring about formal legal and policy changes, the pace of behavior change in the population accelerates [16]. In the case of smoking, entrenched norms and values have yielded, and hopefully will continue to yield, to the sustained efforts of the public health movement to counter them.

Can public health evidence of the detrimental effects of sedentariness induce a social movement that will lead to the changing of values, behavior, and ultimately laws and regulations? Because our modern society is currently structured to promote widespread sedentariness, and because sedentariness is not associated with the extremely high magnitude of health risk as smoking, it may be more difficult than it was with smoking to spur such a social movement. However, as individuals in our population continue to enjoy longer lifespans and as evidence of the benefits of physical activity for maintaining strength, coordination, and ability to perform activities of daily living continues to mount, physical activity throughout life should be come to be seen as one of the best guarantors of a high quality of life in older adulthood.

Even among countries with similar levels of economic and technological development, there is large variation in the importance of bicycling as a means of urban travel. Most northern European countries have comparable *per capita* incomes, political and economic systems, and levels of urbanization as the United States. Yet bicycle use in urban areas in these European countries is far higher than in the United States. The bicycle currently accounts for less than one percent of all urban trips in the United States, while it accounts for 30 percent of all such trips in the Netherlands, 20 percent of such trips in Denmark, and 12 percent of such trips in Germany. Even citizens in the least bicycle-oriented European countries of Italy and France depend on the bicycle for five percent of urban travel.

What accounts for the far higher level of bicycle use in Europe? Certainly it is not due to a lack of alternative transportation options. Auto ownership levels in these European countries are comparable to the United States, and are among the highest in the world. Further, the public transportation systems in northern and western Europe are the most extensive and highest-quality in the world. Europeans are not cycling due to economic necessity: per capita incomes in Sweden, Switzerland, the Netherlands, and Denmark are as high or higher than those in the United States. Climate and topography do not explain the difference in popularity of bicycling between Europe and the United States: the climate is worst in Europe precisely where bicycling is the most prevalent. Finally, bicycling may be thought to be more popular in northern and western European countries because the average trip distance in these countries is less than the average distance in the United States. There is some truth to this: on average, urban trips tend to be about 50 percent longer in the United States than in western Europe. The more decentralized, lower-density urban areas in the United States obviously lead to longer trip distances. However, even in the United States, 49 percent of all urban trips are three miles or less, 40 percent are two miles or less, and 28 percent are one mile or less, and thus are easily covered by bicycle. Thus, the longer average trip distance in the United States hardly accounts for the less than one percent usage of bicycles for urban trips in the United States, and for the over ten-fold difference compared with northern and western European countries.

The main reason for differences in the level of bicycling use is public policy. In the Netherlands, Denmark, Germany, and Switzerland, various levels of government have constructed extensive systems of bikeways and bike lanes with completely separate rights-of-way. Bicyclists are increasingly given right-of-way priority over autos; the police and courts enforce bicycle priority in urban traffic.

The western portion of Germany has had a particularly successful public policy shift that has favored increased bicycle use over the past two decades. This increased use has been achieved in spite of extremely high per capita auto ownership (second-highest in the world after the United States), recent rapid development and suburbanization around German cities, and subsidization of public transportation passes.

Over the past two decades, virtually every German city has implemented a range of policies to promote both bicycling and walking. The city of Muenster has been in the forefront of such policy implementation. Muenster has a large network of integrated bicycle paths, with most paths separated from both auto and pedestrian traffic; this network increased from 145 kilometers (km) to 252 km over the twenty-year period from 1975 to 1995. Muenster has a tree-lined bicycle expressway that encircles the city center. This expressway provides direct connections with major bike routes radiating to outlying parts of the city, its suburbs, and the surrounding countryside, which is also crossed by a dense network of bike paths. Most residential streets in Muenster can be safely used by bicyclists, thanks to traffic-calming measures that give pedestrians and bicyclists right-of-way priority and restrict auto speeds to 30 km per hour (19 miles per hour, mph).

Providing this dense network of bike paths and routes is only part of Muenster's strategy to promote bicycling among its residents. Other policies include: special bike streets, which permit auto traffic but give bicyclists strict priority in right-of-way over the entire breadth of the street; streets that are one-way for cars but two-way for bicyclists; reserved bus lanes that can be used by bicyclists but not by autos; street networks with deliberate dead ends and circuitous routing for cars but direct, fast routing for bikes;

permission for bicyclists to make left and right turns where prohibited for autos; special lanes at intersections that allow bicyclists to pass waiting cars and proceed directly to the front; while cars must stop at a considerable distance from the intersection, and an advance green light for bicyclists at intersections, so they can clear the high-traffic area before the cars get started; permission for bicyclists to ride in auto-free pedestrian zones at certain times of day, when they are uncrowded; comprehensive training in bicycling safety for all school children; frequent surprise inspections by plainclothes police to check for safe working condition of bicycles, to intercept stolen bicycles, and to enforce traffic laws for bicyclists; bike rental and repair facilities at all train stations and at many other transportation nodes throughout the region; and an expansive network of bicycle parking facilities, including sheltered bike racks, theft-proof bike cages, and spacious lockers that can be rented on a monthly or annual basis and provide room for bikes, clothing, and space for changing clothing.

At the same time that German cities have greatly increased incentives for bicyclists, they have sharply increased disincentives for auto drivers. Traffic calming has been initiated in most urban residential neighborhoods in the country; since 1980, most cities have reduced speed limits to 30 km per hour (19 mph) and have further slowed and discouraged auto traffic by narrowing streets, increasing curves, setting up roadway bottlenecks, and installing speed bumps, bollards, and bicycle lanes. In virtually all German cities, there is an extensive network of streets in the town center and main commercial district that is completely off-limits to private autos. One of the most important necessities for auto use is parking, and most German cities have decreased the supply of parking while increasing its price. In Muenster, all free parking has been eliminated in the city core, and the total number of auto parking places has been reduced, forcing auto drivers to park their cars in satellite lots and walk, bike, or take public transportation to the city center. Finally, most cities have a virtual moratorium on new roadway construction. Roadway congestion is a serious problem in many German cities, but the approach commonly taken has been to allow the congestion to discourage more auto use, rather than to build more roads which quickly fill up with traffic (this has been the predominant strategy in the United States).

The combination of carrot-and-stick approaches has proved very effective in Germany in increasing bicycle use. The lesson from this country is that bicycling can be increased even under quite unfavorable circumstances, including high auto ownership, poor climate, and an aging population, with the right public policies.

In the United States, in contrast, very little has been done to promote bicycle use. The few bikeways and bike lanes in American cities are usually uncoordinated, poorly maintained, and, because they are usually not separated from auto traffic, dangerous for bicyclists. Even more seriously, most American auto drivers have little respect for the legal right of bicyclists to share the roads. As a result, bicycling is relatively unsafe. There are over 800 bicyclist fatalities per year in the United States; bicyclists account for two percent of all traffic deaths, but only 0.2 percent of all passenger miles traveled. The danger of bicycling discourages many would-be cyclists in this country. Constructing separate rights-of-way for bicyclists would be one solution; another would be strict enforcement of the legal right of bicyclists to share the road equally with autos.

SUMMARY POINTS

- The diseases linked to sedentariness are major causes of morbidity and mortality in industrialized societies; thus the impact of sedentariness on public health is large.
- Significant health benefits are achievable with moderate amounts of physical activity.
- To substantially reduce the public health burden of disease due to sedentariness, the population distribution of physical activity must be shifted upwards. A "high-risk" strategy that focuses only on the most inactive tail of the distribution will not have a large public health impact.
- Physical activity has proved difficult to modify on a large scale by using individually-focused approaches to behavior change.
- Environmental and policy approaches to increasing physical activity across the population include efforts in increase physical activity within schools and workplaces, offering incentives for physically-active commuting, providing safe paths/routes for bicyclists and walkers and giving priority to such persons over auto drivers, and opening community venues such as malls, school, *etc.* for physical activity programs.

RECOMMENDATIONS

- Strategies to shift the population distribution of physical activity upward should focus on the underlying social determinants of this distribution, rather than on merely attempting to convince individuals to become more active.
- Because people spend a large proportion of their waking time commuting to, and working at, their workplaces, employers can play an important role in increasing physical activity among adults by offering

incentives for physically-active commuting and for participation in physical activity during the work day.
* The combination of carrot-and-stick approaches in some northern European cities to discourage automobile use and encourage bicycle use has proved highly effective; policymakers in the United States, who has done very little to promote walking or bicycling rather than automobile use, should follow the lead of these European cities. Potential benefits include not only increased physical activity levels across the population, but decreased traffic congestion, decreased pollution, and retainment of green spaces around urban areas.

SUGGESTED FURTHER READING

1. U.S. Department of Health and Human Services (1996) *Physical Activity and Health: A Report of the Surgeon General.* Atlanta, GA: U.S. Department of Health and Human Services, Centers for Disease Control and Prevention, National Center for Chronic Disease Prevention and Health Promotion.
2. King A, prevention through physical activity: issues and opportunities. *Health Educ Q* **22:** 499-511.

REFERENCES

1. U.S. Department of Health and Human Services (1996) *Physical Activity and Health: A Report of the Surgeon General.* Atlanta, Georgia: U.S. Department of Health and Human Services, Centers for Disease Control and Prevention, National Center for Chronic Disease Prevention and Health Promotion.
2. McGinnis JM, Foege WH (1993) Actual causes of death in the United States. *JAMA* **270:** 2207-2212.
3. Hahn R, Teutsch S, Rothenberg R, *et al.* (1990) Excess deaths from nine chronic diseases in the United States, 1986. *JAMA* **264:** 2654-2659.
4. Williams C, Carter B, Eng A (1980) The Know Your Body program: a developmental approach to health education and disease prevention. *Prev Med* **9:** 371-83.
5. Bush P, Zuckerman A, Theiss P, *et al.* (1989) Cardiovascular risk factor prevention in black schoolchildren: two-year results of the Know Your Body program. *Am J Epidemiol* **129:** 466-82.
6. Killen J, Telch M, Robinson T, *et al.* (1988) Cardiovascular disease risk reduction for tenth graders: a multiple-factor school-based approach. *JAMA* **260:** 1728-33.
7. Luepker R, Perry C, McKinlay S, *et al.* (1996) Outcomes of a field trial to improve children's dietary patterns and physical activity: the Child and Adolescent Trial for Cardiovascular Health (CATCH). *JAMA* **275:** 768-76.

8. King A, Jeffery R, Fridinger F, *et al.* (1995) Environmental and policy approaches to cardiovascular disease prevention through physical activity: issues and opportunities. *Health Educ Q* **22:** 499-511.
9. U.S. Department of Health and Human Services (1993) *1992 National Survey of Worksite Health Promotion Activities.* Washington, DC: Office of Disease Prevention and Health Promotion, U.S. Department of Health and Human Services.
10. Luepker R, Murray D, Jr DJ, *et al.* (1994) Community education for cardiovascular disease prevention: risk factor changes in the Minnesota Heart Health Project. *Am J Public Health* **84:** 1383-93.
11. Carleton R, Lasater T, Assaf A, *et al.* (1995) The Pawtucket Heart Health Program: community changes in cardiovascular risk factors and projected disease risk. *Am J Public Health* **85:** 777-85.
12. Farquhar J, Foartmann S, Flora J, *et al.* (1990) Effects of communitywide education on cardiovascular disease risk factors: the Stanford Five-City Project. *JAMA* **264:** 359-65.
13. Marcus B, Banspach S, Lefebvre R, *et al.* (1992) Using the stages of change model to increase the adoption of physical activity among community participants. *Am J Public Health* **6:** 424-29.
14. Rose G (1992) *The Strategy of Preventive Medicine.* New York, NY (USA): Oxford University Press.
15. Fortmann S, Flora J, Winkleby M, Schooler C, Taylor C, Farquhar J (1995) Community intervention trials: reflections on the Stanford Five-City Project experience. *Am J Epidemiol* **142:** 576-86.
16. Susser M. The tribulations of trials - interventions in communities (1995) *Am J Public Health* **85:** 156-158.
17. Moritz B (1992) *A Plan to Create a Center for Human Powered Transportation.* Seattle, WA (USA): University of Washington Press.
18. National Park Service (1994) *An Americans' Network of Parks and Open Space: Creating a Conservation and Recreation Legacy.* Washington, DC: U.S. Department of the Interior, National Park Service, National Park System Advisory Board.
19. Princeton Survey Research Associates (1994) *Prevention Magazine's Children's Health Index.* Prevention.
20. U.S. Department of Transportation (1994) *Final Report: The National Bicycling and Walking Study: Transportation Choices for a Changing America.* Washington, DC: U.S. Department of Transportation, Federal Highway Administration
21. Zehnpfenning G (1993) *Measures to Overcome Impediments to Bicycling and Walking: The National Bicycling and Walking Study, case study No. 4.* Washington, DC: U.S. Department of Transportation, Federal Highway Administration

Chapter 19

Sexual Behavior and Cancer Prevention

Charles S. Morrison, Ph.D., Pamela J. Schwingl, Ph.D., Kavita Nanda, M.D., M.H.S., Willard Cates, Jr., M.D., M.P.H.
Family Health International, Research Triangle Park, NC

INTRODUCTION

Unlike tobacco use, a high-fat diet, or environmental pollutants, sexual behavior is typically not thought to be a "cause" of cancer. The long induction time between infection with a sexually transmitted virus and the development of cancer, as well as the rare occurrence of cancer among those age groups with the highest infection rates, may explain why sexual behavior and cancer remain unlinked in the public mind. Moreover, cancer researchers themselves have tended to under-emphasize the role of infections in human cancer etiology [1].

Investigation of the infectious origins of human cancer began in the last century, but only in the last 30 years has convincing evidence emerged that neoplasia can be triggered by viral infections, many of which are sexually transmitted [1]. In the 1980s and 1990s, several sexually transmitted viral infections (STVI) have become established as known or strongly suspected in the etiology of cancer. In 1981, when Sir Richard Doll estimated that viruses play an etiologic role in the induction of approximately ten percent of all fatal malignancies in the U.S., [2] only hepatitis B virus (HBV) was firmly linked with hepatocellular carcinoma. Soon after in the early 1980s, specific types of human papillomavirus (HPV) became implicated as the etiologic agents responsible for cervical and other genital cancers [3]. Later, hepatitis C virus (HCV) became linked with chronic liver disease and hepatocellular carcinoma [4]. In the mid-1980s human immunodeficiency virus (HIV) was associated with Kaposi's sarcoma and intermediate or high-grade B-cell lymphoma. Finally, other oncogenic STVI, including human lymphotropic virus-type 1 (HTLV-1) and human herpesvirus-8 (HHV-8)

G.A. Colditz et al. (eds.), Cancer Prevention: The Causes and Prevention of Cancer - Volume I, 235–251.
© 2000 *Kluwer Academic Publishers.*

emerged as agents in the etiology of adult T-cell leukemia/lymphoma
(HTLV-1) and Kaposi's sarcoma and body cavity-lymphoma (HHV-8) [5].

1.   ASSOCIATION BETWEEN SEXUAL BEHAVIOR
          AND CANCER

The link between sexual behavior and cancer depends on both the
evidence linking a specific virus with a specific cancer and on the evidence
for the transmission of the virus through sexual behavior. Seven viruses are
known to be transmitted through sexual practices and are associated with
increased risks of cancer (Table 19.1).

Table 19.1 Sexually transmitted viral infections (STVI) and associated cancers (adapted from
references [3-5, 13, 14])

Virus	Cancer
Human papillomavirus (HPV): types 16 and 18 (1); types 31 and 33 (2a) some other HPV types (2b)	Cervical intraepithelial neoplasia and carcinoma; vulvar, penile, and anal carcinoma
Hepatitis B virus (HBV) (1)	Hepatocellular carcinoma
Hepatitis C) (1)	Hepatocellular carcinoma
Hepatitis D virus (HDV) (1)	Hepatocellular carcinoma
Human lymphotropic virus-type 1 (HTLV-1) (1)	Adult T-cell leukemia
Human immunodeficiency virus-type 1 (HIV-1) (1)	Kaposi's sarcoma, non-Hodgkin's lymphoma
Human herpes virus (HHV-8)	Kaposi's sarcoma, body cavity lymphoma

Numbers in parentheses represent International Association for Research on Cancer (IARC)
classification of an agent to humans: (1) agent is carcinogenic to humans; (2a) agent is
probably carcinogenic to humans; (2b) agent is possibly carcinogenic to humans; IARC has
not yet classified the carcinogenicity of HHV-8.

1.1   Linking viruses to cancer

Evidence associating HBV and HCV with hepatocellular carcinoma is
particularly strong [4].   Hepatitis B infection is causally related to
approximately 80 percent of hepatocellular carcinoma cases. Hepatitis B
antigenemia (HBsAg) is the key epidemiologic marker of HBV infection,
and an induction period of approximately 20 years exists between initial

infection and tumor diagnosis. About five to ten percent of adults infected with HBV will develop chronic antigenemia. Persistence of the antigen in serum leads to increased risk of severe chronic hepatitis, cirrhosis, and liver cancer, and carriers have a 100-fold risk of developing hepatocellular carcinoma compared with non-carriers [6]. The risk of cancer is also high among babies born to infected mothers, 70 to 90 percent of whom become infected, with a high risk of persistent antigenemia. HCV is less infectious than HBV, but accounts for the majority of nonA-nonB hepatitis cases [7]. Approximately four million Americans have been infected with HCV, and because it can take years for symptoms to develop, HCV may lead to 10,000 deaths annually [7]. Up to 70 percent of those infected with HCV will develop chronic liver disease and about 15 percent will develop cirrhosis of the liver.

A fourth hepatitis virus, HDV is associated with chronic liver disease and hepatocellular carcinoma but depends on co-infection with HBV for replication. Still another recently discovered RNA hepatitis virus, HGV/GBV-C, is currently being investigated for its clinical significance in chronic hepatitis. HGV/GBV-C co-exists in 20 percent of patients with HCV, and is common in HIV-infected women; but whether it exists only as a co-infection with limited pathogenicity remains to be determined [8].

HPV is strongly associated with genital cancers. More than 70 types of human papillomaviruses exist, and of these, over 20 can be sexually transmitted [9]. Women infected with high-risk HPV types 16 or 18 have at least a 50-fold risk of developing cervical intraepithelial neoplasia (CIN) compared with those with no detectable HPV, and over 200 times the risk of developing invasive cancer [10]. More than 90 percent of the estimated 13,700 cases of cervical cancer diagnosed in the U.S. in 1998 are attributable to HPV infection [11].

Other oncogenic viruses associated with cancer include HTLV-1, the etiologic agent of adult T-cell leukemia/lymphoma (ATLL). This cancer occurs almost exclusively in areas where HTLV-1 is endemic (Japan, Caribbean, West Africa) and 90 percent of patients with ATLL are positive for HTLV-1 [5]. Kaposi's sarcoma and non-Hodgkin's lymphoma (NHL) are greatly increased in people with HIV-1, possibly related to the immune dysfunction allowing other STVIs to predominate. Some studies indicate at least a 1000-fold increase in Kaposi's sarcoma and a 100-fold increase in non-Hodgkin's lymphoma among HIV-infected people [5]. Finally, the HHV-8 genome is regularly found in AIDS associated Kaposi's sarcoma, with one study reporting that 83 percent of persons with Kaposi's sarcoma have antibodies against HHV-8 [12]. The HHV-8 genome is also regularly found in HIV-negative homosexual men with Kaposi's sarcoma, and in persons with classic Kaposi's sarcoma [13], and HHV-8 may play a role in AIDS-associated lymphomas [14].

1.2   Evidence for sexual transmission of these viruses

Substantial epidemiologic evidence indicates that the viruses just described are transmitted sexually. For example, hepatitis B infection occurs more frequently among adolescents and adults who have multiple sex partners, longer duration of sexual activity, and a history of sexually transmitted diseases [4]. An estimated 120,000 cases of HBV were sexually transmitted in the U.S. in 1996 [15]. Hepatitis C and D and hepatitis G/GBV-C are transmitted through sexual activity, although hepatitis C is less efficiently spread through sexual activity than HBV [4].

Evidence for sexual transmission of genital HPV is strong. Genital HPV infection has been associated with an early age of first intercourse and multiple sex partners, and is not found in virgins [16]. The prevalence of genital HPV is highest among sexually active young adults [3], and HPV-related c (SIL) and cancer occur more frequently in women with early sexual activity, a greater number of sex partners, and lack of barrier contraceptive use [17]. HPV-related anal cancer is seen primarily in men who practice receptive anal intercourse, especially those who are HIV-positive [18].

HIV transmission has been consistently associated with having sex with an HIV-infected partner, having multiple sex partners, engaging in unprotected intercourse, and having other concurrent sexually transmitted diseases (STDs). In addition, the small number of cases of these infections among children 7 to 14 years of age is strong evidence for transmission of HPV, HBV, and HIV through sexual activity. There is considerable evidence linking homosexual sex and transmission of HHV-8, but the mechanism for transmission remains unknown.

2.   PREVENTION STRATEGIES

Strategies to prevent STVI include both *behavioral and educational interventions* and *biomedical interventions* (Table 19.2). Effective individual and community-focused behavioral interventions have the potential to prevent the full spectrum of infections spread through sexual behavior [19]. Biomedical interventions are generally aimed at preventing specific STVI and their sequelae, including STVI-related cancers.

2.1   Behavioral and Educational Interventions

Substantial evidence exists that both individual and community-level behavioral interventions can be effective in modifying risky sexual behaviors.

Table 19.2. Strategies for prevention of sexually transmitted viral infections (STVI)-related cancers (adapted from references [19-41])

Intervention Type (Level of Focus)	Description	Advantages	Disadvantages
Behavioral/Educational			
Client Counseling (Individual)	Routine counseling by providers to reduce risky behavior	Providers advice trusted; counseling at reproductive health visits appropriate;	Time-consuming; follow-up important; unproven benefit
Counseling and Testing (Individuals/Couple)	Voluntary testing for STVI (mostly HIV), post-test counseling to explain results and reduce risky sexual behavior	Widely available in the U.S.; moderately effective in some groups; appropriate for couples	Duration of impact unclear; quality of counseling variable
Small Group (Individual)	Behavioral skills training (e.g., safer sex negotiation training); social support for behavior change (support groups)	Feasible to conduct; proven effective in various populations; may protect against all STVI	May need to be repeated/updated for sustained behavior change
Training of Peer Leaders (Community)	Change normative sexual behavior by training of opinion leaders to deliver safer sex messages ('diffusion of innovation')	Proven effectiveness; may reach higher-risk individuals who don't volunteer for small groups; impacts on entire community	Generalizability to most vulnerable groups and long-term impact unclear
Mass Media/Social Marketing (Community)	Sexuality and STI prevention education; condom distribution programs	Reaches wide audience at low cost; increases condom sales	More impact on knowledge than behaviors; politically sensitive
School-based education (Community)	Sexuality and STI prevention education; condom distribution programs	Reaches the majority of adolescents; reduces STI and pregnancy rates	Politically sensitive; programs often restricted
Regulatory/Structural (Societal/Structural)1	Regulation of condom distribution, advertising; HIV testing-partner notification	Affects entire society	May infringe on individual rights; politically sensitive
Biomedical			
Prophylactic Vaccines (Individual)	HBV vaccine	Highly effective; prevents infection to client and client's sex partners	High coverage of susceptible groups problematic
Screening/Early Detection (Individual)	Pap smear and visual inspection for CIN; HBsAg and HCsAg testing; HIV testing	Provides basis for early treatment of STVI	Impact on transmission of STVI to sex partners unknown
STVI Treatment (Individual)	Post-exposure HBV prophylaxis; interferon for chronic HBV/HCV carriers; antiviral therapy for HIV; removal of CIN	May prevent some STVI and cancers and other STVI sequelae	Expensive; impact on transmission of STVI to sex partners unknown

Counseling by Health Providers. The U.S. Preventive Services Task Force (USPSTF) [20] recommends that all primary care providers counsel their patients to avoid high-risk sexual behaviors. Key messages for STVI prevention include: delaying the onset of sexual activity; abstaining from sex with individuals not known to be infection-free; and consistent use of latex condoms. Counseling should be client-centered, based on a careful sexual and drug use history including questions about the number and type of sexual partners, history of past STI, use of condoms, and particular high-risk practices (*e.g.*, anal intercourse) [20]. The message should fit the client's perceptions, inform the client of the expected impact of the recommended actions, provide specific information, ask for an explicit commitment from the client, and make use of a combination of educational strategies - including audiovisual aids, written materials, and group classes. This may necessitate using other clinic-based staff or referring clients to local self-help groups [20].

Voluntary HIV testing and counseling has been an important strategy for reducing high-risk sexual behavior in the U.S. Increasing evidence indicates that this intervention has an impact. For example, homosexual men who learn they are HIV-seropositive have generally made greater reductions in risky behavior than those who learned they were seronegative or those who were unaware of their serostatus [21]. Similarly, among blood donors and patients with sexually transmitted diseases who received notification of HIV serostatus and post-notification counseling, significantly fewer men and women reported unsafe sex thereafter [22]. Results from a recently conducted trial in Kenya, Tanzania and Trinidad show that among women and men randomized to receive either voluntary HIV counseling and testing (VCT) or a standardized AIDS information intervention, that those receiving VCT had greater reductions in the prevalence of unprotected intercourse with non-primary partners and with commercial sex partners at 6-month follow-up than did those receiving the AIDS informational intervention [23]. Likewise, studies from Zaire and Rwanda demonstrate that discordant couples who received intensive counseling after notification of HIV test results dramatically increased levels of condom use 18 months (Zaire) [21] and 12 months (Rwanda) [22] after the intervention compared with pre-intervention levels.

Small Group Interventions. Small group interventions have been largely guided by cognitive-behavioral theory. In general, they involve up to 18 hours of contact time, and have focused on condom use skills, sexual assertiveness, safer sex negotiation skills training, eroticizing safer sex, and self-management skills to deal with 'high-risk' situations [19, 22]. Four recent randomized controlled trials provide convincing evidence that cognitive-behavioral interventions aimed at changing the behavior of individuals are effective in reducing self-reported HIV risk behaviors and incident STD. In Project RESPECT, heterosexual HIV-negative patients coming for STD examinations were randomized to enhanced counseling, brief counseling, and didactic messages arms. At three- and six-month follow-up visits, consistent condom use was higher in both the enhanced and brief counseling arms compared with the didactic message arm. At 6 and 12 months, participants in the two counseling arms had significantly lower rates of new STDs (gonorrhea, chlamydia, syphilis, HIV) than those in the didactic messages arm [24]. In the recent NIMH Multisite HIV Prevention Trial, participants randomized to an experimental condition (7 small-group HIV risk reduction sessions) reported fewer unprotected sexual acts, had higher levels of condom use and were more likely to use condoms consistently over a 12-month follow-up period than were participants assigned to the control group (one hour AIDS video and question and answer session) [25]. In a recent trial of a behavioral intervention to prevent STD among minority women, women assigned to a three-session behavioral intervention had lower rates of bacterial STD at both 6 and at 12 months than women assigned to the control (standard counseling) intervention [26]. Finally, a trial among African-American homosexual and bisexual men found that participants randomized to a triple session cognitive-behavioral intervention had greater reductions in unprotected anal intercourse at both 12 and 18 months compared with men randomized to a single session intervention [27]. Thus, high-quality studies have demonstrated the success of cognitive-behavioral interventions in reducing self-reported risk behavior and STD incidence in a variety of populations. However the impact of such individual-level interventions on the maintenance of longer term behavioral changes (>1 year) and on HIV incidence has not been adequately examined. Many prevention experts believe that more intense, sustained and diverse interventions are needed to maintain low-risk behaviors over the long-term [22].

2.1.2   Community-Focused Behavioral Interventions

Peer and Community Opinion Leaders   Community-focused interventions attempt to change behavioral norms either among specific high-risk groups (*e.g.* homosexual men) or across the society as a whole. One successful approach has been the use of peer and community opinion leaders to affect normative sexual behavior ("diffusion of innovation" approach). For example, a community intervention trial compared changes in sexual behavior in four cities where opinion leaders were trained to deliver HIV prevention messages to young homosexual men. At 9 months follow-up, there was a reduction in unprotected anal intercourse in experimental cities, while little change was observed in four control cities not receiving the intervention [22]. A community-level controlled trial in Zimbabwe tested the impact of a workplace HIV peer education program among factory workers. Forty factories were either randomized to HIV testing and counseling alone (control) or HIV counseling and testing plus peer education (intervention). Factory-specific HIV incidence appears to be lower among intervention factories compared to control factories. In addition, individual HIV incidence was lower among workers at the intervention factories compared with control factories [28]. The Centers for Disease Control AIDS Community Demonstration Projects evaluated a theory-based community-level intervention to promote consistent condom and bleach use among high-risk populations in five U.S. cities. In these projects, role-model stories were distributed, along with condoms, by community educators who encouraged behavioral changes among high-risk persons. A quasi-experimental research design demonstrated that, at the community level, consistent condom use increased with both main and non-main sexual partners in intervention as compared with control communities [29].

Mass Media Campaigns   Mass media campaigns using a variety of reinforcing messages have been successful in HIV prevention. A Swiss campaign used household mailings followed by public media advertisements to promote condom use and monogamy. The campaign resulted in increased AIDS knowledge, condom sales and use [22]. Social marketing of condoms has taken place in many African countries and has been associated with dramatic increases in condom sales and use in those countries.

School-Based Interventions   School-based interventions are an important venue for preventing high-risk sexual behavior among adolescents. A 1994 study by the CDC showed that a majority of states and 81 percent of school districts required teaching STI prevention. Almost four-fifths of teachers taught about sexual behaviors that can transmit HIV and other STI, but only about one-third provided instruction about correct condom use [19]. An Institute of Medicine Committee evaluating school-based sexual education classes found that programs that provide information on both abstinence and contraceptive use "appear to be effective in delaying the onset of sexual intercourse and encouraging contraceptive use once sexual activity has begun, especially among younger adolescents" [19].

Although 431 schools in 21 states have condom availability programs as part of STI prevention efforts, these represent only two percent of all public high schools in the U.S. In most schools some form of parental consent is required for student participation. Evaluations of school-based condom distribution programs suggest that the programs protect sexually active students against STI and pregnancy, and do not result in earlier onset of sex or more frequent sexual activity [19].

2.2   Regulatory/Structural Interventions

Unlike many areas of cancer prevention, regulatory approaches have not played a central role in preventing STVI-related cancers. Concerns over intrusion into private sexual choices have raised questions about civil liberties. Nevertheless, in some specific situations, regulatory approaches have been successfully used. In 1984, bathhouses in San Francisco were first regulated by 'monitors' and then later closed by the city government [30]. Some cities have mandated condom availability in high schools [19] and some states mandate partner notification after diagnosis of HIV infection. The most successful structural intervention is Thailand's policy of 100 percent condom use in brothels which appears to be responsible for major declines in STI in Thailand [30]. The incidence of HIV-1 in Thailand has also decreased.

2.3   Biomedical Interventions

2.3.1   Vaccines

The development of both prophylactic and therapeutic vaccines are important measures for the prevention of viral infection and ultimately cancer, and are the most cost-effective medical intervention. Prophylactic vaccines aim to prevent the acquisition of virus, and therefore can be considered to be an individual-level primary prevention strategy. Therapeutic vaccines aim to reduce progression of the viral infection among infected individuals, and thus are considered to be an individual-level secondary prevention strategy. However, by preventing viral shedding in infected individuals and subsequent transmission, therapeutic vaccines can also be considered a population-level primary prevention strategy.

The only effective, currently available prophylactic STVI vaccine is the hepatitis B vaccine. HBV vaccine affords persistent protection against clinical HBV infection and chronic virus carriage for seven to nine years. Use of the vaccine has reduced the incidence of HBV by 90 to 95 percent in homosexual men. In addition, since hepatitis D depends on co-infection with HBV for replication, HBV vaccine is also effective for HDV. Universal vaccination of newborns and 'catch-up' immunization of children and adolescents 0 to 18 years of age, children in populations at high risk for HBV infection (*e.g.,* Alaska Natives, Pacific Islanders, and children who reside in households of first-generation immigrants from countries where

HBV infection is moderately or highly endemic, adolescents, and high-risk adults) is recommended. HBV vaccine programs have successfully been implemented in school-based clinics, primary care clinics, and other clinical settings [19].

While currently available HBV vaccines are safe and efficacious, the three-dose regimen is logistically difficult, has a comparably high rate of nonresponders (five percent in adults), and it is possible that strains of HBV showing mutations of HBsAg could escape immunity induced by the current vaccine. These considerations have intensified efforts to clinically test recently developed combined vaccines and to enhance the immunogenicity of current vaccines [31].

A vaccine to prevent HCV infection is not expected to be developed in the foreseeable future. Without a vaccine, there is an increased probability of developing chronic HCV infection. Thus, the greatest impact on disease burden associated with HCV infection is likely to be achieved by primary prevention strategies to reduce or eliminate risk for transmission. The effectiveness of the HBV vaccine against hepatocellular carcinoma is under investigation.

Both prophylactic and therapeutic HPV vaccines are being developed; however, their development has been complicated by the fact that HPV does not grow in tissue culture, has low antigenicity, and has multiple subtypes. Phase I trials of a prophylactic vaccine for HPV types 6/11 and phase II trials of therapeutic HPV vaccines for women with cervical cancer are currently underway. However, neither persistently high levels of antibody nor protection from cancer have been demonstrated. Prophylactic HSV and HIV vaccines are in development, but are many years away from being clinically available. A phase III trial of VaxGen's gp120 vaccine is currently underway in the United States and Thailand. In Uganda, a vaccine based on a canary pox vector (ALVAC CP 205) is being studied to evaluate immune responses in a phase I design.

2.3.2   Mechanical and Chemical Barriers.

Barrier contraceptives are effective in preventing many STI. Studies from serodiscordant couples convincingly demonstrate that consistent use of male latex condoms is effective in preventing HIV transmission. However apart from HIV, data are sparse on their effectiveness in preventing other STVI (Table 19.3). Epidemiologic modeling has shown that even partial reduction in HPV acquisition can lead to decreases in cervical cancer incidence [32]. *In vitro,* both male latex and polyurethane condoms have been shown to be sufficient barriers to viruses smaller than HPV [33]. However, limited clinical data exist on male latex condom use for the prevention of HPV. Although early case-control studies showed a protective effect of barriers for cervical cancer, more recent cross-sectional and cohort studies are inconsistent for HPV prevention. No studies have examined the effectiveness of condoms for prevention among HPV-discordant couples. The female polyurethane condom is impermeable to HIV, HSV and HBV in laboratory studies [34]. Two human studies suggest that the female condom may reduce bacterial STDs [35, 36], and, if used consistently and correctly, this method should reduce STVI transmission.

Table 19.3 Barrier contraceptive use and prevention of sexually transmitted viral infections (STVI) (adapted from references [19, 32-36])

Type of Barrier	Strength of Evidence	Type STVI & Level of Protection
Male Latex Condom	Strong: Prospective studies of HIV-discordant couples	**HIV:** 90-100% reduction for always vs. some/no use; 50-90% reduction for any *vs.* no use
	In vitro studies only	**HBV:** Impervious barrier to HBV
	Weak: single cross-sectional study	**HSV:** 40% reduction in HSV-2 seropositivity for some *vs.* no use
	Weak for HPV transmission; moderate for CIN, cancer	**HPV:** Inconsistent for HPV transmission; risk of CIN, cancer reduced by 20-50% in most studies
Female Condom	*In vitro* studies only	**HIV:** Impervious barrier to HIV & CMV
Spermicide (N-9)	Randomized-trial, prospective studies	**HIV:** Not shown effective
	In vitro; cross-sectional; case-control studies	**HPV:** No inactivation of HPV *in vitro*; risk of CIN, cervical cancer reduced by 20-70% in most studies
	In vitro only	**HSV:** Inactivates HSV in vitro
Diaphragm (with Spermicide)	Moderate: cross-sectional, case-control studies	**HPV:** Risk of CIN, cervical cancer reduced by 20-70% in most studies.
Cervical Cap	No evidence	

HIV = human immunodeficiency virus; HBV = hepatitis B virus; HPV = human papilloma virus; CIN = cervical intraepithelial neoplasia; CMV = cytomegalovirus

The efficacy of spermicides for preventing STVI has not been demonstrated. Spermicides containing nonoxynol-9 (N-9) inactivate *in vitro* many sexually transmitted pathogens including HIV and HSV by destroying the viral outer envelope membrane. However, N-9 may not inactivate HPV which has no envelope membrane. Moreover, *in vitro* microbicidal activity does not translate into *in vivo* effectiveness. The highest quality human studies of different doses of N-9 to prevent HIV transmission have not demonstrated any effect. Although several case-control studies of spermicide use and cervical cancer show a protective effect, limited data exist for HPV.

Similar to spermicides, the efficacy of other barrier methods has not been proven. Diaphragms used with spermicides protect against some bacterial STI; they have also been associated with reduced risk of cervical cancer. However, limited evidence exists that diaphragms prevent HPV transmission. No studies have examined the effect of the cervical cap or male polyurethane condoms on the transmission of cancer-related STVI.

2.3.3   Early Identification and Screening.

Routine screening for HBV infection in the general population is not recommended. In the interest of preventing mother-to-infant transmission, however, screening for HBsAg is recommended for pregnant women during their first prenatal visit, and persons determined to be at high risk of sexually transmitted diseases should be screened to assess eligibility for vaccination. The CDC recommends that persons with selected medical conditions, and prior recipients of transfusions or organ transplants be screened for HCV. In addition, health care workers with occupational exposures and children born to HCV-positive women should also be screened for HCV. Since early treatment of HCV with interferon is associated with a higher rate of resolved infection, early identification of HCV is important.

Invasive squamous cervical cancer is preceded by preneoplastic lesions that can be identified by screening, and then treated. The primary method of screening for cervical intraepithelial lesions and cancer is the *Papanicolaou* (Pap) test. Routine screening with Pap testing is currently recommended for all women who have ever been sexually active or have reached the age of 18, and who have a cervix. Where resources exist, Pap testing should begin with the onset of sexual activity and should be repeated every three years or tailored to sexual risk. Despite the low sensitivity of the Pap, cervical cancer screening programs have had remarkable success in decreasing cervical cancer mortality over the last 30 years [20, 32].

Several new technologies for improving the sensitivity of cervical cytology screening have recently been developed. These include liquid-based monolayer preparations, computerized primary screening, and 100 percent computerized re-screening of initially normal slides. HPV testing for high-risk subtypes has also been suggested for primary screening because it does not require a pelvic exam for sample collection. However, these new technologies are associated with high costs, and only marginal cancer prevention benefit due to the increased detection and treatment of transient HPV infections and low-grade cervical lesions [32]. Women with low-grade squamous intraepithelial lesions (LSIL) and atypical squamous cells of undetermined significance (ASCUS) on cytology are often referred for further diagnosis and treatment because some will have high-grade lesions, even though the majority of ASCUS will regress. For these women, adjunctive screening for HPV to identify those at high risk of underlying high-grade lesions is promising [37]. Another technique for primary cervical cancer screening in settings where Pap testing is not available is visual inspection of the cervix after acetic acid application. In a recent study in Zimbabwe, this promising technique had higher sensitivity than the Pap test [38]. However, this technique has low specificity, is difficult to quality control, and has not yet been shown to reduce incidence or mortality from cervical cancer.

The value of early identification of acute HIV infection has become more important with the availability of highly active anti-retroviral therapy (HAART). Combined with HIV viral load measurements and CD4 T-cell counts, use of anti-viral therapies can reduce the HIV "setpoint" to provide a better disease prognosis.

2.3.4   Curative Therapeutic Agents.

Curative therapeutic agents for viral STDs are limited. Current treatment of HBV and HCV infections includes limited courses of alpha interferon aimed at clearance of viral markers and remission induction [39]. In patients with chronic hepatitis C, combination therapy with Ribavirin and interferon is now FDA-approved for treatment in patients who relapse after treatment with interferon [40], and may soon be approved for initial therapy [41]. Post-exposure HBV prophylaxis (HBIG, hepatitis B immune globulin along with the HBV vaccine), has a combined efficacy of about 75 percent in protecting susceptible persons from primary infection. IG is not effective for postexposure prophylaxis of HCV.

Treatment options for women with biopsy confirmed high-grade cervical squamous intraepithelial lesions include ablation or excision. Therapy is aimed at removing precancerous tissue rather than curing HPV infection. Treatments for genital condyloma include chemical or physical destruction, and are associated with high recurrence rates. Theoretically, treatment of either SIL or condyloma could decrease the reservoir of virus, but no evidence exists that treatment affects HPV transmission risk. This is likely due to persistent HPV in normal adjacent mucosa and skin. Evaluation and treatment of partners, and post-treatment use of condoms have not been shown to affect recurrence rates. Recently developed immune modifiers such as imiquimod may be more effective at eliminating the virus, but have not been adequately investigated.

A combination of antiviral therapies is available for the treatment of HIV infection. Nucleoside and non-nucleoside reverse transcriptase inhibitors used together with viral protease inhibitors have reduced viral loads, increased immune competence, and improved clinical symptoms and may reduce infections. HIV viral load measurements are now being used to calibrate anti-viral therapies to provide optimal disease prognosis.

Improved detection and treatment of bacterial STI has been demonstrated to effectively reduce HIV transmission [19]. In addition, treatment for such infections in persons co-infected with HIV may reduce HIV genital shedding and subsequent HIV transmission to sex partners.

CONCLUSIONS

The association between some cancers (*e.g.* hepatocellular, cervical, other genital) and sexual behavior is strong. This suggests that clinicians, researchers, and policymakers need to more fully recognize STVIs as causes of cancer. Effective behavioral strategies including test-based client counseling, small group interventions, school-based STVI education, training of community opinion leaders, mass media, and social marketing can reduce risky sexual behaviors. In addition, the hepatitis B vaccine should be widely promoted as a primary prevention strategy to reduce HBV infection. Other biomedical interventions including early detection and treatment of STVI offer substantial promise in the prevention of STVI-associated cancers. Combination behavioral and biomedical STVI prevention strategies will be necessary to reduce viral prevalence in communities, akin to using combination therapies to attack viral infections and cancers in individuals.

SUMMARY POINTS

- STVI are important and preventable causes of cancer.
- Sexual behaviors engaged in early in life may affect cancer risk many years later.

- Primary prevention of STVI acquisition can be enhanced by delaying the onset of sexual activity; abstaining from sex with individuals not known to be infection-free; consistently using latex condoms, and being vaccinated against HBV.
- Secondary prevention of some STVI-related cancers is possible through screening, early detection, and early treatment.

RECOMMENDATIONS

- Health providers should proactively inquire about risky sexual behaviors and provide client-centered counseling to reinforce safer sexual practices.
- Community leaders should be recruited to help change sexual norms and promote healthier sexuality.
- Policymakers must provide leadership and resources to make healthy sexual behaviors a standard part of cancer prevention strategies.

SUGGESTED FURTHER READING

1. Institute of Medicine (1997) *The Hidden Epidemic: Confronting Sexually Transmitted Diseases.* Washington, DC: National Academy Press.
2. Choi KH, Coates TJ (1994) Prevention of HIV infection. *AIDS* **8**: 1371-1389.
3. Holmes KK, ed. (1999) *Sexually Transmitted Diseases, Third Edition.* New York, NY (USA): McGraw Hill.

REFERENCES

1. zur Hausen H. Viruses in human tumors – reminiscences and perspectives (1996) *Adv Cancer Res* **68**: 1-22.
2. Doll R, Peto R (1981) The causes of cancer: quantitative estimates of avoidable risk of cancer in the United States today. *J Natl Cancer Inst* **66**: 1196-1308
3. International Agency for Research on Cancer Ad Hoc Working Group (1995) Human Papillomaviruses. In: *IARC Monograph Evaluating Carcinogenic Risks in Humans. Volume 64.* Lyon, France: IARC.
4. International Agency for Research on Cancer Ad Hoc Working Group (1994) Hepatitis Viruses. In: *IARC Monograph Evaluating Carcinogenic Risks in Humans, Vol 59.* Lyon, France: IARC.

5. International Agency for Research on Cancer Ad Hoc Working Group (1996) Human Immunodeficiency Viruses and Human T-Cell Lymphotropic Viruses. In: *IARC Monograph Evaluating Carcinogenic Risks in Humans, Vol 67* Lyon, France: IARC.

6. Evans AS, Mueller NE (1990) Viruses and cancer - causal associations. *Ann Epidemiol* **1**: 71-92.

7. Centers for Disease Control (1998) Recommendations for prevention and control of Hepatitis C virus (HCV) infection and HCV-related chronic disease. *MMWR Morb Mortal Wkly Rep* **47**(RR-19): 1-39.

8. Chow WC, Ng HS (1997) Hepatitis C, E and G virus – three new viruses identified by molecular biological technique in the last decade. *Ann Acad Med* **26**: 682-686.

9. Stoler MH (1996) A brief synopsis of the role of human papillomaviruses in cervical carcinogenesis. *Am J Obstet Gynecol* **175**: 1091-1098.

10. Lorincz AT, Reid R, Jenson AB, *et al.* (1992) Human papillomavirus infection of the cervix: relative risk associations of 15 common anogenital types. *Obstet Gynecol* **79**: 328-337.

11. American Cancer Society (1998) *Cancer Facts and Figures.* Altanta, GA: American Cancer Society.

12. Sitas F, Carrara H, Beral V, *et al.* (1999) Antibodies against Human Herpesvirus 8 in black South African patients with cancer. *N Engl J Med* **340**: 1863.

13. Moore PS, Chang Y (1995) Detection of herpesvirus-like DNA sequences in Kaposi's sarcoma in patients with and without HIV infection. *N Engl J Med* **332**: 1181-1185.

14. Cesarman E, Chang Y, Moore PS, *et al.* (1995) Kaposi's sarcoma-associated herpesvirus-like DNA sequences in AIDS-related body-cavity-based lymphomas. *N Engl J Med* **332**: 1186-1191.

15. Cates W (1999) Estimates of the incidence and prevalence of sexually transmitted diseases in the United States. *Sex Transm Dis* **26**(Suppl): S2-S7.

16. Rylander E, Ruusuvaara L, Almstromer MW, *et al.* (1994) The absence of vaginal human papillomavirus 16 DNA in women who have not experienced sexual intercourse. *Obstet Gynecol* **83**: 735-737.

17. Stone KM, Zaidi A, Rosero-Bixby L, *et al.* (1995) Sexual behavior, sexually transmitted diseases, and risk of cervical cancer. *Epidemiology* **6**: 409-414.

18. Palefsky J (1991) Human papillomavirus infection among HIV-infected individuals. Implications for development of malignant tumors. *Hematol Oncol Clin North Am* **5**: 357-370.

19. U.S. Institute Of Medicine (1997) *The Hidden Epidemic: Confronting Sexually Transmitted Diseases.* Washington, DC: National Academy Press.

20. U.S. Preventive Services Task Force (1996) *Guide to Clinical Preventive Services.* Baltimore, MD: Williams & Wilkins.

21. Higgins DL, Galavotti C, O'Reilly KR, *et al.* (1991) Evidence for the effects of HIV-antibody counseling and testing on risk behaviors. *JAMA* **266**: 2419-2429.

22. Choi KH, Coates TJ (1994) Prevention of HIV infection. *AIDS* **8**: 1371-1389.

23. Coates T, Sangiwa, Balmer D, *et al.* (1998) Voluntary HIV Counseling and Testing (VCT) *Reduces Risk Behavior in Developing Countries: Results from the Voluntary Counseling and Testing Study.* Geneva, Switzerland: 12th Int Conf AIDS, June 28-July 3.

24. Kamb MK, Fishbein M, Douglas JM, *et al.* (1998) Efficacy of risk-reduction counseling to prevent human immunodeficiency virus and sexually transmitted diseases. *JAMA* **280**: 1161-1167.

25. NIMH Multisite HIV Prevention Trial Group (1998) The NIMH Multisite HIV Prevention Trial: reducing HIV sexual risk behavior. *Science* **280**: 1889-1894.

26. Shain RN, Piper JM, Newton ER, *et al.* (1999) A randomized, controlled trial of a behavioral intervention to prevent sexually transmitted disease among minority women. *N Engl J Med* **340:** 93-100.
27. Peterson JL, Coates TJ, Catania J, *et al.* (1996) Evaluation of an HIV risk reduction intervention among African-American homosexual and bisexual men. *AIDS* **10:** 319-325.
28. McFarland W, Machekano R, Mzezewa V, *et al.* Impact of a workplace peer education program on HIV incidence in Zimbabwean factories. (Submitted for publication).
29. CDC AIDS Community Demonstration Projects Research Group (1999) Community-level HIV intervention in 5 cities: final outcome data from the CDC AIDS Community Demonstration Projects. *Am J Public Health* **89:** 336-345.
30. Sweat MD, Denison JA (1995) Reducing HIV incidence in developing countries with structural and environmental interventions. *AIDS* **9**(Suppl A): S251-257.
31. Jilg W (1998) Novel hepatitis B vaccines. *Vaccine* **16**(Suppl S): S65-S68.
32. McCrory DC, Matchar DB, Bastian LA, *et al.* (1999) Evaluation of cervical cytology. *Evidence Report/Technology Assessment No. 5. (Prepared by Duke University under Contract No. 290-97-0014.) AHCPR Publication No. 99-E010.* Rockville, MD (USA): Agency for Health Care Policy and Research.
33. Lytle CD, Routson LB, Seaborn GB, *et al.* (1997) An *in vitro* evaluation of condoms as barriers to a small virus. *Sex Transm Dis* **24:** 161-164.
34. Costello Daly C, Helling-Geise GE, Mati JK, Hunter DJ (1994) Contraceptive methods and the transmission of HIV: implications for family planning. *Genitourin Med* **70:** 110-117.
35. Fontanet AL, Saba J, Chandelying V, *et al.* (1998) Protection against sexually transmitted diseases by granting sex workers in Thailand the choice of using the male or female condom: results from a randomized controlled trial. *AIDS* **12:** 1851-1859.
36. Soper DE, Shoupe D, Shangold GA, *et al.* (1993) Prevention of vaginal trichomoniasis by compliant use of the female condom. *Sex Transm Dis* **20:** 137-139.
37. Manos MM, Kinney WK, Hurley LB, *et al.* (1999) Identifying women with cervical neoplasia: using human papillomavirus DNA testing for equivocal Papanicolaou results. *JAMA* **281:** 1605-1610.
38. University of Zimbabwe/JHPIEGO Cervical Cancer Project (1999) Visual inspection with acetic acid for cervical-cancer screening: test qualities in a primary-care setting. *Lancet* **353:** 869-873.
39. Hoofnagle JH, Di Bisceglia AM (1997) The treatment of chronic viral hepatitis. *N Engl J Med* **336:** 347-356
40. Hutchison JG, Gordon SC, Schiff ER, Shiffman ML, Lee WM Rustgi VK, *et al.* (1998) Interferon alfa-2b alone or in combination with ribavirin as initial treatment for chronic hepatitis C. *N Engl J Med* **339:** 1485-1492.
41. Davis GL, Estaban-Mur R, Rustgi V, Hoefs J, Gordon SC, Trepo C *et al.* (1998) Interferon alfa-2b alone or in combination with ribavirin for the treatment of relapse of chronic hepatitis C. *N Engl J Med* **339:** 1493-1499

Chapter 20

Reducing Alcohol Intake

William DeJong, Ph.D. and Laura Gomberg, M.S.
Department of Health and Social Behavior, Harvard School of Public Health, Boston, MA and Education Development Center, Inc., Newton, MA

INTRODUCTION

Alcohol contributes to a wide range of medical and health problems, including certain cancers. Use of alcoholic beverages interacts with tobacco smoking in the causation of cancers of the upper respiratory and gastro-intestinal tracts. In addition, alcohol alone is implicated in cirrhosis-mediated hepatocellular cancer and cancer of the upper alimentary tracts, including the oral cavity, pharynx, larynx, esophagus, and liver, and may also cause cancer of the breast and the large bowel [1, 2].

To minimize cancer risk, heavy alcohol consumption should be avoided. Current guidelines define "moderate" drinking as two or fewer drinks per day for men and no more than one drink per day for women [3]. Women in particular should be cautious about their level of alcohol consumption since alcohol may be involved in the etiology of breast cancer [4]. Indeed, women who are at high risk for breast cancer, for example, because of family history, should avoid drinking alcohol entirely [1].

1. AN ENVIRONMENTAL APPROACH TO PREVENTION

Recent alcohol control efforts in the U.S. have been motivated primarily by concerns about youth drinking and the role of alcohol in homicides, suicides, and traffic crashes. What has emerged from this work is a clearer understanding that measures to reduce average alcohol consumption in the

253

general population are an effective means of reducing the percentage of people consuming at excessive levels, who are at greatest risk for long-term alcohol-related problems, including cancer [5].

Previously, efforts to reduce alcohol problems were guided by the paradigm of interventive medicine, which focuses on the identification and treatment of alcoholics or dependent drinkers in need of care [6]. An unavoidable shortcoming of this approach is that many people who would benefit from intervention will not be identified through traditional screening methods. Even so, this approach has a common-sense appeal: resources are directed to extreme drinkers, while leaving unaffected the majority of drinkers not identified as being at special risk.

Despite its appeal, the interventionist approach is limited in what it can achieve. A chief reason is that the negative consequences of drinking, while more probable among diagnosed alcoholics, are also found among non-dependent drinkers. Prevention experts have noted, in fact, that the majority of alcohol-related problems associated with acute intoxication are caused by non-dependent drinkers, whose vast numbers greatly exceed those of dependent drinkers [5, 7].

The search for an alternative strategy is informed by the observation, described by Edwards and his colleagues [5], of "a relationship between the overall level of alcohol consumption in society and population rates of diverse types of damage, including somatic diseases resulting from long-term heavy drinking, accidents following acute intoxication, and criminal violence and suicide" (p. 102). An implication of this relationship is that a moderate change in alcohol consumption by the population as a whole might greatly reduce the prevalence of heavy drinking and the number of related problems [6].

The question, then, is how to bring about a population-wide change in alcohol consumption. Alcoholism and problem drinking are commonly viewed in the U.S. as problems that arise out of human weakness. Accordingly, traditional prevention efforts have been directed at individuals, primarily in the form of educational messages designed to increase awareness about the dangers of heavy alcohol consumption. Such education programs are an insufficient preventive measure, for they leave unaltered the many societal factors that drive alcohol consumption and its negative consequences.

Recent prevention work in public health has been guided by a social ecological framework, which recognizes that health-related behavior is affected through multiple levels of influence: intrapersonal factors, interpersonal processes, institutional factors, community factors, and public policy [8]. In the case of alcohol consumption, several factors contribute to heavy alcohol consumption, including advertising that portrays drinking as a means to achieve popularity and social acceptance; liquor stores that fail to check for proof-of-age identification; bars that offer "happy hours" and other low-price promotions or serve intoxicated patrons; and lax enforcement of local, state, and federal laws.

Momentum is now building for a more comprehensive prevention approach, one that moves beyond traditional educational messages about the dangers of alcohol abuse to bring about changes in the environment in which people make decisions about their alcohol consumption. At the core of this environmental approach is a thoughtful analysis of the physical, social, economic, and legal environment that affects alcohol use, followed by outcome-driven strategic planning for institutional, community, and public policy change that reshapes the environment in order to discourage high-risk drinking [9]. As described below, evaluation studies have shown that community-based prevention projects that focus on environmental change can reduce alcohol consumption and alcohol-related problems [10, 11].

2.   AN OVERVIEW OF PREVENTION STRATEGIES

2.1   School-Based Education

The best school-based education programs to reduce alcohol consumption by youth are similar to those found to be effective in smoking prevention, with a focus on changing perceived norms about alcohol consumption, recognizing social pressures to drink, and teaching specific skills for resisting those pressures. Developed primarily for elementary and middle school students, the strongest programs include homework assignments with parents, use of interactive teaching methods, and repeat or "booster" sessions as children grow older [12]. As is the case for smoking prevention, most educators endorse the idea that alcohol education should be part of a comprehensive school health curriculum, rather than a stand-alone program [11].

2.2   Mass Media Campaigns

Mass media campaigns have a potentially important role to play in reducing alcohol consumption. Nearly all U.S. national campaigns have focused on drunk driving prevention, however, not on alcohol consumption *per se*, with youth-oriented campaigns by the National Council on Alcoholism and Drug Dependence and the U.S. Department of Health and Human Services being notable exceptions. These campaigns have relied for the most part on donated airtime. While voters in California, Massachusetts, and other states have approved increased tobacco excise taxes to fund anti-tobacco media campaigns, a similar California referendum to increase alcohol excise taxes failed to pass in 1990.

Media campaigns directed to youth should emphasize many of the same themes recommended for anti-tobacco campaigns: (1) present peer role models who are independent, mature, and popular and have made the decision not to drink; (2) create reactance against the marketing strategies used by alcohol companies to influence young people; (3) focus on consequences of alcohol use that are immediate and have a high probability of occurrence; and (4) teach youth how to recognize social pressures to use alcohol and demonstrate specific techniques for resisting those pressures. As is the case with tobacco, mass media campaigns can also be used to enhance school and community programs, encourage public debate on policy initiatives to reduce alcohol consumption, and publicize new laws and regulations or increased enforcement [13].

2.3   Social Norms Marketing Campaigns

Several prevention programs on college and university campuses have used mass media campaigns to try to change the social environment regarding alcohol consumption. Principal among these efforts has been social norms marketing campaigns. These campaigns are grounded in the observation that students tend to overestimate the number of their peers who drink heavily [14]. To the extent this misperception drives normative expectations about alcohol use, and to the extent those expectations drive actual consumption, it is important that steps be taken to correct the misperception [15].

Campaign planners have hypothesized that telling students about the true level of alcohol consumption will correct misperceptions, change normative expectations, and then reduce both students' intention to engage in high-risk drinking and their subsequent alcohol consumption. Although more definitive research is needed, preliminary evaluation results suggest that this strategy may be effective in changing perceived norms of alcohol consumption and in changing actual levels of consumption on campus [16]. Whether such a campaign might work in the general population has not yet been tested.

2.4   Restrictions on Alcohol Advertising

Few prevention advocates have called for outright bans on alcohol advertising, but have instead pushed for advertising reform that would moderate its influence on youth, problem drinkers, and other vulnerable populations. One suggested reform, for example, is to end beverage alcohol advertising that portrays drinking as a means to achieve popularity or social acceptance, sexual appeal, or social or financial status [17]. Prevention advocates have renewed calls for the Federal Communications Commission to require television and radio stations to run prevention counter-advertising in proportion to the amount of paid alcohol advertising that the stations carry. Another proposal is to require broadcast ads for alcohol to include warning information, similar to what is presently required for container warning labels. Local marketing is also of concern. Several jurisdictions have moved to prohibit "happy hours" and other reduced-price alcohol promotions.

2.5   Increased Alcohol Excise Taxes

The demand for alcohol is price sensitive, meaning that as alcohol becomes more expensive, consumption drops. For this reason, prevention advocates have promoted increased alcohol excise taxes as an effective strategy for reducing alcohol-related problems. According to one recent review of the literature, heavy and dependent drinkers appear to be as responsive to price as more moderate drinkers [18].

Alcohol excise taxes have not kept pace with inflation, nor have they been equalized for alcohol content across the categories of beer, wine, and distilled spirits. Prevention advocates have called for substantial excise tax increases for beer and wine to match the levels by alcohol content now applied to distilled spirits and for all alcohol excise taxes to be indexed to inflation.

Increased excise taxes serve another function: they provide revenue that may be designated to fund comprehensive, community-based campaigns for effective alcohol control. Just as excise taxes on cigarettes and legal settlements arising from state-sponsored lawsuits have been used to fund state-level tobacco control programs, alcohol excise taxes may also be used to provide an infrastructure on which alcohol control programs may be built. Thus, alcohol excise taxes may both directly influence alcohol intake by providing a price barrier to accessing alcohol, and by contributing funds for other community or state-level prevention programming.

To create a climate of support for higher alcohol excise taxes, prevention advocates should increase public understanding of the following facts: (1) alcohol is an addictive drug; (2) alcohol has a sizeable impact on mortality, morbidity, and economic productivity; and (3) higher alcohol excise taxes are a way to compensate for alcohol's costs to society and to protect youth.

2.6   Restrictions on Alcohol Availability

Prohibition was a failed experiment in the U.S. It succeeded in reducing alcohol-related problems but eventually lost public support because of the continued demand for alcohol products and the underground economy that developed to supply them [19]. In more recent years, the U.S. and other countries have implemented several measures to control the availability of alcohol, based on the idea that making access to alcohol less convenient will discourage underage drinking and excessive consumption. Such measures include restricting sales to government-run monopolies, limiting the number and location of alcohol outlets to reduce their density, and restricting the hours and days of sale, all of which have been demonstrated to reduce consumption levels [18].

Minimum drinking age laws are another key measure for reducing alcohol availability among youth. In the U.S., when President Reagan signed the National Minimum Drinking Age Act of 1984, the states were required to raise their minimum drinking age to 21. Any state that failed to comply by 1986 risked the withholding of federal highway funds. All 50 states complied. According to the National Highway Traffic Safety Administration, age 21 laws across the country have saved over 16,000 lives since 1975 [20].

Lax enforcement of the age 21 law continues to be a weak link in community-based prevention. An increased law enforcement presence, including the use of "decoy" operations, is key. There are other measures to consider that could enhance compliance with the law: (1) use of distinctive and tamper-proof licenses for drivers under age 21; (2) "use and lose" laws that impose driver's license penalties on minors who purchase or are found in possession of alcohol; (3) keg registration or other limits on large container sales; and (4) increased penalties for illegal service to minors [21].

2.7   Responsible Beverage Service

Responsible beverage service (RBS) programs have three goals: (1) to prevent alcohol service to minors, (2) to reduce the likelihood of drinkers becoming intoxicated; and (3) to prevent those who are impaired from driving [22]. Evaluations of formal programs to train managers and servers in RBS have shown them to be effective. Customers benefit from the lower risk environment, which creates a positive social outing. Alcohol outlets benefit by training their staff in RBS practices, which decreases liability and improves business. The community benefits from decreased alcohol-related problems. RBS programs can be installed by individual alcohol outlets, but they are more effective when implemented community-wide.

3.   **COMMUNITY-BASED PREVENTION
       CAMPAIGNS**

Alcohol prevention advocates are learning that a comprehensive approach works best. The wisdom of such an approach has been reinforced by new research demonstrating the potential power of community-based coalitions to eliminate mixed message environments that invite irresponsible alcohol use.

One group of investigators worked with three experimental communities, two in California and one in South Carolina, to organize citizen-led programs for more effective community control of alcohol [10]. The programs entailed three key elements: (1) changes in local zoning ordinances to reduce the density of alcohol sales outlets, (2) a community-wide program for responsible beverage service, and (3) enhanced police enforcement of the DUI and age 21 laws. The responsible beverage service program centered around the development of alcohol service policies by bars and restaurants, coupled with training of alcohol beverage servers. Clerks at alcohol sales outlets also received training in how to check for legal proof of age. Enforcement of the age 21 law was enhanced through police officer training and increased budget allocations. Police also conducted monthly sobriety checkpoints to apprehend drunk drivers and used passive alcohol sensors during routine traffic stops. In the program communities, relative to three comparison communities, alcohol sales to minors were cut by half, and there was a 10 percent reduction in nighttime traffic crashes involving a single vehicle (a surrogate measure for alcohol-related crashes).

Encouragement is also found in a recent evaluation of Project Northland, a community-wide prevention program conducted in 24 school districts in northeastern Minnesota [11]. The program targeted the class of 1998, which was in sixth-grade when the study began in 1991. The intervention has four key components: (1) social-behavioral curricula in the schools; (2) peer leadership programs; (3) parental involvement and education programs; and (4) community-wide task forces to deal with local policy and enforcement issues. After three years, students in the intervention school districts reported less onset and prevalence of alcohol use than did students in comparison districts. The defining characteristic of the Northland project is the comprehensiveness of its approach, which has led to changes in public policy and a consistent no-use message for youth.

CONCLUSIONS

Alcohol remains the drug of choice for American young people. Among high school seniors, the reported prevalence of "binge drinking" (five or more drinks in a row) declined from 41 percent in 1983 to 28 percent in 1993, but then increased to 30 percent in 1995 [23]. Heavy alcohol consumption, far beyond the accepted guidelines for "moderate" drinking, remains a significant problem among adults, too. Thus, the challenge of reducing alcohol-related problems through lower alcohol consumption remains a formidable one.

Fortunately, there is a great deal known about how good prevention work can be done. What these last few years have taught, however, is that the fight against underage drinking and alcohol abuse cannot be put on "automatic pilot" or simply relegated to the schools alone. The entire community must remain vigilant, active, and focused, even when alcohol usage trends become favorable. The most dangerous time, perhaps, is when policy makers or the public begin to think that the problem is solved and the public agenda turns elsewhere.

The future of alcohol control is a comprehensive, community-based approach that includes the following: (1) formation and support of local coalitions that work for change in the physical, social, economic, and legal environment that shapes alcohol consumption; (2) rigorous and well-publicized enforcement of existing laws and regulations; (3) mass media campaigns to communicate moderate drinking social norms and expectations; (4) education programs to support individual change and to gain widespread support for new alcohol-control policies; and (5) installation of systems for early identification, referral, and treatment of people with alcohol-related problems.

SUMMARY POINTS

- School-based prevention education needs to be reinforced through a community-based coalition that seeks restrictions on irresponsible alcohol advertising and marketing, strict enforcement of laws to reduce youth access, and new policies to reduce alcohol availability, including higher excise taxes.
- In addition to providing direct prevention messages, mass media campaigns can be used to shift social norms regarding alcohol consumption, enhance school and community programs, encourage public debate on policy initiatives to reduce alcohol consumption, and publicize new laws and regulations or increased enforcement efforts.

- Community-wide responsible beverage service (RBS) programs can be effective in preventing alcohol service to minors, decreasing the number of patrons who become intoxicated, and preventing those who are impaired from driving.

RECOMMENDATIONS

- Alcohol control programs should go beyond awareness and education to bring about basic change at the institutional, community, and public policy level to create an environment that discourages underage drinking and excessive alcohol consumption.
- Public health advocates should work for a wide range of policy initiatives to reduce the availability of alcohol, strongly enforce minimum age laws, eliminate irresponsible advertising and marketing practices, and require responsible beverage service programs.
- Public health advocates should look to increased alcohol excise taxes to fund comprehensive community-based campaigns for effective alcohol control.

SUGGESTED FURTHER READING

1. Edwards G, *et al.* (1994) *Alcohol Policy and the Public Good.* New York, NY (USA): Oxford University Press.
2. U.S. Department of Health and Human Services (1997) *Secretary's Youth Substance Abuse Prevention Initiative: Resource Papers.* Rockville, MD: U.S. Department of Health and Human Services, Substance Abuse and Mental Health Services Administration, Center for Substance Abuse Prevention.
3. U.S. Department of Health and Human Services (1997) *Ninth Special Report to the U.S. Congress on Alcohol and Health.* Bethesda, MD (USA): U.S. Department of Health and Human Services, Public Health Service, National Institute on Alcohol Abuse and Alcoholism.

REFERENCES

1. Colditz G, DeJong W, Hunter D, Trichopoulos D, Willett W, eds. (1996) Harvard Report on Cancer Prevention (Vol. 1): Causes of Human Cancer. *Cancer Causes Control* 7 (Suppl).

2. Ringborg U (1998) Alcohol and risk of cancer. *Alcohol Clin Exp Res* **22**(Suppl): 323S-328S.
3. *Healthy Women, Healthy Lifestyles: What You Need to Know about Alcohol and Illicit Drugs*. (1997) Rockville, MD: U.S. Department of Health and Human Services, Substance Abuse and Mental Health Services Administration, Center for Substance Abuse Prevention.
4. Smith-Warner SA, Spiegelman D, Yaun SS, *et al.* (1998) Alcohol and breast cancer in women: a pooled analysis of cohort studies. *JAMA* **279:** 535-540.
5. Edwards G (1994) *Alcohol Policy and the Public Good.* New York, NY (USA): Oxford University Press.
6. Rose G (1992) *The Strategy of Preventive Medicine.* Oxford (UK): Oxford University Press.
7. Mangione TW, Howland J, Lee M. Alcohol and work: results from a corporate drinking study. In: Isaacs SL, Knickman JR, eds. (1998) *To Improve Health and Health Care, 1998-1999.* San Francisco, CA (USA): Jossey-Bass Publishers.
8. Stokols D (1996) Translating social ecological theory into guidelines for community health promotion. *Am J Health Promot* **10:** 282-298.
9. DeJong W, Vince-Whitman C, Colthurst T, *et al.* (1998) *Environmental Management: A Comprehensive Strategy for Reducing Alcohol and Other Drug Use on College Campuses.* Washington, DC: U.S. Department of Education, Higher Education Center for Alcohol and Other Drug Prevention.
10. Holder HD, Saltz RF, Grube JW, *et al.* (1997) A community prevention trial to reduce alcohol-involved accidental injury and death: overview. *Addiction* **92**(Suppl 2): 155-172.
11. Perry CL, Williams CL, Veblen-Mortenson S, *et al.* (1996) Project Northland: Outcomes of a communitywide alcohol use prevention program during early adolescence. *Am J Public Health* **86:** 956-965.
12. Kumpfer K (1997) What works in the prevention of drug abuse: Individual, school, and family approaches. In: U.S. Department of Health and Human Services. *Secretary's Youth Substance Abuse Prevention Initiative: Resource Papers.* Rockville, MD (USA): U.S. Department of Health and Human Services, Substance Abuse and Mental Health Services Administration, Center for Substance Abuse Prevention.
13. DeJong W, Russell A (1995) MADD's position on alcohol advertising: a response to Marshall and Oleson. *J Public Health Policy* **16:** 231-238.
14. DeJong W, Atkin CK (1995) A review of national television PSA campaigns for preventing alcohol-impaired driving, 1987-1992. *J Public Health Policy* **16:** 59-80.
15. Perkins HW, Wechsler H (1996) Variation in perceived college drinking norms and its impact on alcohol abuse: a nationwide study. *J Drug Issues* **26:** 961–974.
16. Perkins HW, Berkowitz AD (1986) Perceiving the community norms of alcohol use among students: some research implications for campus alcohol education programming. *Int J Addict* **21:** 961–976.
17. Haines MP, Spear S (1996) Changing the perception of the norm: a strategy to decrease binge drinking among college students. *J Am Coll Health* **45:** 134–140.
18. Stewart K. Environmentally oriented alcohol prevention policies for young adults (1997) In: U.S. Department of Health and Human Services. *Secretary's Youth Substance Abuse Prevention Initiative: Resource Papers.* Rockville, MD (USA): U.S. Department of Health and Human Services, Substance Abuse and Mental Health Services Administration, Center for Substance Abuse Prevention
19. Heath DB (1996) The war on drugs as a metaphor in American culture. In: Bickel WK, DeGrandpre RJ, eds. *Drug Policy and Human Nature: Psychological Perspectives on the*

Prevention, Management, and Treatment Illicit Drug Abuse. New York, NY (USA): Plenum Press.

20. National Highway Traffic Safety Administration (1997) *Traffic Safety Facts 1996: A Compilation of Motor Vehicle Crash Data from the Fatal Accident Reporting System and the General Estimates System.* Washington, DC: U.S. Department of Transportation, National Highway Traffic Safety Administration, National Center for Statistics and Analysis.

21. DeJong W, Hingson R (1998) Strategies to reduce driving under the influence of alcohol. *Annu Rev Public Health* **19:** 359-378.

22. Mosher JF (1991) *Responsible Beverage Service: An Implementation Handbook for Communities.* Palo Alto, CA (USA): Health Promotion Resource Center, Stanford University.

23. National Institute on Drug Abuse (1997) *Preventing Drug Use Among Children and Adolescents: A Research-Based Guide.* Bethesda, MD (USA): U.S. Department of Health and Human Services, Public Health Service, National Institute on Drug Abuse.

Chapter 21

Maximizing Cancer Risk Reduction Efforts: Addressing Multiple Risk Factors Simultaneously

Karen M. Emmons, Ph.D. and Elyse Park, Ph.D.
Dana-Farber Cancer Institute, and Harvard School of Public Health, Boston, MA

INTRODUCTION

As other chapters in this book aptly demonstrate, it is well documented that lifestyle behaviors such as smoking, low consumption of fruits and vegetables, lack of physical activity, sun exposure, and unprotected sex, contribute significantly to cancer morbidity. The recent Harvard Report on Cancer Prevention [1] concluded that at least one-half of all cancer deaths can be linked to modifiable behaviors. Further, failure to adhere to cancer screening guidelines can lead to increased cancer morbidity. In the case of both skin and colorectal cancer, screening can detect pre-malignant precursors, and thus failure to be screened can lead to increased cancer morbidity.

Significant gains have been made in improving the health behaviors of the U.S. population. For example, average fruit and vegetable consumption has increased significantly [2]. There has been a dramatic reduction in smoking prevalence in the U.S. over the past 20 years, as well a significant change in social norms related to smoking [3, 4]. An increasingly intolerant attitude towards smoking is evidenced by the large increases in restrictions on public smoking, local regulations regarding smoking, and restriction of smoking in both public and private sector workplaces. Increasingly, the public's attention is being drawn to the importance of sun protection and physical activity, both through national media campaigns [5], and through commercial advertising campaigns focused on selling products to enhance health (*e.g.,* sunscreen, athletic shoes, and equipment). Recent research has led to the discovery of human papilloma virus (HPV) as a primary cause of

G.A. Colditz et al. (eds.), Cancer Prevention: The Causes and Prevention of Cancer - Volume I, 265–279.
© 2000 *Kluwer Academic Publishers.*

cervical cancer, and efforts have begun to educate women about strategies for reducing risk of contracting this preventable cause of cancer.

Despite the increased focus on prevention, the U.S. population still does not have a high level of adherence to cancer prevention guidelines. About 25 percent of the U.S. adult population smokes and only 20 to 30 percent of adults meet or exceed the recommended guidelines for consumption of fruit and vegetables [6-8]. Between 24 to 29 percent of the U.S. adult population report that they do not participate in any physical activity; only about 22 percent of the population reports participating in sustained leisure time activity [9, 10]. About 75 percent of U.S. adults do not regularly use sunscreen at recommended levels during maximal recreational sun exposure [11]. Prevalence of risk factors for cervical cancer, including smoking, having multiple lifetime sexual partners and lack of pap screening tests are unacceptably high [12, 13].

1.   EFFECTIVE APPROACHES TO RISK REDUCTION

There has been a large body of research focused on reducing the prevalence of behavioral risk factors for cancer and identifying the most effective strategies for achieving lasting behavior change. Comprehensive intervention strategies that combine individual change programs, environmental strategies, and policy initiatives are considered to be necessary to make significant and lasting changes in most health behaviors [14, 15]. For example, states that have developed strong tobacco control programs have experienced significant reductions in smoking prevalence, compared to states that have not undertaken such efforts [16-18]. Seventeen states are participating in The American Stop Smoking Intervention Study (ASSIST), a National Cancer Institute demonstration trial targeting policy and population-based tobacco control interventions. Cigarette consumption has been reduced significantly in ASSIST states compared to non-ASSIST states [19]. Media-based interventions and tobacco excise taxes are typically cornerstones of state-level interventions [20].

The importance of environmental interventions is underscored by dietary interventions that target a variety of settings, including schools and workplaces [21]. Most dietary interventions target individual food consumption behavior, and also utilize environmental interventions to increase access to healthy food choices. Many restaurants now utilize point-of-purchase strategies to identify healthy alternatives in their menus, and the National Cancer Institute's 5-A-Day campaign has engaged many supermarket chains in actively promoting fruit and vegetable consumption. Physical activity is another area in which environmental and policy initiatives are likely to be of great importance. Given the large numbers of families in which both parents work or the primary care provider works, many people find little time for exercise. An additional challenge is that, among low-income populations, safe opportunities to exercise are quite limited. Therefore, environmental strategies that provide more opportunities for physical activity in daily life (*e.g.,* sidewalks and bike paths), and those that promote both physical activity as a form of transportation and provide easy opportunities for physical activity (*e.g.,* providing and promoting use of safe, well-lit stairwells), are likely to play an important role in efforts to increase the prevalence of physical activity in the U.S. To date, there have been few evaluations of such interventions [22]. Regulatory and environmental interventions have also been proposed as an important strategy for the prevention of sexually-transmitted cancers, although there has been relatively little emphasis on these types of strategies for a variety of sociopolitical reasons [23]. When utilized, regulatory strategies appear to be quite effective [24].

Effective strategies for encouraging change in behavioral cancer risk factors are available, although continued effort is needed to develop strategies that achieve larger and more lasting effects, and that are cost-effective [14, 25].

2. PREVALENCE OF MULTIPLE RISK FACTORS FOR CANCER

Much of the research focused on behavioral risk factors for cancer has focused on risk factors as separate entities, without consideration of either the impact that having one risk factor (*e.g.* smoking) may have on the likelihood of changing other risk factors (*e.g.* physical inactivity), or the intervention implications of targeting multiple behaviors simultaneously. Further, although the chronic disease risk conferred by each behavioral risk factor independently is significant, disease risk increases even further among individuals who have more than one risk factor [26-31].

There have been several reports on the prevalence of multiple risk factors for chronic disease. An examination of risk factor data collected among women on the Behavioral Risk Factor Surveillance System (BRFSS) revealed that 30 percent of respondents had two or more risk factors for cardiovascular disease (risk factors included hypertension, high blood cholesterol, diabetes, overweight, and current smoking) [32]. The finding that the prevalence of multiple CVD risk factors increased in 1995, compared with 1992, was of particular concern. Multiple risk factor prevalence was highest among older women, black women, those with less education, and those experiencing cost as a barrier to care. A second study based on 1993 BRFSS data revealed important differences among women in multiple risk factor prevalence based on age and ethnicity. Risk factors studied included smoking, obesity, diabetes, heavy alcohol consumption, sedentary lifestyle, seat belt use, consumption of fruit and vegetables, mammography, colorectal screening, and immunizations. Among women ages 18 to 49, after adjusting for education and income, the odds ratio of having three or more risk factors was 1.9 for white women, 2.2 for black women, and 3.4 for American-Indian women, compared to the referent group of Asian women. Similar trends were found in women ages 50 to 64, although the odds ratios were substantially higher than that found among the younger women (2.3, 5.1, and 7.0, respectively). Asians and Pacific Islanders had the lowest prevalence for multiple risk factors, for 7 of the 11 individual risk factors.

Studies conducted among defined populations have revealed similar results. For example, a study of adults working in manufacturing settings revealed that less than ten percent of the sample had none of the studied risk factors, which included smoking, physical inactivity, and consumption of less than five servings of fruits and vegetables per day; about one-third of the workers had one of these risk factors, about half had two risk factors, and 15 percent had all three [33]. It has been found that risk factors tend to cluster, in that smokers are more likely to have multiple behavioral risk factors, and individuals who do not smoke are less likely to have other risk factors [34-40]. Important relationships have been found in how people think about their different health behaviors. People who rate the *negative* consequences of smoking highly are also more likely to rate the *positive* benefits of exercise highly [41]. In addition, individuals who feel confident in their ability to engage in regular physical activity are also more confident in their ability to quit smoking.

Additional research has revealed that, when risk factors co-occur, they are largely unchanging under naturalistic conditions [42, 34]. A study addressing longitudinal change in multiple risk factors over a two and a half year observation period found that over 60 percent of manufacturing workers had two or more risk factors at baseline, and that there was only a small, but significant reduction in the overall mean number of risk factors reported at the worksite level by the final assessment [33]. However, when movement within risk factor categories was examined, there was considerable movement over time; between 25 percent to 48 percent of individuals with varying numbers of risk factors at baseline reduced their risk factor index score by follow-up. Of note, there was also considerable regression in risk factor scores over time, with 13 percent of the sample experiencing an increase in their risk factor score over the study period. Individuals who had

0 or 1 risk factor at baseline were especially vulnerable to relapse. Closer examination of the relationship between risk factors indicated that individuals who did not change a risk factor were more likely to have the other two risk factors. This was true for each of the three risk factors when examined separately. However, the level of change in the risk factor index scores did not vary based on whether the target risk factor was changed, suggesting that change in the risk factors was occurring independently. Examination of demographic and cognitive factors that might predict change in risk factor status did not reveal any significant predictors of change.

There are also a few studies available that examine clustering of cancer *screening* behaviors. For example, breast self-examinations are more frequently performed by women who also have regular Pap smear tests [43]. Having had a mammography screening has also been found to be associated with recency of clinical breast examination, and Pap smear testing, and regularity of breast self-examination [44-46]. Screeners were less likely to smoke and more likely to exercise [47].

3.   TRACKING OF MULTIPLE RISK FACTOR PREVALENCE FROM YOUTH TO ADULTHOOD

Recent data suggests that multiple behavioral risk factors are also prevalent in adolescents [42]. Several studies have demonstrated that cancer risk factors begin to cluster in adolescence, and that these health behavior patterns continue into adulthood [48-50]. Among youth, low levels of physical activity have been found to be associated with cigarette smoking, marijuana use, lower fruit and vegetable consumption, greater television watching, and failure to wear a seat belt [42]. As early as sixth grade, healthy eating and physical activity patterns emerge that appear to be related [49]. Beginning in eighth grade, students who have lower activity patterns and make fewer healthy food choices have a higher smoking prevalence. A dose-dependent relationship has been found between increasing levels of cigarette smoking and increased frequency of binge drinking among students grades five to twelve [51]; the likelihood of using drugs also increased with frequency of cigarette smoking.

One study indicated that a multidimensional risk structure, producing five behavioral clusters, underlies adolescent health behavior [52]. Perceived poor academic performance, no participation in sports, and low fruit and vegetable consumption comprised one cluster; not participating in aerobic activity comprised another. One cluster consisted of self-destructive behaviors including injection drug use, steroid use, suicidal behavior, cocaine and crack use, fighting, and carrying a weapon. Another grouping involved unsupervised swimming, using smokeless tobacco, riding a motorcycle without a helmet and unsafe dieting. The last group was behaviors of normative adolescent risk taking including smoking, drinking, marijuana use, and driving drunk or riding with a drunk driver. In intervening to change or prevent adolescent risk behavior, different approaches are needed for different sets of behaviors; this seems particularly applicable to behaviors involving preventive action and behaviors involving health risk.

The association between multiple risk factors has been observed to strengthen over time, particularly during early to late adolescence [53]. Behavior patterns demonstrated in the sixth grade consistently increased throughout high school; students separated into high and low-risk behavior groups and maintained this ranking, over time. The transition from adolescence into young adulthood involves further changes in health behaviors, primarily in the direction of increasing cancer risk [50, 54]. Patterns of co-occurrence of risk behaviors have been documented [50, 55-58].

4.   THE IMPACT OF MULTIPLE RISK FACTOR INTERVENTIONS FOR CANCER PREVENTION

For the past several years, there has been an increased emphasis on changing multiple risk factors for cancer in defined populations (*e.g.*, worksite-based interventions for diet and smoking), rather than focusing interventions exclusively on one risk factor. However, despite the multiple risk factor intervention focus, outcome evaluations tend to target change in each behavioral risk factor as a separate entity [14, 59]. There are several reasons why it is important to begin to more systemically address the relationships between behavioral risk factors in the context of intervention research, and to examine the associated impact of change in multiple risk factors on cancer morbidity and mortality. First, as noted earlier, behavioral cancer risk factors are highly interrelated; as a result, intervention on one behavior is likely to effect others, whether it is an intentional component of the intervention or not. Second, many of the target behaviors for cancer prevention can be classified as either cessation or acquisition behaviors (*e.g.*, smoking cessation *vs.* initiation of physical activity); these two types of behaviors may have counter-acting reinforcement properties, and therefore be utilized simultaneously to initiate and sustain the change process. Finally, cognitions about the change process have been found to be related across risk factors [60], which suggests that there may be considerable economy of scale in targeting multiple risk factors simultaneously.

5.   WORKSITE MULTIPLE RISK FACTOR INTERVENTIONS

Worksites offer an important opportunity to implement multiple risk factor interventions. Emmons, *et al.* [61] evaluated the impact of a two and half year worksite-based intervention on change in multiple risk factor status among 1267 employees in 24 manufacturing worksites. The intervention targeted fruit and vegetable consumption, physical activity, and smoking (details on the intervention and the study methodology are provided elsewhere [59]. A *categorical risk factor index* was computed in order to evaluate the relationships between the three risk factors [34, 59]. The risk factor index categorizations were based on standard guidelines for preventive health behaviors, including smoking status (smoker *vs.* nonsmoker), consumption of fewer than five servings of fruits and vegetables per day, and exercising less than 20 minutes three times per week. Subjects were assigned a score of 1 if they had a risk factor and a score of 0 if they did not have that risk factor. The three individual risk factor scores were then summed to yield the categorical multiple risk factor score (0 = no risk factors; 3 = all risk factors). Because the categorical risk factor index may ultimately mask more subtle behavior changes over time, a second multiple risk factor index was developed that treats each of the risk factors as a continuous variable, based on the approach of Gomel and colleague [62]. Thus, it was possible to examine the number of fruits and vegetables consumed per day and minutes per week engaged in regular exercise. In order to obtain a continuous assessment of smoking risk, we utilized number of cigarettes smoked per day, given that there is a linear relationship between amount smoked and health risk; nonsmokers were assigned a score of "0" for the smoking risk factor. Each risk factor variable was then standardized separately to produce a z-score for each participant; a constant was added to the smoking risk factor score (baseline constant =-.37581; final constant = -.30103) in order for nonsmokers to receive a score of "0" on this variable [62]. A *standardized multiple risk factor index score* was then obtained by summing the individual risk factor z-scores. Outcome analyses revealed significantly greater decreases in both the categorical and standardized multiple risk factor index for the intervention condition, compared to controls [61].

A cardiovascular risk reduction program was run with twenty-eight worksites in Australia [62, 63]. The worksites were randomized into one of four conditions: health risk assessment, risk factor education, behavioral counseling, or behavioral counseling plus incentives. At the 12-month follow-up, the behavioral counseling condition yielded significantly more change on two measures of multiple risk factors (a multiple logistic function equation and a composite standardized outcome measure), compared to the other conditions.

There is evidence available to suggest that participation in an intensive physical activity program as part of a smoking cessation intervention yields increased smoking cessation and maintenance rates [64, 65]. These results suggest that physical activity can be an important strategy for enhancing smoking cessation rates. It also appears that leisure time activity may increase among smokers who quit [66, 67]. Results from the British Family Heart Study revealed that a family-centered risk reduction program led to a 16 percent reduction in coronary risk scores [68].

5.1   Multiple Risk Factor Interventions in Primary Care Settings

Physicians are in a unique role to impact on multiple cancer risk factors among their patients. Their own attitudes, beliefs and personal health practices may affect physician-counseling behavior. In a sample of 134 community-based primary care physicians, the relationship between self-reported physician counseling behavior across four targeted preventive behaviors – smoking, diet, skin cancer and mammography was examined [69]. Confidence was the most consistent indicator of physicians' delivery of the counseling for all four behaviors. Another study investigated frequency of physicians' advice for twelve cancer risk behaviors including smoking, nutrition, sun protection, physical activity, and screening examinations [70]. Frequency of physician advice was high for female screening behaviors and lowest for skin examination and sigmoidoscopy. Older patients, with poorer perceived health were more likely to receive counseling. Similar findings have been documented in other studies, as has the general finding that only a relatively small portion of patients at risk of developing cancer receives preventive interventions across risk factors delivered [71]. Overall, very few studies have been conducted to examine multiple risk factor interventions in primary care settings. This is an area where substantial research is needed.

CONCLUSIONS

There have been several recent recommendations that health promotion interventions should focus on identifying effective interventions for reducing multiple risk factor prevalence [72, 73, 40]. Intervention strategies that have been found to be effective for targeting individual risk factors may also work well for targeting multiple risk factors simultaneously. However, the outcome evaluations of multiple risk factor intervention trials are typically based on change in single risk factors, and thus there is a relatively limited body of literature available from which to evaluate the outcomes of such interventions on multiple risk factor profiles. Consequently, there are many questions that remain about how to best effect change on multiple risk factors.

Key questions that need to be addressed through further research include an examination of whether multiple risk factors should be addressed simultaneously (*e.g.*, target change in diet and physical activity at the same time) or sequentially (*e.g.*, once dietary goals have been met, then work on physical activity goals). In the context of sequential interventions, the optimal order in which risk factors should be addressed is currently not known (*e.g.*, is it best to start with physical activity or with dietary changes?). Further, it is unclear which risk factor combinations would lead to the best outcomes. Several studies have demonstrated relationships between diet and physical activity. Other studies have documented the relationship between smoking and physical inactivity, and at least one study has documented increased smoking cessation outcomes among women who were also enrolled in a physical activity program. Studies are needed that determine the optimal number of risk factors that should be targeted, and the types of risk targets that yield the best outcomes. Evaluations of long-term outcomes are also needed to determine if multiple risk factor interventions have differential effects on long-term maintenance of behavior change, and whether changes in multiple risk factors are more or less vulnerable to relapse. The cost-effectiveness of multiple risk factor interventions also needs to be demonstrated.

Another area, which has not been the focus of much evaluation, is the role of race and ethnicity in risk factor clustering. It is important to understand how individuals' cultural backgrounds may influence prevalence of multiple cancer risk behaviors [74]. Research is also needed to determine the best channels for delivering multiple risk factor interventions. A number of interventions have been conducted in worksites and schools, and these settings may be particularly well suited to such interventions because they can include both individual and environmental/policy interventions. Research on adolescent health behaviors suggests that further work is needed to determine the optimal strategies for reducing prevalence of multiple risk factors in children and adolescents. School-based health education programs should be coordinated to infuse multiple healthy behaviors throughout the curriculum, instead of presented as single health behavior topics (*e.g.*, physical activity in gym class, nutrition in home economics) [53, 22].

It has been recommended that physician-delivered interventions begin to address multiple risk factors [72], although integrated approaches that can be applied with most patients are needed. Clinical care practice guidelines have traditionally been focused on individual risk factors [75], and thus may not be helpful for health care providers in implementing multiple risk factor interventions. The trend of health care toward HMOs and managed care systems could potentially lead to more effective implementation and monitoring of preventive services targeting multiple risk factors [76]. Managed care services are under pressure to demonstrate higher screening and early detection rates, and higher rates of delivery of smoking cessation interventions. Health care quality implementation mechanisms, such as the HEDIS report card, may be one mechanism for beginning to incorporate a multiple risk factor approach into primary care delivery. HEDIS is a report on the performance of HMOs and includes estimates for the delivery of screening mammography, Pap tests, and advising smokers to quit. HEDIS reports may be an ideal mechanism for tracking the co-occurrence of risk factor interventions it the health care setting, and for encouraging providers to consider multiple risk factor counseling [77]. Future research should also examine the effectiveness of brief interventions, such as those that can be delivered *via* channels such as the primary care setting on multiple risk factor change.

SUMMARY POINTS

- There is emerging evidence that suggests that multiple risk factor interventions may be effective strategies for improving overall cancer risk in U.S. adults.
- Further research is needed to determine the optimal intervention approaches, the cost-effectiveness of multiple risk factor interventions, and the long-term impact of multiple risk factor change on cancer morbidity and mortality.

RECOMMENDATIONS

- Further work is needed to determine how to best improve upon the level of effectiveness of existing interventions, and to disseminate the best strategies.
- Considerable research is needed to determine how best to impact on multiple behavioral risk factors simultaneously, which would maximize both public health resources and impact on disease prevention.
- By working together with communities to develop and implement initiatives to maximize community members' health behaviors across

risk factors, public health researchers can make a significant impact on cancer risk in the U.S.

SUGGESTED FURTHER READING

1. Colditz GA, DeJong D, Hunter DJ, Trichopoulos D, Willett WC, eds. (1996) Harvard Report on Cancer Prevention. Volume 1. Causes of Human Cancer. *Cancer Causes Control* 7(Suppl): 1-59.
2. Emmons KM, Linnan L, Shadel W, Marcus BH, Abrams DB (1999) The Working Healthy Trial: A worksite health promotion program targeting physical activity, diet, and smoking. *J Occup Environ Med* 41(7): 545-555.
3. Emmons KM, Shadel WG, Linnan L, Marcus BH, Abrams DB (1999) A prospective analysis of change in multiple risk factors for cancer. *Cancer Res Therapy Control* 8: 15-23.

REFERENCES

1. Colditz GA, DeJong D, Hunter DJ, Trichopoulos D, Willett WC, eds. (1996) Harvard Report on Cancer Prevention. Volume 1. Causes of Human Cancer. *Cancer Causes Control* 7(Suppl): 1-59.
2. U.S. Dep. Agriculture ARS (1996) Food consumption, prices and expenditures, 1996: annual data 1970-1994. *Stat Bull. No. 928.*
3. Centers for Disease Control and Prevention (1991) Cigarette smoking among adults–United States, 1991. *MMWR Morb Mortal Wkly Rep* 42: 230-33.
4. Centers for Disease Control and Prevention (1996) Cigarette smoking among adults–United States. *MMWR Morb Mortal Wkly Rep* 45: 588-590.
5. Abroms L, Jorgenson CJ, Emmons KM, *et al.* Gender differences in young adults' attitudes towards sun protection (submitted for publication).
6. Serdula MK, Coates RJ, Byers T, *et al.* (1995) Fruit and vegetable intake among adults in 16 states: results if a brief telephone survey. *Am J Public Health* 85: 236-39.
7. Subar AF, Heimendinger J, Krebs-Smith SM, *et al.* Five A Day for better health: a baseline study of American's fruit and vegetable consumption. National Cancer Institute, 1995a.
8. Subar AF, Heimendinger J, Patterson BH, *et al.* (1995) Fruit and vegetable intake in the United States: the baseline survey of the Five A Day for Better Health Program. *Am J Health Promot* 9: 352-60.
9. National Center for Health Statistics, Adams PF, Benson V (1991) *Current estimates from the National Health Interview Survey, 1990. Vital and Health Statistics, Series 10, No. 181.* Hyattsville, MD: U.S. Department of health and Human Services, Public Health Service, Centers for Disease Control, National Center for health Statistics, DHHS Publication No. (PHS) 92-1509.

10. National Center for Health Statistics, Piani AL, Schoenborn CA (1993) *Health Promotion and Disease Prevention: United States, 1990.* Vital and Health Statistics, Series 10, No. 185. Hyattsville, MD: U.S. Department of Health and Human Services, Public Health Service, Centers for Disease Control and Prevention, National Canter for Health Statistics, DHHS Publication No. (PHS)93-1513.

11. Banks B, Silverman R, Schwartz R, *et al.* (1992) Attitudes of teenagers toward sun exposure and sunscreen use. *Pediatrics* **89:** 40-42.

12. Perez-Stable EJ, Marin G, Marin BV (1994) Behavioral risk factors: a comparison of Latinos and non-Latino whites in San Francisco. *Am J Public Health* **84:** 971-6.

13. Sugarek NJ, Deyo RA, Holmes BC (1988) Locus of control and beliefs about cancer in a multi-ethnic clinic population. *Oncol Nurs Forum* **15:** 481-486.

14. Sorensen G, Emmons KM, Hunt MK, *et al.* (1998) Implications of the results of community intervention trials. *Annu Rev Public Health* **19:** 379-416.

15. Ockene JK, Emmons KM, Mermelstein R, *et al.* Functions related to the maintenance of smoking cessation. (In press).

16. Emmons KM, Kawachi I, Barclay G (1997) Tobacco control: a brief review of its history and prospects for the future. *Hematol Oncol Clin North Am* **11:** 177-195.

17. Hu T, Sung H, Keeler TE (1995) Reducing cigarette consumption in California: Tobacco taxes vs. an anti-smoking media campaign. *Am J Public Health* **85:** 1218-1222.

18. Harris JE, Connolly GN, Brooks D, Davis B (1996) Cigarette smoking before and after an excise tax increase and an anti-smoking campaign: Massachusetts, 1990-1996. *MMWR Morb Mortal Wkly Rep* **45:** 966-970.

19. Manley MW, Pierce JP, Gilpin EA, *et al.* (1997) Impact of the American Stop Smoking Intervention Study (ASSIST) on cigarette consumption. *Tob Control* **6**(Suppl 2): S12-S16.

20. DeJong W (1997) Prevention of Tobacco Use. *Cancer Causes Control* **8**(Suppl): S5-S8.

21. Glanz K (1997) Dietary Change. *Cancer Causes Control* **8**(Suppl): S13-S16.

22. Gortmaker S, Mariani A, Peterson K, *et al.* (1997) Exercise. *Cancer Causes Control* **8**(Suppl): S17-S19.

23. Morrison C, Schwingl PJ, Cates W Jr (1997) Sexual behavior and cancer prevention. *Cancer Causes Control* **8**(Suppl): S21-S25.

24. Sweat MD, Dennison JA (1995) Reducing HIV incidence in developing countries with structural and environmental interventions. *AIDS* **9**(Suppl A): S251-257.

25. Baranowski T, Davis M, Resnicow K, *et al.* Gimme 5 fruit and vegetables for fun and health: outcome evaluation. *Am J Health Promot* (In press).

26. Berglund G, Eriksson KF, Israelsson B, *et al.* (1996) Cardiovascular risk groups and mortality in an urban Swedish male population: the Malmo Preventive Project. *J Intern Med* **239:** 489-97.

27. Taylor V, Robson J, Evans S (1992) Risk factors for coronary heart disease: a study in inner London. *Br J Gen Pract* **42:** 377-80.

28. Sebastian JL, McKinney WP, Young MJ (1989) Epidemiology and interaction of risk factors in cardiovascular disease. *Prim Care* **16:** 31-47.

29. Kannel WB (1989) Risk factors in hypertension. *J Cardiovasc Pharmacol* **13**(Suppl 1): S4-10.

30. Anderson KM, Wilson PWF, Odell PM, *et al.* (1991) An updated coronary risk profile. A statement for health professionals. *Circulation* **83:** 356.

31. Criqui MH, Barrett-Connor E, Holdbrook MJ, *et al.* (1980) Clustering of cardiovascular disease risk factors. *Prev Med* **9:** 525.

32. Greenlund KJ, Giles WH, Keenan NL, *et al.* (1998) Prevalence of multiple cardiovascular disease risk factors among women in the United States, 1992 and 1995: the Behavioral Risk Factor Surveillance System. *J Womens Health* **7**: 1125-33.

33. Emmons KM, Shadel WG, Linnan L, *et al.* (1999) A prospective analysis in multiple risk factors for cancer. *Cancer Res Therapy Control* **8**: 15-23.

34. Emmons KM, Marcus BH, Linnan L, *et al.* (1994) Mechanisms in multiple risk factor interventions: Smoking, physical activity, and dietary fat intake among manufacturing workers. *Prev Med* **23**: 481-89.

35. Perkins KA, Rohay J, Meilahn EN, *et al.* (1993) Diet, alcohol, and physical activity as a function of smoking status in middle-aged women. *Health Psychol* **12**: 410-15.

36. Morabia A, Wynder EL (1990) Dietary habits of smokers, people who never smoked, and ex-smokers. *Am J Clin Nutr* **52**: 933-37.

37. Klesges RC, Eck LH, Isbell TR, *et al.* (1990) Smoking status: effects on the dietary intake, physical activity, and body fat of adult men. *Am J Clin Nutr* **51**: 784-89.

38. Marks BL, Perkins KA, Metz KF, *et al.* (1991) Effects of smoking status on content of caloric intake and energy expenditure. *Int J Eat Disord* **10**: 441-49.

39. Dallongeville J, Maracaux N, Fruchart JC, *et al.* (1998) Cigarette smoking is associated with unhealthy patterns of nutrient intake: a meta-analysis. *J Nutr* **128**: 1450-57.

40. Simoes EJ, Byers T, Coates RJ, *et al.* (1995) The association between leisure-time physical activity and dietary fat in American adults. *Am J Public Health* **85**: 240-44.

41. King T, Marcus BH, Pinto B, *et al.* (1996) Cognitive-behavioral mediators of changing multiple behaviors: smoking and a sedentary lifestyle. *Prev Med* **25**: 684-691.

42. Pate RR, Heath FW, Dowda M, *et al.* (1996) Associations between physical activity and other health behaviors in a representative sample of U.S. adolescents. *Am J Public Health* **86**: 1577-1581.

43. Murray M, McMillan C (1993) Health beliefs, locus of control, emotional control and women's cancer screening behavior. *Br J Clin Psychol* **32**: 87-100.

44. Pearlman DN, Rakowski W, Ehrich B, *et al.* (1996) Breast cancer screening practices among black, Hispanic, and white women: reassessing differences. *Am J Prev Med* **12**: 327-37.

45. Pearlman DN, Rakowski W, Ehrich B (1996) Mammography, clinical breast exam, and pap testing: correlates of combined screening. *Am J Prev Med* **12**: 52-64.

46. Rakowski W, Pearlman D, Rimer BK, *et al.* (1995) Correlates of mammography among women with low and high socioeconomic resources. *Prev Med* **24**: 149-58.

47. Rakowski W, Rimer BK, Bryant SA (1993) Integrating behavior and intention regarding mammography by respondents in the 1990 National Health Interview Study of Health Promotion and Disease Prevention. *Public Health Rep* **108**: 605-24.

48. Hedberg VA, Bracken AC, Stashwick CA (1999) Long-term consequences of adolescent health behaviors: implications for adolescent health services. *Adolesc Med* **10**: 137-51.

49. Kelder SH, Perry CL, Klepp KI, *et al.* (1994) Longitudinal tracking of adolescent smoking, physical activity, and food choice behaviors. *Am J Public Health* **84**: 1121-26.

50. Baranowski T, Cullen KW, Basen-Engquist K, *et al.* (1997) Transitions out of high school: time of increased cancer risk? *Prev Med* **26**: 694-703.

51. Torabi MR, Bailey WJ, Majd-Jabbari M (1993) Cigarette smoking as a predictor of alcohol and other drug use by children and adolescents: evidence of the "Gateway Drug Effect." *J School Health* **63**: 302-6.

52. Basen-Engquist K, Edmundson EW, Parcel GS (1996) Structure of health risk behavior among high school students. *J Consult Clin Psychol* **64**: 764-75.

53. Lytle LA, Kelder SH, Perry CL, *et al.* (1995) Covariance of adolescent health behaviors: the class of 1989 study. *Health Educ Res* **10**: 133-46.

54. Dinger MK, Waigandt A (1997) Dietary intake and physical activity behaviors of male and female college students. *Am J Health Promot* **1**: 360-62.

55. Emmons KM, Wechsler H, Dowdall G, *et al.* (1998) Predictors of smoking among U.S. college students. *Am J Public Health* **88**: 104-7.

56. Zabin LD (1984) The association between smoking and sexual behavior among teens in U.S. contraceptive clinics. *Am J Public Health* **74**: 261-3.

57. Millstein SG, Irvins CE Jr, Adler NE, *et al.* (1992) Health Risk Behaviors and Health Concerns Among Young Adolescents. *Pediatrics* **89**: 422-8.

58. Fisher M, Rosenfeld WD, Burk RD (1991) Cervicovaginal human papillomavirus infection in suburban adolescents and young adults. *J Pediatr* **119**: 821-5.

59. Emmons KM, Linnan LA, Shadel WG, *et al.* (1999) The Working Healthy Project: a worksite health promotion trial targeting physical activity, diet, and smoking. *J Occup Environ Med* **41**: 545-555.

60. King TK, Matacin M, Bock BC, *et al.* (1997) *Body Image Evaluations in Women Smokers.* Poster presentation. Miami, FL: The 31st annual meeting of the Association for the Advancement of Behavior Therapy, November.

61. Emmons KM, Shadel WG, Linnan L, *et al.* The impact of a worksite health promotion intervention on multiple risk factors for cancer. (Submitted for publication).

62. Gomel MK, Oldenburg B, Simpson JM, *et al.* (1997) Composite cardiovascular risk outcomes of a work-site intervention trial. *Am J Public Health* **87**: 673-76.

63. Gomel M, Oldenburg B, Simpson JM, *et al.* (1993) Work-site cardiovascular risk reduction: a randomized trial of health risk assessment, education, counseling, and incentives. *Am J Public Health* **83**: 1231-38.

64. Marcus BH, Albrecht AE, King TK, *et al.* (1999) The efficacy of exercise as an aid for smoking cessation in women: a randomized controlled trial. *Arch Intern Med* **159**: 1229-34

65. Marcus BH, Albrecht AE, Niaura RS, *et al.* (1991) Usefulness of physical exercise for maintaining smoking cessation in women. *Am J Cardiol* **68**: 406-7.

66. French SA, Hennrikus DJ, Jeffery RW (1996) Smoking status, dietary intake, and physical activity in a sample or working adults. *Health Psychol* **15**: 448-454.

67. Perkins AK, Rohay J, Meilahn EN, *et al.* (1993) Diet, alcohol, and physical activity as a function of smoking status in middle-aged women. *Health Psychol* **12**: 410-415.

68. Family Heart Study Group (1994) Randomised controlled trial evaluating cardiovascular screening and intervention in general practice: principal results of British family heart study. *Br Med J* **308**: 313-20.

69. Park E., DePue JD, Goldstein MG, *et al.* (1998) Predisposing attitudes to physicians counseling behaviors across multiple cancer risk factors. Poster presentation at the Society for Behavioral Medicine Nineteenth Scientific Sessions, April.

70. Park E, Goldstein M, DePue J, *et al.* (1999) *Predictors of Cancer Prevention Counseling Behavioral Risk Factors.* San Diego, CA: Presentation at the Society for Behavioral Medicine.

71. Heywood A, Sanson-Fisher R, Ring I, *et al.* (1994) Risk prevalence and screening for cancer by general practitioners. *Prev Med* **23**: 152-59.

72. Ockene JD, McBride PE, Sallis JF, *et al.* (1997) Synthesis of lessons learned from cardiopulmonary preventive interventions in healthcare practice settings. *Ann Epidemiol* **7**: S32-S45.

73. Berglund G, Eriksson KF, Israelsson B, *et al.* (1998) Cardiovascular risk groups and mortality in an urban Swedish male population: the Malmo Preventive Project. *J Intern Med* **236:** 489-97.

74. Hahn RA, Heath GW, Chang MH (1994) Cardiovascular disease risk factors and preventive practices among adults - United States, 1994: a behavioral risk factor atlas. *MMWR Morbid Mortal Wkly Rep* **47:** 35-69.

75. Fiore MC, Bailey WC, Cohen SJ, *et al.* (1995) *Smoking cessation: Clinical Practice Guideline No. 18.* Bethesda, MD: U.S. Department of Public Health and Human Services, Public health Service, Agency for Health Care Policy and Research, AHCPR #96-0692.

76. McIntosh H (1995) Managed care takes control of prevention and control. *J Natl Cancer Inst* **87:** 955-58.

77. Use of clinical preventive services by adults aged <65 years enrolled in health-maintenance organizations – United States, 1996 (1998) *MMWR Morb Mortal Wkly Rep* **47:** 613-19.

Chapter 22

Prevention of Work-Related Cancers

Anthony D. LaMontagne, Sc.D., M.A., M.Ed. and David C. Christiani, M.D., M.P.H., M.S.
Dana-Farber Cancer Institute, Boston, MA, Occupational Health Program, Harvard School of Public Health, and Harvard Medical School,Boston MA

INTRODUCTION

The first discovered cause of cancer also spurred some of the first preventive interventions. Soon after his 1775 report of excess scrotal cancers in young chimney sweeps, Percival Pott made some suggestions to prevent such cancers. He recommended that chimney sweeps, who usually swept naked so as not to soil their only set of clothes, be given a second set of clothes and not be allowed to sweep naked. He also recommended that sweeps be allowed to wash after cleaning each chimney. The interventions recommended by Pott and others were opposed in England well into the next century, and excess scrotal cancers among chimney sweeps continued [1, 2]. Pott's recommendations were heeded in nearby Holland, however, and scrotal cancers among chimney sweeps decreased [1]. During the same time period in Germany, Sweden, and other parts of continental Europe where sweeping techniques (from above as opposed to from inside), protective clothing, and personal hygiene measures were far superior, scrotal cancers among chimney sweeps were virtually absent.

The lessons of Pott's intervention efforts are as relevant today as they were over 200 years ago. They represent the crux of public health practice: observation, inference, action, and evaluation. In Pott's case, it was an astute clinician's observation that led to the inference that chimney sweeping was associated with scrotal cancers. Today, a range of other possible observers also exist, including workers, health and safety professionals, and regulators. It was not until the early 1900s that the *cause* of scrotal cancer in

G.A. Colditz et al. (eds.), Cancer Prevention: The Causes and Prevention of Cancer - Volume I, 281–300.
© 2000 *Kluwer Academic Publishers.*

chimney sweeps was determined to be absorption of polycyclic aromatic hydrocarbons. Specific knowledge of cause, while always desirable, is not always necessary to effect prevention. Pott's recommendations for action were made on the basis of the best available evidence at the time, and erred in favor of protecting the public's health. In retrospect, we know Pott's recommendations were well conceived. A set of complementary intervention strategies were devised, including clinical measures, primary prevention in the workplace, and regulatory or other policies aimed at ensuring the universal implementation of appropriate preventive measures for all workers in all workplaces. As well as providing a compelling historical anecdote, Pott's story introduces the essential elements of workplace cancer prevention that will be outlined below in this brief overview of the subject.

1. THE PREVENTION OF WORK-RELATED CANCERS

Work-related cancers are highly preventable. Reasons for this include: (1) the availability of well-developed methodologies for exposure prevention and control; (2) the defined social and physical structure for intervention provided by the workplace; (3) the involuntary and undesirable nature of hazardous exposures, which generally precludes the challenges of overcoming addictions or deeply embedded behavioral or social norms (in contrast, for example, to tobacco use); and (4) knowledge of many specific occupational carcinogens as well as many specific jobs and industrial processes that have been associated with excess cancer incidence [3].

Work-related cancers are further distinguished in that the primary responsibility for their prevention rests not with the workers who are affected by such cancers but with the manufacturers and distributors of carcinogenic substances and with the companies who use these substances. These principles are embodied in the U.S. public policies of strict product liability and the Occupational Safety and Health Act of 1970.

Strict product liability states that a material or device manufacturer is strictly liable for physical harm caused by their product to users and consumers. Strict product liability is the basis of 'toxic tort' lawsuits brought by workers due to cancers and other diseases alleged to result from workplace exposures [4]. For example, tens of thousands of suits have been brought by workers against the manufacturers of asbestos (Workers' Compensation laws preempt workers from suing their employers directly, such that they can only sue third parties under strict product liability). The extent to which strict product liability encourages preventive efforts has yet to be systematically assessed, but likely plays an important role in the U.S.

The Occupational Safety and Health Act of 1970 states that "Each employer shall furnish to each of his employees employment and a place of employment which are free from recognized hazards that are causing or are likely to cause death or serious physical harm to his employees" [Public Law 91-596, Section 5(a) (1)]. Thus public law places the primary responsibility for safety and health squarely on the employer. As discussed in further detail below, workers, healthcare providers, and others also have important roles that complement those of the employer in the prevention of work-related cancers.

Prevention strategies for work-related cancers, then, can be broadly divided into three categories: (1) those that should be applied to prevent potentially carcinogenic substances from being marketed and distributed; (2) those that apply in the workplace where potential carcinogens are in use; and (3) public policy interventions aimed at ensuring universal implementation of pre-market and workplace prevention strategies. These are outlined in turn below, with threads of policy included in the first two as well as the last sections.

2. CARCINOGEN IDENTIFICATION

Carcinogen recognition or identification is the enabling step for prevention. Carcinogens can be identified by testing of materials to determine carcinogenicity before or after they enter into commerce, from presenting patients (clinical case series), by epidemiologic study, or by disease surveillance (Table 22.1). Clearly, prediction of carcinogenicity is the most desirable from a preventive perspective. Clinical and epidemiologic identification are discussed in detail in Chapter 5 on the occupational causes of cancer in this volume. Thus, they are discussed only briefly with respect to their essential role in cancer prevention, followed by a more in-depth discussion of pre-market testing and surveillance.

Table 22.1 Strategies for the identification of occupational carcinogens

Strategy	Responsible and Contributing Stakeholders
Pre- and post-market laboratory testing	Chemical manufacturers and distributors, government
Clinical detection	Healthcare providers, workers, unions, employers
Epidemiologic study	Researchers, public health professionals, workers, unions, employers, government
Exposure and disease surveillance	Public health professionals, healthcare providers, workers, unions, government, employers

2.1   Clinical and Epidemiologic

From Percival Pott's time through the 1970s, most occupational carcinogens were initially identified by astute clinicians. These were typically reported as case series [3, 5]. Historically, case series have been the main source of hypotheses for formal epidemiologic study, and were the foundation upon which today's field of occupational and environmental epidemiology was built [5]. More recently, however, clinical identification plays a smaller role in epidemiologic hypothesis generation for a number of reasons [5]. To some degree, complementary means of identification have also developed in recent decades to offset the decrease in clinical identification. These include laboratory testing, prediction of carcinogenicity based on structural similarity to known carcinogens (so-called 'structure-activity relationships'), and disease surveillance systems. Nevertheless, it appears that occupational cancer epidemiology efforts are not commensurate with the continuing extent of the problem [3, 6-8]. An estimated six to ten percent of all cancers are attributable to occupational exposures, representing tens of thousands of preventable deaths each year [8]. The lack of societal concern about occupational cancers is attributable to many factors, including: (1) the majority of the most easily identified occupational carcinogens may be known (*e.g.,* those that cause rare tumors at low doses); (2) there is a dearth of exposure data on workplace carcinogens; and (3) our disease surveillance systems are generally weak on detecting occupational cancers and other diseases. As has been demonstrated by innovative investigators, some of these challenges can be surmounted with new methods for exposure assessment, expanded sample sizes in epidemiologic studies, and better integration of occupational epidemiology with public health surveillance efforts [9]. These same methods offer promise for assessing the complex risk-enhancing as well as protective interactions between occupational and non-occupational exposures (such as tobacco use and dietary patterns). Ongoing epidemiologic efforts are needed to support prevention and control interventions from the workplace to the national policy level.

2.2   Laboratory testing

An essential complement to *post hoc* clinical or epidemiologic identification of occupational carcinogens is the prediction of carcinogenicity and other adverse health effects through pre-market laboratory testing. Numerous *in vitro* and *in vivo* laboratory tests of genotoxicity and carcinogenicity have been developed for this purpose. Such tests are ideally conducted before a substance is introduced into commerce; however, they are also useful for further assessing suspect humans carcinogens [3, 5]. For examples, case series and early epidemiologic studies for both vinyl chloride (angiosarcoma of the liver) and beta-naphthylamine (bladder cancer) were supported by subsequent demonstration of the clear carcinogenicity of these substances in animal studies.

The U.S. government has been conducting a testing program for determining the carcinogenicity of chemicals since 1961. The program was initiated at the National Cancer Institute (NCI), and since 1978, has been conducted as the National Toxicology Program (NTP). NTP conducts animal and other carcinogenesis tests and periodically publishes a comprehensive list of known and suspected human carcinogens in its Biennial Report on Carcinogens (Eighth Edition published in 1998, see http://ntp-server.niehs.nih.gov/). Despite the fact that this is probably the largest such testing program in the world, the NTP can test the carcinogenicity of only a couple of dozen new chemicals each year. Yet, each year, roughly 1000 new chemicals enter commercial markets. In the U.S. free market system, those who bring toxic substances to market – and thus may profit – are supposed bear the cost and responsibility of proving their safety. This principle is reinforced by strict product liability (described above), which should provide further incentive for industry testing efforts. Thus, a system appears to be in place to ensure that manufacturers and distributors of potentially hazardous substances conduct the bulk of pre-market testing. However, as described in detail below, this system is not working.

Because voluntary industry efforts to conduct pre-market testing were deemed inadequate, the U.S. government intervened in the form of the Toxic Substances Control Act (TSCA) of 1976. TSCA (15 U.S.C., section 2601(b)) stated that:

> "It is the policy of the United States that... adequate data should be developed with respect to the effect of chemical substances and mixtures on health and health and the environment and that the development of such data should be the responsibility of those who manufacture and those who process such chemical substances and mixtures."

TSCA gave the Environmental Protection Agency (EPA) the authority to require chemical testing and to impose controls as necessary. The authority of the Act to require pre-market testing, however, has been hampered by numerous weaknesses of the law and has been woefully underutilized [4, 10]. The TSCA also requires reporting of industry studies to the EPA to provide early warning of potential hazards. To date, however, voluntary hazard reporting by industry has been poor.

In a recent move to an "incentive" rather than a regulatory approach to getting companies to report testing data, the EPA granted amnesty (*i.e.*, drastically reduced fines) to companies that had not reported new data to the EPA, as required.   The results were striking: 11,000 never-published scientific studies from 120 companies were handed in to the EPA, including some studies indicating that chemicals on the market today could pose a "substantial risk of injury to health or to the environment" [11].   The drastically reduced penalties for non-reporting still netted a total of over $22 million in fines, but represented the non-collection of hundreds of millions of taxpayer dollars.   Among the studies was one conducted in 1985 that showed an association between a rare type of nasal cancer and exposure to formaldehyde. It was conducted at the same time that the U.S. Occupational Safety and Health Administration (OSHA) was developing a formaldehyde standard and the carcinogenicity of formaldehyde was being hotly debated. In 1985, the EPA was grappling with over whether to classify formaldehyde as a possible human carcinogen, which it did do in 1987.   These findings indicate the need for much stronger measures to ensure both the conduct of testing *and* the timely reporting of results.

Following the passage of TSCA, the National Research Council (NRC) conducted an extensive review to assess the status of toxicity testing efforts [12].   The NRC randomly selected 100 chemicals with production volume greater than one million pounds per year and extrapolated the results of this random sample to the 3000 high production volume chemicals then in use. The NRC concluded that 78 percent of the high production chemicals in U.S. commerce lacked even "minimal toxicity information", a disappointing state of affairs given the ongoing regulatory and other efforts to increase testing.

In the 15 years since the NRC conducted its initial review of pre-market testing efforts, one might reasonably expect that there has been significant progress in this area.   To address this question, the Environmental Defense Fund (EDF) recently replicated the NRC's study [10].   The EDF selected a random sample of chemicals that were *both* high production volume *and* had already been identified as subjects of regulatory attention (approximately 500 of the 75,000 chemicals that the EPA listed as being made in the U.S. in 1996), which EDF described as *high priority* chemicals (thus, the EDF study should err in favor of *overstating* the availability of toxicity information). The results show strikingly little progress since the early 1980s: 71 percent of the sampled high priority chemicals do not meet the minimum data requirements for human toxicity screening set by the Organization for Economic Cooperation (OECD), an international organization made up of the world's 19 wealthiest countries, including the U.S.   This minimum data set includes acute toxicity, repeated dose toxicity, genetic toxicity (*in vitro* and *in vivo*), reproductive toxicity, and development toxicity.   While only 25 percent have not been tested for genetic toxicity, carcinogenicity tests have not been conducted on 63 percent of high priority chemicals.

This continuing lack of toxicity information shows inadequate societal commitment to preventing carcinogenic substances from entering into commerce. As well as raising concerns about health hazards in the workplace, this information deficit raises concerns for consumers and the environment. In addition, ignorance of hazard precludes the development of appropriate workplace control strategies for potential carcinogens that do enter into commercial use. Concerted voluntary efforts, renewed regulatory efforts, and new strategies will be required to narrow this shameful deficit in toxicity testing information.

3. WORKPLACE PREVENTION AND CONTROL STRATEGIES

The prevention and control of exposure to occupational carcinogens is most instructively viewed through the continuum from the source (*e.g.,* raw material or by-product), through dispersion of the carcinogen (*e.g.,* through air), to the target of the carcinogen (*i.e.,* the worker) (Figure 22.1). The goal is to be as far upstream in the causal pathway as possible: preventing exposure (primary prevention) is far more effective and desirable than treating clinical or even pre-clinical disease (secondary and tertiary prevention). In addition, interventions at or near the source of exposure also can help to prevent community exposures through environmental emissions, consumer goods, and the food supply. This continuum is codified in the "hierarchy of controls"-a comprehensive set of exposure prevention and control measures used by occupational health professionals [13]. While the hierarchy provides a prioritized approach to prevention and control, it is often appropriate to combine multiple control strategies.

A complementary prevention framework is the "4 E's": education, engineering/technology, enforcement/regulation, and economic incentives. Some add a fifth "E" for epidemiology/surveillance. This approach was developed by the National Highway Traffic Safety Administration and provides an example of a safety perspective to complement industrial hygiene's 'hierarchy'. While interventions closer to the source are still preferred in this approach, the general strategy is to use as many of the 4 or 5 together as possible. While the hierarchy focuses on the locus of the workplace, the "4 E's" also includes carcinogen identification and policy, which in this chapter are expanded in the sections preceding and following this section on prevention in the workplace. Below, we outline the hierarchy of controls with examples that could also be viewed through the "4 Es" framework.

Effectiveness	Prevention Level	Prevention Target	Hierarchy of Controls
Most Effective	Primary	Control at the Source of Hazard	Elimination Substitution Use Reduction
	Primary	Controlling Dispersion	Engineering Controls (e.g., local exhaust ventilation, process enclosure) Exposure Assessment Administrative Controls (e.g., workplace policies and procedures)
	Primary	Control at the Worker	Safe Work Practices Personal Protective Equipment Biological Monitoring for absorption of a toxicant
	Secondary	Control at the Worker	Pre-clinical medical exams/screening Biological monitoring for effects of absorbed toxicants
Least Effective	Tertiary	Control at the Worker	Diagnosis Therapy Rehabilitation

Figure 22.1 Prevention frameworks

3.1 Control at the Source of Exposure

The first and most effective strategy in the hierarchy of controls is hazard elimination or substitution. The information needed to evaluate the health hazards of a new material or a potential substitute should be available from pre-market toxicology testing such that the introduction of substitutes does not create new hazards. For example, perchloroethylene - a chlorinated organic solvent that has been shown to be carcinogenic in animal studies - is widely used as a dry cleaning agent. Both use reduction technologies and safer substitutes are currently being piloted in dry cleaning establishments around the country [14]. In another example, a process was developed in which small plastic beads are air-blasted at the surface of airplanes to remove old paint, thus eliminating the need for carcinogenic methylene chloride-based paint strippers and cutting the time of removing paint by 80 percent [13].

3.2   Controlling Dispersion

Where carcinogens cannot be eliminated or substituted, process changes and engineering controls can be used to reduce worker exposures to the lowest feasible level. For example, after the discovery in the early 1970s that vinyl chloride monomer exposure was associated with angiosarcoma of the liver in exposed production workers, an OSHA standard was passed in 1975 that reduced the occupational exposure limit from 200 ppm to 1 ppm. In response to this mandate, vinyl chloride reactor systems were redesigned as enclosed systems, which not only met the 1 ppm exposure limit, but also increased productivity and reduced production costs [15]. Local exhaust ventilation can also be adapted to capture carcinogenic emissions in the path between the source and the worker. For instance, the carcinogen ethylene oxide is widely used in hospitals to sterilize heat- and moisture-sensitive medical devices. Since the passage of a 1984 OSHA regulatory standard for ethylene oxide, however, most EtO sterilizers have been manufactured with built-in local exhaust ventilation that greatly reduces exposures [16].

Other means of controlling dispersion include wetting hazardous dusts to prevent suspension in air, the use of safe work practices, and the implementation of appropriate policies and procedures. Whatever means are used, it is crucial to periodically assess exposure levels. Those known or suspected carcinogens that are regulated by OSHA include requirements for exposure monitoring as well as exposure limits in their respective OSHA standards. Voluntary guidelines for exposure monitoring and exposure limits are also available for many non-regulated carcinogens, from groups such as the National Institute for Occupational Safety and Health (NIOSH: see www.cdc.gov/niosh) and the American Conference of Government Industrial Hygienists (ACGIH: see www.acgih.org).

3.3   Control at the Worker

At the level of the worker, the most important interventions are training and education: training in hazard recognition and the appropriate use of engineering and other exposure controls, and participatory education to help workers become active participants in health and safety in their workplaces [13]. Supervisors and managers also need training and education to improve understanding of their roles and responsibilities, and in turn, their effectiveness in fulfilling those roles. Workers, unions, supervisors, and managers can work jointly to protect health and safety through meaningful participation on health and safety committees. The use of personal protective equipment is appropriate to protect workers only where engineering or other exposure controls closer to the source are not feasible [13].

3.4   Pre-clinical Medical Screening or Surveillance

Pre-clinical medical screening or surveillance refers to conducting tests or exams on individuals who may be exposed to hazardous chemicals in the workplace but who show no clinical signs or symptoms of exposure-related disease. For many occupational diseases, detection and initiation of treatment at pre-clinical or early stages can slow or reverse the course of disease (secondary prevention). However, early detection can improve the clinical course of only a few work-related cancers, and thus it plays a minor role in the control of work-related cancers [17]. Pre-clinical screening can be used to prevent the occurrence of cancers through bio-monitoring for markers of susceptibility or the absorption of carcinogens, if coupled with exposure assessment and timely exposure control interventions. Bio-monitoring can also be used to detect early exposure-associated biological effects with known or suspected relationships to cancers. While these technologies are rapidly developing, their effectiveness in conveying survival or quality-of-life benefits to affected patients have yet to be established.

Healthcare providers in all contexts - ranging from specific occupational screenings to primary care - play a crucial, albeit indirect role in occupational cancer prevention through the collection of patients' occupational histories. [3, 5, 18] For example, broad-based improvements in occupational history-taking would strengthen the preventive role of existing surveillance systems (*e.g.,* cancer registries), enhance the detection of new occupational carcinogens, improve the feasibility of occupational epidemiology studies, and support compensation claims for work-related cancers. The continuing deficit in occupational history-taking in general medical practice hampers the detection and thus the prevention of work-related cancers and other diseases. Improved and expanded medical education efforts in this area are needed to rectify this situation. [3, 18].

Although clinical detection of work-related cancers usually confers only limited benefits to affected persons, it still plays an important role in the larger framework of prevention. First, early detection of sentinel occupational disease cases should lead to timely exposure control interventions to prevent cancers in workers in similar jobs [17]. Second, as described above, clinical detection often leads to epidemiologic study. In the U.S., epidemiologic evidence is almost always required to justify the development of occupational regulations for carcinogens [19]. Such regulations, or standards, typically mandate a series of primary and secondary preventive measures following the hierarchy of controls described above. Thus, epidemiologic study (bottom of Figure 22.1) feeds back to stimulate primary preventive interventions (top of Figure 22.1) at the policy and practice level.

4. PUBLIC POLICY

Public policies aimed at preventing or controlling work-related cancers are most conveniently divided into federal, state, and international.

4.1 Federal - OSHA

Ideally, the hierarchy of controls would be implemented voluntarily in all workplaces. However, the history of work-related cancer and other diseases has amply demonstrated the need for regulatory pressure. [3, 19] For example, bladder cancer excesses among aromatic amine dye workers were first documented in an 1895 case report, yet bladder cancers from worker exposures to these substances continue to occur into the 1990s in the U.S. [5, 20]. In fact, using the best available hazard surveillance data, NIOSH found that there was an increase in the number of workers potentially exposed to bladder carcinogens from the 1970s to the 1980s [21].

OSHA was created in 1970 to develop and enforce workplace health and safety standards. OSHA's first set of substance-specific standards targeted fourteen carcinogens, requiring that exposures be reduced to the lowest feasible level using strict exposure controls. Substance-by-substance rulemaking, however, was very slow and inefficient. In 1977, the General Accounting Office estimated that at the prevailing rate it would take OSHA 100 years to regulate the known occupational hazards at that point in time. Many of the same scientific and policy issues arose with each carcinogen rule-making (*e.g.*, level of mechanistic, animal, or epidemiologic evidence required for action).

To address these issues, OSHA promulgated a generic carcinogen policy in 1980 [19]. The Policy detailed a prioritization scheme for known and suspected carcinogens, stated that appropriately-conducted animal experiments could be adequate for regulation even in the absence of epidemiologic data, and determined that limits would be set at the lowest feasible level.   This broad-based, proactive approach was effectively abandoned in 1980, however, after a court challenge to the recently promulgated benzene standard. In a decision that spurred the rapid growth of risk assessment, the Supreme Court ruled that OSHA had to prove that exposures to benzene at the proposed level posed a "significant risk" to employees. "Significant risk", the Supreme Court opinion further stated, "was somewhere in the range of 1/1000 extra lifetime mortality risk". Thus OSHA's well-conceived effort to develop an aggressive occupational cancer prevention policy was derailed, leaving a quantitative risk assessment emphasis and a set of inconsistent and incomplete carcinogen policies to this day [19].

In the 1980s, OSHA's standard-setting for carcinogens and other hazardous chemicals slowed considerably.   OSHA regulated two new workplace carcinogens - ethylene oxide in 1984 and formaldehyde in 1988 - and revised the standards for benzene (after further epidemiologic study and quantitative risk assessment, the benzene standard struck down by the Supreme Court 1980 was passed in 1987) and asbestos (lowering the exposure limit to the level recommended ten years earlier by a joint OSHA and NIOSH committee). A significant gain for workplace cancer prevention in the 1980s, however, was OSHA's Hazard Communication, or "right-to-know" standard.   Hazard Communication established the principle that employees had a right to know about the hazards of materials in their workplace. This included requirements for labeling of hazardous substances, worker training and education, and the listing of NTP and International Agency for Research on Cancer (IARC) classifications of materials on publicly available Material Safety Data Sheets.   While Hazard Communication was a major advance in terms of worker access to information, the standard imposed no exposure limits or other direct protections, and thus represents a much less effective approach to cancer prevention than the Generic Carcinogen Policy of 1980.

In the 1990s, OSHA regulation of workplace carcinogens continues to be slow and hampered by political and other pressures. For example, a final standard on methylene chloride was promulgated in 1997 after almost a decade of OSHA rulemaking and was then immediately challenged in court by industry. The continuing risk assessment emphasis imposed on OSHA dominates   a   cumbersome   and   inefficient   rule-making   process, overshadowing the original emphasis on exposure control embodied in OSHA's first carcinogen standards.   The risk-based exposure limit for asbestos, for example, has been lowered four times through laborious rule-making procedures since it was first set in 1970, while substances such as vinyl bromide and vinylidine chloride (close chemical relatives of vinyl chloride) and para- and meta- toluidine (benzidine-related aromatic amines) await initial rulemaking.

Both OSHA and NIOSH, OSHA's research and development counterpart, have been chronically under-funded and politically hampered in their efforts to prevent and control work-related cancers and other diseases [7, 22]. NIOSH is currently expanding its internal and extramural intervention research programs, ranging from intervention selection and development through effectiveness evaluation, to better demonstrate the need for and impact of interventions ranging from toxics use reduction to national regulatory standards [23]. Practically-oriented intervention research will support the development of maximally effective interventions that are minimally burdensome on industry. Improved support for both OSHA and NIOSH are needed in order to fully realize the prevention of work-related cancers.

4.2   Federal - Bans

The Toxic Substances Control Act (TSCA) described above also grants the EPA authority to ban especially harmful substances. In practice, the banning of substances has been rarely used: only nine chemicals have been removed from commerce or restricted in use under TSCA [10]. Strikingly, this short list does not include asbestos - the occupational carcinogen with the widest known impacts to date. Because of its ability to cause various cancers and other diseases, the EPA initiated efforts in 1984 to phase out asbestos use in the U.S. [4]. The EPA's effort was first rejected by the Office of Management and Budget on a cost-benefit basis, and has been tied up since then in litigation. As a result of these efforts, asbestos use has been greatly restricted but not totally banned in the U.S. By contrast, in the 1980s and 1990s several European countries banned the use of asbestos [24]. Strengthening of TSCA or new regulatory measures are needed to further develop this important policy option. In the interim, aggressive investigation of safer substitutes for known carcinogens - which often makes economic as well as public health sense - would help offset the weakness of the U.S. banning mechanism.

4.3   Federal/State - Surveillance

Improved population-based characterization of patterns of occupational carcinogen exposures and occupational cancers is needed to guide preventive efforts and to support preventive policy development. Yet, occupational disease surveillance systems in the U.S. are poorly developed at the government, industry, and union levels; and state and federal exposure surveillance systems are even less developed [23, 25]. To date, most planning and advocacy efforts have focused on improving disease surveillance [26]. NIOSH has led the development of several innovative state-based occupational disease surveillance systems, some of which are relevant for occupational cancers (*e.g.*, the National Occupational Mortality System). At the federal level, existing incomplete systems such as the Bureau of Labor Statistics Annual survey and OSHA Integrated Management Information System on occupational exposures are severely limited by various design problems [26]. Even small steps such as implementing the systematic collection of detailed occupational histories in existing cancer registries would constitute a significant improvement in the national system [22].

From a prevention perspective exposure surveillance systems hold the potential to identify intervention priorities and demonstrate impacts much sooner and more efficiently than surveillance for work-related cancers. Indeed, demonstration of achievement of stated performance goals by federal government agencies (*e.g.*, OSHA, NIOSH) is becoming increasingly important for Congressional budget authorizations under the Government Results and Performance Act (GPRA), further emphasizing the appropriateness of exposure- over disease surveillance results to demonstrate OSHA and NIOSH progress on five-year performance objectives [25]. Comparing two nationwide cross-sectional exposure, NIOSH found that there was an overall *increase* in the proportion of workers exposed to occupational carcinogens from the 1970s to the 19080s, although there was also an increase in the proportion of appropriate exposure control measures in place for potentially exposed workers in the 1980s [21]. Though no broad-based national exposure survey has been conducted in the 1990s, NIOSH is currently developing expanded plans for a continuous national exposure surveillance system. Such a system would greatly expand opportunities for exposure prevention and control. Finally, exposure surveillance can be readily practiced at the plant level as well as by government or other large entities [27]. Plant-level exposure surveillance provides for the most timely and efficient feedback to primary prevention to control exposures to carcinogens as well as other hazardous agents.

4.4   State - Toxics Use Reduction Initiatives

In the 1990s, more than ten states have passed toxics use reduction laws that mandate or encourage the reduction of toxics use in industry and provide free information and consulting on use reduction technologies and safer substitutes [13]. These programs are purposefully integrated in targeting both reduction of occupational exposures inside plants and environmental exposures in surrounding communities. The 1989 Massachusetts Toxics Use Reduction Act (TURA) was one of the first such policies developed (see http://turi.uml.edu). [13, 14] Since the passage of TURA in 1989, Massachusetts has experienced a 20 percent reduction in the use of toxic chemicals in affected industries. The strong primary prevention orientation of toxics use reduction initiatives provides a hopeful example of new policy developments.

4.5 State - Workers' Compensation

Only a very small percentage of occupational cancers and other diseases are compensated under Workers' Compensation in the U.S. This is enabled in part by the other missing pieces needed (*e.g.*, disease surveillance) to provide a fully functional occupational health system in the U.S. Thus, Workers Compensation policy for the most part fails to either compensate or contribute to the prevention of work-related cancers. By contrast, conservative estimates of total economic costs for fatal occupational diseases show that the greatest losses are caused by cancers, accounting for $9.4 billion in 1992 - fully half of the economic costs of all occupational diseases [28]. Thus, the financial responsibility for occupational cancers is shifted away from Workers' Compensation - where it properly belongs - and exists as a 'hidden tax' in future Medicare and other public expenses [28]. Most importantly, the failure of the compensation and healthcare systems to recognize the costs of occupational cancers precludes recognition of the substantial economic benefits that would result from their prevention.

However small, some hopeful signs of reform exist. For example, several states have adopted presumptive cancer policies for firefighters whereby certain cancers are presumed to have resulted from occupation (*e.g.*, lung) provided certain conditions are met (*e.g.*, worker was not a smoker). Illinois and Wisconsin adapted such policies in the last year. In a related vein, New Mexico recently adopted a resolution urging the U.S. Congress to pass legislation ensuring fair compensation to all uranium miners who have contracted lung cancer and other diseases as a result of their employment (still far short of compensation). Other options for improving occupational cancer compensation include apportionment according to etiologic fractions (*e.g.*, for lung cancers in asbestos-exposed workers who were smokers) and integrating compensation of occupational disease into a national healthcare system [24]. More creatively, some state Workers' Compensation systems have channeled premiums into small primary prevention programs, reasoning that dollars spent on prevention will go much further in addressing occupational disease problems than dollars spent on compensation. Although the level of such funding is small in relation to the size of the problem, it is a move in a positive direction from tertiary to primary prevention (Figure 22.1).

4.6   International

This chapter has thus far focused on the occupational cancer prevention in the U.S. Rapidly industrializing countries face even greater challenges [28]. Public policy pressures and economic globalization have led in some cases to the export of hazardous industries from developed countries to the developing world, a situation reminiscent of the increases in smoking in developing countries that have paralleled decreases in developed countries. For example, declining asbestos production and use in response to regulation in developed countries has been paralleled by rapid increases in developing countries in Asia, Africa, and South America. [24, 29]   To stem the recurrence of the developed world's occupational cancer experience in the world's rapidly industrializing nations, coordinated international efforts are required.

5.   INTEGRATING THE PREVENTION OF WORK- AND LIFESTYLE-RELATED CANCERS

Workers with the highest occupational exposures also tend to have higher cancer and other health risks from non-occupational exposures, such as smoking, poor diet, and low socioeconomic status [30, 31]. These exposures can interact in various ways in the causation of cancer. In addition to being the locus of occupational health efforts, the worksite has been a traditional venue for health promotion interventions targeting personal and social behaviors that increase cancer and other health risks [3, 31].   Low educational status, for example, is one of the strongest risk factors for smoking and also predisposes to employment in higher exposure jobs. Only recently, however, have cross-disciplinary efforts been made to integrate health promotion and occupational health protection [32].

From a health promotion perspective, integrating occupational health concerns with health promotion interventions will likely increase the appeal and credibility of such programs to blue collar workers - one of the most challenging groups to affect with health promotion interventions. This point was made clear in the recent Working Well trial, a large randomized, controlled worksite intervention study conducted in four centers in the U.S. Only one of the study centers integrated occupational health into the intervention targeting tobacco control and diet. That study center was the only one of the four to observe a significant increase in smoking cessation rates [31]. For occupational health, integration with health promotion provides a significant new channel for reaching workers with occupational health messages.

From the worker perspective, job risks and life risks are integrated day-to-day. However, interventionists should attend carefully to the important and delicate distinction between employers being primarily responsible for providing a safe and healthy workplace and employees having primary control over personal and social behaviors. Increasing integration of health promotion, occupational health protection, and other disease prevention efforts will lead to increasingly comprehensive and effective cancer prevention programs. Opportunities for further improvement in this area include: building stronger partnerships with workers and unions; increasing communication among workers, employers, and public health professionals; and improving cross-training among public health disciplines.

CONCLUSIONS

Work-related cancer is highly preventable. Primary prevention of work-related carcinogenic exposures coupled with health promotion interventions are essentially the only tools available for addressing this continuing public health problem. Very few evidence-based tools are available for reducing work-related cancer mortality through secondary or tertiary preventive efforts. Most opportunity for the direct control of exposure to carcinogens in the workplace rests with employers and those who manufacture and distribute carcinogenic substances. Workers, as individuals, also have a role to play in following safe work practices and participating in health and safety activities. Unions, as representatives of workers, have also played a considerable role in stimulating management prevention and control efforts, despite representing a small percentage of American workers. Healthcare providers play essential roles in primary and secondary prevention, and as worker/patient advocates. Government plays an essential role through the dissemination of hazard control information, the promulgation of occupational health standards, and the support of occupational health research and professional training. After a strong start with the creation of OSHA in the 1970s, government and societal efforts to prevent work-related cancers have stalled. Yet, work-related cancer continues to be a large public health problem. Ample strategies are available to identify occupational carcinogens, and prevent and control carcinogenic exposures in the workplace. Yet, Percival Pott's legacy has yet to be fulfilled. The principal barriers to the prevention of work-related cancers today are more political and economic than scientific and medical. Significant increases in societal commitment, political will, and resources are needed to better prevent the thousands of work-related cancers that continue to occur in the U.S. each year.

SUMMARY POINTS

- Occupational cancers are highly preventable through pre-market screening and the application of a systematic hierarchy of controls in the workplace.
- Manufacturers, employers, workers, unions, health care providers, and occupational health professionals all play important roles in workplace cancer prevention.
- Regulatory standard-setting and enforcement are an essential complement to voluntary occupational cancer prevention efforts.
- Occupational cancer prevention efforts must be supported by a fully functional national occupational health system in order to realize their full potential.
- The integration of work-related and lifestyle-related intervention efforts could improve the overall effectiveness of workplace cancer prevention efforts.

RECOMMENDATIONS

- Expanded efforts in pre-market testing are needed to prevent the introduction of carcinogenic substances into general commerce.
- Epidemiologic studies continue to be needed to characterize and control exposures to recognized carcinogens, to identify new occupational carcinogens, and to characterize the interactions between workplace carcinogenic exposures and non-occupational exposures to carcinogenic as well as protective factors.
- Approaches that emphasize controlling workplace carcinogenic exposures to the extent feasible using the hierarchy of controls should be more broadly applied in both workplace and regulatory interventions.
- Expanded efforts in occupational health surveillance, particularly exposure surveillance, are needed to better characterize carcinogenic exposures and to support timely and effective primary prevention.
- Renewed political and budgetary support for OSHA and NIOSH are needed in order to adequately protect workers from preventable work-related cancers.

SUGGESTED FURTHER READING

1. Stellman JM, Stellman SD (1996) Cancer and the workplace. *CA-A Cancer Journal for Clinicians* **46**(2): 70-92.
2. Stellman JM, ed. (1998) *Encyclopaedia of Occupational Health and Safety*. Geneva, International Labour Organization, Volume 4.
3. DiNardi SR, ed. *The Occupational Environment: Its Evaluation and Control*. Fairfax, VA (USA): American Industrial Hygiene Association Press.
4. Levy BS, Wegman DH, eds. *Occupational Health: Recognizing and Preventing Work-Related Disease, Fourth Edition*. Boston: Little, Brown, and Company, (In press).
5. Halperin W, Baker EL, eds. (1992) *Public Health Surveillance*. New York, NY (USA): Van Nostrand Reinhold.

REFERENCES

1. Murray L (1995) Occupational health. In: Blumenthal D, Ruttenber AJ, eds. *Introduction to Environmental Health*. Second Edition ed. New York, NY (USA): Springer Publishing Company, Inc, pp. 275-319.
2. Waldron HA (1983) A brief history of scrotal cancer. *Br J Industrial Med* **40**: 390-401.
3. Landrigan P, Markowitz S, Nicholson W (1995) Cancer prevention in the workplace. In: Greenwald P, Kramer SK, Weed DL, eds. *Cancer Prevention and Control*. New York, NY (USA): Marcel Dekker, Inc., pp. 393-410.
4. Ashford N, Caldart C (1996) *Technology, Law and the Working Environment*. Washington, D.C.: Island Press.
5. Sellers C (1997) Discovering environmental cancer: Wilhelm Hueper, post-World War II epidemiology, and the vanishing clinician's eye. *Am J Public Health* **87**: 1824-1835.
6. Infante P (1991) Viewpoint: prevention versus chemophobia: a defence of rodent carcinogenicity tests. *Lancet* **337**: 538-540.
7. Landrigan P (1993) Cancer research in the workplace. In: President's Cancer Panel Meeting. Bethesda, MD (USA): National Institutes of Health, pp. 224-232.
8. Leigh JP, Markowitz SB, Fahs M, *et al.* (1997) Occupational injury and illness in the United States. Estimates of costs, morbidity, and mortality. *Arch Intern Med* **157**: 1557-1568.
9. Siemiatycki J (1995) Future etiologic research in occupational cancer. *Environ Health Perspect* **103**(Suppl 8): 209-215.
10. EDF (1997) *Toxic Ignorance: The Continuing Absence of Basic Health Testing for Top-Selling Chemicals in the United States*. New York, NY (USA): Environmental Defense Fund.
11. Lavelle M (1997) EPA's Amnesty has become a mixed blessing. *Natl Law J* **1997**: A1-A18.
12. Council NR (1984) *Toxicity Testing--To Determine Needs and Priorities*. Washington DC: National Academy Press.

13. Wegman DH, Levy BS (1995) Preventing occupational disease. In: Wegman DH, Levy BS, eds. *Occupational Health: Recognizing and Preventing Work-Related Disease.* Boston, MA (USA): Little, Brown, and Company, pp. 83-101.

14. Ellenbecker MJ (1996) Engineering controls as an intervention to reduce worker exposure. *Am J Industrial Med* **29:** 303-307.

15. OTA (1985) Chapter 5: Technologies for Controlling Work-Related Illness. In: *Preventing Illness and Injury in the Workplace.* Washington, DC: US Congress, Office of Technology Assessment, pp. 175-185.

16. LaMontagne AD, Kelsey KT (1998) OSHA's renewed mandate for regulatory flexibility review: in support of the 1984 ethylene oxide standard. *Am J Ind Med* **34:** 95-104.

17. Cone JE, Rosenberg J (1990) Medical surveillance and biomonitoring for occupational cancer endpoints. *Occup Med* **5:** 563-581.

18. Institute of Medicine (1988) *Role of the Primary Care Physician in Occupational and Environmental Medicine.* Washington, D.C.: National Academy Press.

19. Robinson JC, Paxman DG (1991) Public health and the law: OSHA's four inconsistent carcinogen policies. *Am J Public Health* **81:** 775-780.

20. Michaels D (1995) When science isn't enough: Wilhelm Hueper, Robert A.M. Case, and the limits of scientific evidence in preventing occupational bladder cancer. Int J Occup Environ Health **1:** 278-288.

21. Griefe A, Halperin W, Groce D, O'Brien D, Pedersen D, Myers JR, Jenkins L (1995) Hazard surveillance: its role in primary prevention of occupational disease and injury. *Appl Occup Environ Hyg* **10:** 737-742.

22. Infante PF (1995) Cancer and blue-collar workers: who cares? *New Solutions* **5:** 52-57.

23. NIOSH (1996) *National Occupational Research Agenda.* Bethesda, MD: U.S. Public Health Service, Centers for Disease Control, National Institute for Occupational Safety and Health.

24. Karjalainen A (1997) Asbestos--a continuing concern. *Scand J Work Environ Health* **23:** 81-82.

25. Gomez MR (1997) Recommendations for optimizing the usefulness of existing exposure databases for public health applications. *Am Ind Hyg Assoc J* **58:** 181-2.

26. Markowitz SB (1998) The role of surveillance in occupational health. In: Rom WN, ed. *Environmental and Occupational Medicine.* Philadelphia, PA (USA): Lippincott-Raven Publishers, pp. 19-29.

27. LaMontagne AD, Herrick RF, Van Dyke MV, Martyny JW, Ruttenber AJ (2000) Exposure databases and exposure surveillance: promise and practice. *Am Ind Hyg Assoc J* (In press).

28. Fahs MC, Markowitz SB, Leigh JP, *et al.* (1997) A national estimate of the cost of occupationally related disease in 1992. *Ann NY Acad Sci* **837:** 440-455.

29. Pearce N, Matos E, Vainio H, Boffetta P, Kogevinas M, eds. (1994) *Occupational Cancer in Developing Countries.* Lyon: International Agency for Research on Cancer.

30. Walsh D, Jennings SE, Mangione T, *et al.* (1991) Health promotion versus health protection? Employees' perceptions and concerns. *J Public Health Policy* **12:** 148-164.

31. Sorensen G, Himmelstein JS, Hunt MK, *et al.* (1995) A model for worksite cancer prevention: integration of health protection and health promotion in the Wellworks project. *Am J Health Promot* **10:** 55-62.

32. Heaney C, Goldenhar L (1996) Worksite health programs: working together to advance employee health. *Health Educ Q* **23:** 133-136.

Chapter 23

Socioeconomic Status

Kimberly Lochner Sc.D. and Ichiro Kawachi, M.D., Ph.D.
Harvard Center for Society and Health and Department of Health and Social Behavior, Harvard School of Public Health, Boston, MA

INTRODUCTION

Socioeconomic disadvantage – whether measured by low income, low educational attainment or low occupational status – has been consistently linked with higher overall cancer incidence and mortality [1]. Despite the wealth of evidence supporting this link, little progress has been made in reducing socioeconomic disparities in cancer. With few exceptions, these disparities have persisted over time, and in some cases, they appear to be widening [2]. A broad set of explanations has been set forth to account for the greater burden of cancer incidence and mortality among individuals of lower socioeconomic status (SES), including diminished access to preventive and curative health care services as well as exposure to a range of carcinogens in residential and occupational settings.

Whenever SES is discussed in the context of cancer etiology, it is often incorrectly assumed that nothing can be done about addressing socioeconomic disparities short of advocating major social revolution. Since epidemiologists cannot eliminate poverty, it is argued, they should stick to dispensing practical advice on steps that individuals can take to reduce their personal risk of cancer, *e.g.*, stopping smoking, or joining a health club [3]. Yet, as we shall argue in the following chapter, several interventions do exist by which policy makers can attempt to break the link between socioeconomic disadvantage and cancer risk. The types of intervention available to reduce socioeconomic disparities in cancer risk can be classified under the various "levels" of prevention: primary, secondary, and tertiary.

G.A. Colditz et al. (eds.), Cancer Prevention: The Causes and Prevention of Cancer - Volume I, 301–311.
© 2000 *Kluwer Academic Publishers.*

Primary prevention strategies address the socioeconomic disparities in the underlying causes of cancer (*e.g.,* exposure to passive smoking). Secondary prevention refers to the early detection and treatment of cancer. Various forms of cancer screening fit this category. Finally, tertiary prevention refers to strategies that address socioeconomic disparities in access to specialized, curative services which may prolong survival as well as limit the degree of disability and the impact on quality of life associated with cancer diagnosis. Each of these strategies is discussed in turn, beginning with the case for tertiary prevention. Clearly, the scope for abating socioeconomic disparities in cancer broadens as we move further upstream along the chain of events from improving survival, to early detection, to preventing incidence.

1.   TERTIARY PREVENTION: IMPROVING ACCESS TO CURATIVE AND PALLIATIVE SERVICES

Early studies comparing indigent with nonindigent cancer patients found that those of lower socioeconomic status had poorer prospects of survival [4]. Current evidence indicates that the overall 5-year cancer survival rate of poor Americans, regardless of race, is about 10 percent to 15 percent lower than that of middle class Americans [5]. While delay in diagnosis (*i.e.,* unequal access to secondary prevention) is frequently invoked to explain lower cancer survival among poor individuals, this cannot completely account for their survival disadvantage. SES differences in survival have been noted to persist even after adjustment for stage of disease [6].

Although the intervening mechanisms leading to reduced survival chances among the socioeconomically disadvantaged have not been fully elucidated, unequal access to curative and palliative treatment is a likely factor. In one study, for example, non-small-cell lung cancer patients who were not covered by private insurance were less likely to receive surgery than patients with private insurance, even after adjusting for relevant clinical factors such as age, functional status, and stage of disease [7]. Even among patients who did not receive surgery, those with private insurance were more likely to receive *other* oncological services such as radiation or chemotherapy, again after adjusting for relevant clinical factors [7]. Consistent with such patterns of unequal access to treatment services, Greenwald *et al.* [8] reported significantly lower survival rates among lower income patients newly diagnosed with non-small-cell lung cancer, as tracked by the Fred Hutchinson Cancer Research Center's Cancer Surveillance

System. Presumably, this difference could not be accounted for by unequal access to screening, since no reliable method exists to detect lung cancer at an early stage.

The impact of unequal access to tertiary care is often further compounded by the lack of continuity in health care and fragmentation of services among socioeconomically disadvantaged populations. Intervention projects in recent years have begun to focus on improving the delivery of tertiary health care to correct this disparity. For example, the "patient navigator model" has been adopted in several hospital settings to improve access to diagnosis and treatment for economically disadvantaged and low literacy populations. In this model, a "navigator", who is a patient advocate, is appointed to assist individuals with the personal, medical, and social problems that arise in their interactions with the health care system. The "patient navigator" also plays a critical role in ensuring access to follow-up services [9].

In summary, although socioeconomic disparities in cancer prognosis is likely to reflect a complex interaction of delayed diagnosis, inadequate health insurance coverage, unequal treatment by health care providers, incomplete compliance with therapeutic regimens, as well as other as yet unidentified factors (*e.g.*, low literacy, poor social support), current evidence suggests that practical steps can be taken to remove some of the more obvious obstacles that prevent low SES patients from receiving the optimal standard of care, thereby improving their chances of survival.

2.   SECONDARY PREVENTION: IMPROVING ACCESS TO CANCER SCREENING

Screening for early detection of cancer remains one of the mainstays of the public health approach to cancer prevention. It has been estimated that screening could prevent 15 to 30 percent of all deaths from breast cancer among women over 40 and virtually all deaths from cervical cancer [10].

However, lower SES women have been consistently shown to be less likely to receive regular Pap smear or mammogram screening, and consequently to present at a more advanced stage of disease compared to higher SES women [11]. In 1990, the year that the Breast and Cervical Cancer Prevention Act of 1990 authorized the Centers for Disease Control to provide breast and cervical cancer screening services to underserved women, only 27 percent of poor women 50 years and older had received a mammogram in the past two years compared with 53.5 percent of non-poor women – a staggering difference of 26.5 percentage points. By 1994, recent use of mammography among poor women had increased to 44.5 percent while among non-poor women it had risen to 64.9 percent - a difference of

20.4 percentage points. The *Healthy People 2000* goal is for 60 percent of women in this age group to have received a mammogram within the past two years, a target which affluent women have evidently exceeded. As shown in Figure 23.1, lower income women still fall far short of this goal: a fact which is true for both white and black women (data not shown) [12].

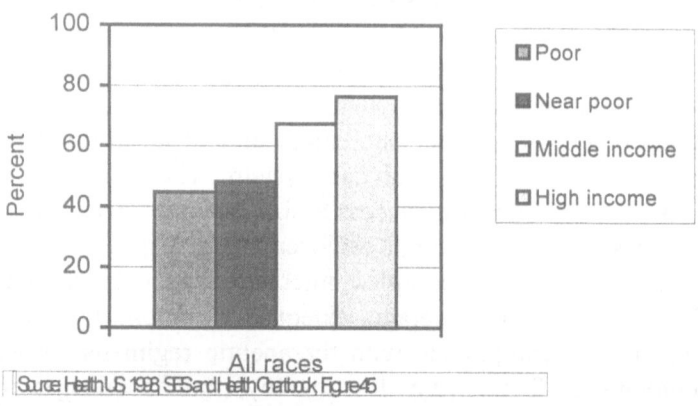

Figure 23.1 Mammography within the past 2 years among women 50-years of age and over, by family income: United States, 1993-1994

There are several remediable reasons why lower SES women lack adequate screening for breast and cervical cancer. One obvious barrier is cost. Lack of health insurance coverage as well as restrictions on Medicaid reimbursement rates prohibit access to screening services among the poor [13]. The impact of cost on screening uptake has been demonstrated by interventions targeted at overcoming the cost barrier. For example, intervention programs in Newark, New Jersey [14] and Long Island, New York [15] that provided free or reduced-cost screening for cervical and breast cancer, respectively, demonstrated improved screening utilization among socioeconomically disadvantaged women.

Policy makers may ask who is going to provide the resources needed to finance screening services for underserved populations during an era of fiscal constraint. Yet evidence suggests that the affluent receive *too frequent* screening, even as the poor receive too little. On current estimates, over half (54 percent) of the eligible women in the United States are screened annually with Pap smears. By contrast, some 22 percent of women have not been screened at all in the past ten years. These women tend to be older, uninsured, lower SES, or otherwise at higher risk of cervical cancer. If 54 percent of the women who are currently annually screened were to be switched to a three-year screening schedule, Colditz has estimated that the protection against cervical cancer would decrease only slightly among these women, from 93.5 percent to 90.8 percent. The same women would require 30 fewer tests each between the ages 20 to 65. By allocating those resources to ensure that the 22 percent of the population previously screened every ten years is now screened every three years, society could reap a substantial gain in their protection from cervical cancer (from 64 percent to 90.8 percent), whilst increasing their lifetime Pap screens from five to fifteen years. At the population level, such a strategy translates into fewer cases of cervical cancer (an overall 4.4 percent reduction), and about half the current number of Pap smears performed.

Although lack of health insurance and cost considerations pose significant obstacles to screening, it is important to recall that socioeconomic disadvantage is also associated with a multitude of other barriers, including: personal factors (lack of knowledge, lack of health literacy, low self efficacy), time constraints (inability to take time off work, lack of transportation and child care), as well as failure of physician referral and fragmentation of services [17]. As well, the settings where low income women receive their medical care, such as hospital emergency rooms or clinics, often fail to give priority to cervical cancer and other forms of screening [18].

Strategies to overcome these barriers and to improve breast and cervical cancer screening rates range from community-based programs targeted to low SES patient populations – such as media campaigns, literature distribution, and mobile mammography vans – to primary care practice-based programs, such as patient reminder systems and counseling. Thus far, evaluations of primary care-based interventions have yielded positive results. For example, an intervention where nurse practitioners offered breast and cervical cancer screening to low income women during routine visits resulted in a substantially increased uptake of screening compared with a control setting which used only a physician reminder system [19].

An individual's use of screening services may also be profoundly influenced by the socioeconomic characteristics of the neighborhood in which they live. Thus, not only are preventive health services less likely to be located in poor neighborhoods, but the concentration of socioeconomic disadvantage in such settings may intensify other barriers to screening uptake, such as the absence of community norms about getting screened, as well as lack of shared knowledge about the benefits of screening. Shared information about why, how, and where to get screened constitute the *social capital* of a community, which may be lacking in disadvantaged neighborhoods [20].

Using data from the Surveillance Epidemiology and End Results (SEER) program, one study found that women living in a socioeconomically disadvantaged neighborhood had a 60 percent greater chance of being diagnosed with invasive cervical cancer and a 51 percent greater chance of being diagnosed with invasive breast cancer, taking into account individual factors, such as race/ethnicity and age [21]. Although this study did not directly address screening practices, the later-stage of cancer diagnosis among women residing in disadvantaged communities suggests that strategies to improve screening uptake should be targeted to low SES *neighborhoods* as well as to low SES *individuals*.

3.   PRIMARY PREVENTION: LIFESTYLE CHANGE THROUGH REGULATORY INTERVENTION

Screening is an example of what Geoffrey Rose termed the "high risk" strategy of prevention. In other words, the strategy targets the high risk "tail" of the population distribution of risk (*i.e.,* identifying those who have detectable, early stage cancer), whilst leaving unchanged the underlying distribution of risk from whence the cases arose [22]. As Rose pointed out, the greatest scope for prevention is likely to occur through implementing "population-based" strategies of prevention, *i.e.,* strategies aimed at shifting the underlying distribution of risk in populations. In the example of cervical cancer, this may include strategies to shift the underlying distribution of sexual practices (for example, encouraging the use of barrier methods of contraception). It is important to note that the various approaches to prevention – primary, secondary, tertiary, as well as "high risk" and "population-based" – are not mutually exclusive. Eliminating socioeconomic disparities in cancer risk will inevitably require action at all levels.

Epidemiology has identified a multitude of lifestyle "risk factors" for cancer. Socioeconomic variations in cancer risk can often by "explained" by differential exposure to such risk factors. From this, it is often assumed that eliminating the SES gradient in cancer risk is a matter of educating individuals to adopt health-promoting lifestyles. However, such a view ignores the reality that socioeconomic disparities in several risk factors have been widening over time as a result of the selective uptake of health advice by the affluent, advantaged members of society. For example, despite decades of progress in reducing tobacco use, smoking prevalence among low SES Americans persists at levels up to three times higher than the most educated, affluent segments. As a result, the socioeconomic gap in smoking has actually widened over time, even as more Americans succeed in quitting each year. It is unlikely, then, that progress in reducing the socioeconomic disparity in tobacco-related cancers will be achieved through individually targeted interventions, such as providing smoking cessation services or nicotine replacement therapy. The experience of clinical trials of individual behavior modification has shown just how difficult this task can be, especially among low income populations [23].

Instead, the greatest opportunity for reducing socioeconomic disparities in smoking behavior is likely to come through implementing population-based preventive measures such as raising excise taxes, banning workplace second-hand smoke exposure, and restricting tobacco advertising (which are often deliberately targeted toward the poor) [1].

The successful implementation of prevention policies requires the presence of three key ingredients: the scientific knowledge base, political will, and appropriate social strategies [24]. In the case of tobacco control, it has proved difficult to mobilize the political will to raise cigarette excise taxes at the federal level given the dependence of politicians on campaign donations contributed by the tobacco industry. Consequently, the most innovative tobacco control programs in this country have been left to State-level initiatives. California and Massachusetts, followed by Arizona and Oregon, have each provided examples where ballot-led initiatives resulted in the creation of comprehensive cancer control programs funded through state excise taxes on tobacco. Raising the excise tax on cigarettes is known to be one of the most effective means of reducing tobacco use in low income populations. Data from the CDC indicate that people with low incomes, racial and ethnic minorities, and youth, are the groups most responsive to cigarette price increases. In particular, smokers with incomes below the family median income were more likely quit smoking in response to price increases than smokers with higher family incomes.

Policies other than cigarette excise tax increases and advertising restrictions can also influence smoking behavior among low SES groups. As knowledge about the hazards of environmental tobacco smoke (ETS) has increased, restrictions on smoking in several arenas have been implemented – public places, restaurants, government and private-sector work sites. Studies indicate that work site smoking restriction policies not only reduce exposure to ETS but also encourage active smokers to quit. National data from the 1992-93 Current Population Survey indicate that 81.6 percent of all indoor workers have some type of workplace smoking policy and 46 percent of Americans work where there is a 100 percent smoke-free policy. However, wide socioeconomic disparities persist across workplaces with regard to their smoking restriction policies. Thus, only 21 percent of food service workers reported working in a smoke-free workplace compared with

81 percent of health care professionals [25]. Similarly, according to the 1990-91 Adult Use of Tobacco Survey in California, white-collar workplaces were twice as likely to have formal smoking restriction policies compared to blue-collar workplaces.

Communities have also pursued tobacco control policies through their local Boards of Health – for example, by enforcing bans on vending machines, prohibiting the placement of cigarette billboards near schools, and regulating counter-top displays of tobacco products in retail stores. Here again, socioeconomic disparities have arisen due to the differential ability of communities to organize and pass local ordinances. Communities that are high in stocks of social capital – where citizens are equipped with the knowledge and requisite civic skills to manipulate the political system to their advantage – are more likely to garner outcomes that promote the health of their residents.

CONCLUSION

Despite notable progress in the prevention of cancer, there has been limited progress in reducing, let alone eliminating, socioeconomic disparities in risk. Of the three ingredients required to translate public health knowledge into action, building the political will to create sustained change has proved the most difficult (the other two being building the knowledge base and developing appropriate social strategies). Though some are quick to ascribe political indifference to the sheer magnitude of the problem at hand, public health must share some of the blame for not publicizing the disparities in cancer risk more widely. Thus, cancer surveillance systems, such as state tumor registries, routinely fail to collect information on socioeconomic status. Even in the rare instances where such information is collected, it is seldom analyzed or publicized. An egregious practice in the United States has been to treat "race" as a proxy for socioeconomic status, thereby encouraging the widespread but erroneous belief that inequalities in cancer risk are somehow rooted in genetic differences, and that consequently, nothing can be done to remedy the disparities. As we have tried to argue, the majority of cancer disparities are amenable to practical interventions; and moreover, they do not require large-scale social revolution.

Eliminating social disparities in cancer will ultimately require the cooperation of different segments of society – government, communities, businesses – to address the differential exposure of Americans to cancer risk. Yet the wide and persistent gulf in the health achievement of citizens across the socioeconomic spectrum is something that no democratic society ought to tolerate.

SUMMARY POINTS

- Despite long-standing evidence demonstrating higher cancer incidence and poorer survival among lower SES populations, little progress has been made in reducing socioeconomic disparities in cancer.
- It is often erroneously assumed that reducing socioeconomic disparities in cancer will require the elimination of poverty, or some other large-scale social revolution.
- The majority of the excess burden of cancer among socioeconomically disadvantaged populations arise through factors that are in fact amenable to primary, secondary, and tertiary prevention.
- Several interventions are possible within the health care sector to reduce SES disparities in cancer, *e.g.,* improving access to screening (secondary prevention), or improving access to tertiary oncology services.
- Tertiary and secondary prevention strategies, while important components of efforts to improve cancer survival among the disadvantaged, do not address the underlying distribution of risks that leads to the higher incidence of cancer among the poor.
- The primary prevention of cancer risk among lower SES populations therefore remains an important goal. This means addressing the differential exposure to cancer risks in workplaces and residential settings, through regulatory change.

RECOMMENDATIONS

- Federal and state agencies need to routinely collect, analyze, and report socioeconomic disparities in cancer risk. Such monitoring and surveillance is an essential prerequisite of building the political will to create change.
- The greatest scope for prevention lies in population-based strategies that seek to shift the population distribution of cancer risk. Often, these shifts come about through changes in social norms created by the regulatory environment, *e.g.,* workplace smoking bans, restrictions on cigarette advertising. Wherever possible, policy

makers should explore the options for implementing population based prevention strategies. Such an approach often has the double advantage of addressing the underlying forces that give rise to socioeconomic disparities in cancer risk.

SUGGESTED FURTHER READING

1. Kogevinas M, Pearce N, Susser M, Boffetta P, eds. (1997) *Social Inequalities and Cancer. IARC Scientific Publications* No. 138. Lyon, France International Agency for Research on Cancer.
2. Berkman LF, Kawachi I, eds. (2000) *Social Epidemiology.* New York, NY (USA): Oxford University.

REFERENCES

1. Lochner K, Kawachi I (2000) Socioeconomic status. In: Hunter D, Colditz G, eds. *Cancer Prevention: the Causes and Prevention of Cancer*, Volume 1, Section 1. Dordrecht, The Netherlands: Kluwer Academic Publishers.
2. Faggiano F, Partanen T, Kogevinas M, Pearce N, *et al.* (1997) Socioeconomic differences in cancer incidence and mortality. In: Kogevinas M, *et al.*, eds. *Social Inequalities and Cancer Lyon:* IARC Scientific Publications; No. 138, pp. 65-176.
3. Rothman KJ, Adami HO, Trichopoulos D (1998) Should the mission of epidemiology include the eradication of poverty? *Lancet* **352**: 810-813.
4. Linden G (1969) The influence of social class in the survival of cancer patients. *Am J Public Health* **59**: 267-274.
5. Freeman HP (1989) Cancer in the socioeconomically disadvantaged. CA Cancer J Clin **39**: 266-79.
6. Cella D (1991) Socioeconomic status and cancer survival. J Clin Oncol **9**: 1500-09.
7. Greenberg ER, Chute CG, Stukel T, Baron JA, *et al.* (1988) Social and economic factors in the choice of lung cancer treatment. *N Engl J Med* **318**: 612-17.
8. Greenwald H (1996) Explaining reduced survival among the disadvantaged. *Milbank Q* **74**: 215-38.
9. Black BL, Ades TB (1994) American Cancer Society urban demonstration projects: models for successful intervention. *Semin Oncol Nurs* **10**: 96-103.
10. CDC. The National Breast and Cervical Cancer Early Detection Program. http://www.cdc.gov/nccdphp/dcpc/nbccedp/about.htm (accessed June 1999).
11. Mandelblatt J, Andrews H, Kerner J, Zauber A, *et al* (1991) Determinants of late stage diagnosis of breast and cervical cancer: the impact of age, race, social class, and hospital type. *Am J Public Health* **81**: 646-49.
12. Pamuk E, Makuc D, Heck K, Reuben C, Lochner K (1998) *Socioeconomic Status and Health Chartbook. Health, United States.* Hyattsville, MD (USA): National Center for Health Statistics.

13. Pamies R, Woodard L (1992) Cancer in the socioeconomically disadvantaged populations. *Prim Care* **19**: 443-50.
14. Holland B, Foster J, Louria D (1993) Cervical cancer and health care resources in Newark, New Jersey, 1970-1988. *Am J Public Health* **83**: 45-48.
15. Lane D, Polednak A, Burg M (1992) Breast screening practices among users of county-funded health centers vs women in the entire community. *Am J Public Health* **82**: 199-203.
16. Colditz GA, Hoaglin DC, Berkey CS (1997) Cancer incidence and mortality: the priority of screening frequency and population coverage. *Milbank Q* **75**: 147-173.
17. Kiefe CI, McKay SV, Halevy A, Brody BA (1994) Is cost a barrier to screening mammography for low-income women receiving Medicare benefits? *Arch Int Med* **154**: 1217-1224.
18. Marcus AC, Crane LA, Kaplan CP, Goodman KJ, *et al.* (1990) Screening for cervical cancer in emergency centers and sexually transmitted disease clinics. Obstet Gynecol **75**: 453-55.
19. Mandelblatt J, Traxler M, Lakin P, *et al.* (1993) A nurse practitioner intervention to increase breast and cervical cancer screening for poor, elderly, black women. J *Gen Int Med* **8**: 173-78.
20. Kawachi I, Kennedy BP, Lochner K (1999) Social capital and self-rated health: a contextual analysis. *Am J Public Health* **89**: 1187-1193.
21. Breen N, Figueroa J (1996) Stage of breast and cervical cancer diagnosis in disadvantaged neighborhoods: a prevention policy perspective. *Am J Prev Med* **12**: 319-26.
22. Rose G (1992)*The Strategy of Preventive Medicine*. New York, NY (USA): Oxford University Press.
23. Syme SL (1998) Social and economic disparities in health: thoughts about intervention. *Milbank Q* **76**: 493-505.
24. Atwood K, Colditz GA, Kawachi I (1997) From public health to prevention policy: placing science in its social and political contexts. *Am J Public Health* **87**: 1603-1606.
25. Gerlach KK, Shopland DR, Hartman Am, Gibson JT, *et al.* (1997) Workplace smoking policies in the United States: results from a national survey of more than 100,000 workers. *Tob Control* **6**: 199-206.

Chapter 24

Population-Level Change in Risk Factors for Cancer

Graham A. Colditz, M.D., Dr.P.H. A. Lindsay Frazier, M.D., and Glorian Sorensen, Ph.D
Channing Laboratory, Department of Medicine, Brigham and Women's Hospital and Harvard Medical School; Harvard School of Public Health; Dana-Farber Cancer Institute, Boston, MA

INTRODUCTION

The greatest promise for cancer prevention rests on the ability to change multiple and often interrelated behaviors that have been shown to increase cancer risk. It has been conservatively estimated that through lifestyle changes, over 50 percent of cancer could be prevented [1]. This estimate assumes that the lifestyles associated with low cancer incidence could be followed by most of the population. However, changes in lifestyle are difficult and all the population will not move to the low risk categories that underlie estimates of the percentage of cancer that is truly preventable. A more realistic goal is that we gradually shift the entire distribution of risk factors across the population, as has happened for instance with total fat intake and egg consumption. Over time, as the message that saturated fat is related to coronary heart disease the entire population distribution has shifted in the United States; everyone eats less. For example, whole milk consumption has decreased from an average of 213 pounds per day in 1970 to 78 pounds per day in 1993. Why this approach will work is the result of thinking promulgated by Rose. Here we review the potential benefit of moderate and achievable changes in diet and physical activity in terms of reducing the burden of cancer in the United States.

Rose advocates the need for population approaches to prevention of chronic disease [2]. He emphasizes that when the relation between a lifestyle factor or biological predictor of risk is continuous, the majority of cases attributable to the exposure will likely arise in those who are not classified as being at high risk. He illustrates this with examples of blood pressure and

313

G.A. Colditz et al. (eds.), Cancer Prevention: The Causes and Prevention of Cancer - Volume I, 313–323.
© 2000 *Kluwer Academic Publishers.*

rates of coronary heart disease. Specifically, even small changes in blood pressure at the population level can translate into large reduction in the rates of coronary disease and stroke. Law and colleagues illustrate this point and estimate that a three percent reduction in blood pressure for the whole population (a decrease of 4 mm Hg systolic blood pressure) would produce a 25 percent reduction in the number of people classified as hypertensive. Similarly, a five percent reduction in blood pressure would produce a 30 percent reduction in stroke [3]. To reduce the risk of disease in the population substantial benefits can be achieved by a small reduction for all members of the society rather than just focusing on the high-risk groups.

Building on the public health approach to prevention of cardiovascular disease, Cook and colleagues explore the potential benefits for the U.S. population examining changes in diastolic blood pressure across the whole population as opposed to major treatment interventions for those with hypertension [4]. They estimate that a decrease as small as two percent in diastolic blood pressure for the whole population would produce a 17 percent decrease in the prevalence of hypertension, a six percent decrease in the risk of coronary heart disease, and a 15 percent decrease in the risk of stroke and transient ischemic attack. This, a population prevention strategy for those 35 to 65 years of age would therefore reduce CHD incidence more than medical treatment of all those with diastolic blood pressure greater than 95 mm Hg. They conclude that in the U.S. today, population level interventions that would reduce the intake of sodium, through reduction in the salt content in manufactured food, for example, would produce a greater reduction in coronary disease than the current treatment approach. Indeed, because of growing public awareness of risk factors for heart disease, population wide trends in cardiovascular risk factors show continuing improvement and the rate of coronary heart disease incidence and mortality continues to decrease [5].

When we consider population approaches to cancer prevention, we must address the etiologic process, which covers a different time course and sequence from coronary heart disease. Although cardiovascular disease is the end point of the chronic process of atherosclerosis, treatment focuses on the reversal and subsequent prevention of the acute thrombotic process of myocardial infarction. Cancer, on the other hand, is the result of a long process of accumulating DNA damage, leading late in the process to clinically detectable lesions such as *in situ* and invasive cancer. For example, studies of the progression in colon cancer from first mutation to invading malignancy suggest that DNA changes accumulate over a period of as long as 40 years. The goal of cancer prevention is to arrest this progression; different interventions interrupt carcinogenesis at different points in the process. Further, most cancers do not have a late "acute" event, analogous to thrombosis, which can be prevented with medical interventions.

The fact that different interventions will impact at different points along this developmental process that can stretch over nearly half a century has implications for when we can expect to see pay-off in terms of lower cancer rates. Research has demonstrated that those who initiate smoking during early adolescence greatly increase risk of lung cancer even when one controls for dose and duration of smoking [6-8]. If we could delay the age at which most adolescents first start to smoke, we would probably substantially reduce lung cancer rates [9], but this benefit will not be observable for 20 to 40 years after the intervention. Adult cessation, on the other hand, will reduce risk more rapidly [10], but fails to address the continuing recruitment of the next generation of smokers. Recent declines in the incidence of lung cancer among younger men and women in the United States reflect reductions in the rate of smoking among younger adults [11]. Other lifestyle interventions may act as preventive early in the DNA pathway to cancer. For example, aspirin and folate appear to act early in the pathway inhibiting colon cancer [12, 13]. We do not consider these or similar strategies here.

Targeting populations through community-based interventions represents an 'upstream' approach for reducing behaviors and ultimately lowering cancer incidence and mortality. That is, these approaches address the conditions that contribute to and sustain the high incidence of cancer in the population [14]. Community-based strategies are particularly important for risks that are widely diffused in the population; in such cases, individual strategies would simply be too costly and ultimately would be less effective [15].

Community-based interventions aim to reduce risk related behaviors among individuals, reduce exposures in the environment that are health hazards, and increase utilization of preventive services offered through health care providers.

The recent reduction in smoking prevalence provides an instructive example of population level changes. Numerous changes in tobacco policies as outlined in this book reflect and contribute to decreasing social acceptability of smoking, including increasing restrictions on smoking in workplaces, health care facilities and other public places; increased taxation; and restricted youth access through the banning of vending machines; and regulation of point-of-purchase advertising on tobacco sales to youth. These changes in social norms have contributed to decreased uptake by adolescents, and enhanced support for quitting.

Another example of changing social norms comes from the national efforts in Australia to reduce sun exposure and subsequent risk of melanoma and other skin cancers. In addition to messages aimed in individuals, efforts of the Sunsmart Program have included the Australian cancer societies working with local communities to modify regulations pertaining to children's play areas, requiring the use of shade cloth to reduce ultraviolet light exposure. Collaborations with architects have also led to the introduction of an annual award for design of Sunsmart buildings, and regulatory changes have removed all sales taxes from sunscreen products. Marketing of sunprotective clothing has also been promoted by the cancer societies.

In contrast with these public health interventions, controlled trials of population based studies have also been evaluated, largely in the United States. Numerous studies have tested the effectiveness of population-based cancer prevention and control interventions in an array of settings, including in entire communities, worksites, schools, churches, and the media. Several large-scale community based studies have focused on smoking cessation, including American Stop Smoking Intervention Trial, ASSIST [16]; Community Intervention Trial for smoking cessation, COMMIT [17]). Fruit and vegetable consumption has also been addressed (5-A-Day for Better Health), as has breast cancer screening (Breast Cancer Screening Consortium), and multiple behavioral risk factors through workplace settings (Working Well [18]). These studies are in varying stages of implementation, analysis, and reporting.

The results of these trials underline several important accomplishments. For example, COMMIT provides promising evidence that community-based interventions may be particularly important in reducing smoking among less educated smokers. COMMIT was a randomized, controlled community-based intervention trial that included eleven matched pairs of communities across North America, and was designed to test the effectiveness of multifaceted, four-year community-based intervention to encourage smokers, particularly heavy smokers, to achieve and maintain cessation. A significant intervention effect was observed among light to moderate smokers, and the effect appeared to be greater for the less educated subgroup. However, there was no intervention effect on heavy smokers.

Taken as a group, the 5-A-Day Interventions suggest that interventions targeted through specific channels, such as worksites or schools, can effectively increase fruit and vegetable consumption [19]. This program also supports the feasibility of a pubic-private partnership and provides a useful model for other translational initiatives. Provider-initiated interventions have contributed to modest reduction in smoking [20], but the effectiveness of such interventions is likely to grow with increased availability of nicotine replacement therapy [21].

1.   FUTURE DIRECTIONS

Concerns remain regarding the effectiveness of community based interventions. Overall, the size of the effects observed in these research-based interventions has been small. Numerous explanations have been offered to account for this, including inappropriateness of the intervention being tested, interventions offered over too short a time period, or with too little intensity, deferred effects of interventions, or the inclusion of too few communities [22, 23]. From a methodologic consideration that runs across all primary prevention trials, we must also consider the impact of secular trends in the general population or comparison group. It is noteworthy that the intervention group has often achieved substantial change that is greater than, though not significantly different from the comparison group, which enrolled in the trial but failed to obtain the intensive intervention.

Interpretation of the apparently small effects in population level change also deserves consideration. A small population wide change translates into substantial benefit. Take for example physical activity and colon cancer. The prevalence of physical activity has been stable or decreasing over the recent past [24]. In 1994, 30 percent of the U.S. population reported no leisure-time physical activity[25]. Another 54 percent are somewhat active but still fail to meet the current recommendations of engaging in light to moderate physical activity for at least 30 minutes per day [24, 26].

The relation between physical activity and colon cancer shows a significant dose response relation in many studies and, therefore, we assume a linear dose response for these calculations [27]. This relation is seen among those who already are active as well as among those who are inactive [27].

We estimate that if the entire population increased their level of physical activity by 30 minutes of brisk walking per day (or the equivalent energy expenditure = 15 MET hours per week) we would observe a 15 percent reduction in the incidence of colon cancer. The reduction in colon cancer is predicted for both men and women as the magnitude of the relation between leisure-time physical activity and colon cancer is comparable across gender [27]. For the entire U.S. population this increase in activity translates to approximately 14,340 cases prevented per year. This assumes that even those who are already active increase their levels. If, on the other hand, the 22 percent of the population who already met the year 2000 goals do not undertake any additional increase in their activity, then the benefits for the total population are substantially truncated. Further reduction in the benefit is seen if the 36 percent of the population with no current physical activity are the only focus of the prevention strategy.

2.   FRUIT AND VEGETABLES AND LUNG CANCER

For fruit and vegetable intake we note that the population intake is continuous. Estimates from the 1989 to 1991 Continuing Surveys of Food

Intakes by Individuals (CSFII) suggest that the mean population intake of fruit and vegetables is 4.2 servings per day (SE=0.06) and that 32 percent of adults consume five servings or more of fruit and vegetables [28]. While smokers may consume fewer servings of fruits and vegetables per day than nonsmokers, and the majority of the protective benefit against lung cancer is through countering the adverse effects of smoking, we nevertheless estimate the overall population benefit.

Based on data from Steinmetz and colleagues we accept the linear dose-response as reported from the prospective follow-up of women in Iowa [29]. These results are consistent with numerous other studies of diet and lung cancer supporting a ten percent reduction in risk for each serving of fruit and vegetables consumed per day [30]. We estimate that the reduction in risk is ten percent per serving of fruit and vegetables per day. Again this benefit extends for increasing intake beyond the current goal of five servings per day. That is, if all the population increased their daily intake of fruit and vegetables by one serving per day, we would reduce the number of lung cancer cases by ten percent, or approximately 17,150 cases prevented per year.

Alternatively, if all of the US population attained the year 2000 goal of five servings of fruit and vegetables per day [31] then we might have a 20 percent decrease in lung cancer among the 70 percent of the population who were initially below the year 2000 goal and no reduction in risk among the 32 percent of the population already meeting the goal. The overall population benefit is therefore 14 percent (0.2 x 0.7). This estimate assumes that the 8 percent of the population who do not consume any vegetables also do not consume any fruit, and that 15 percent consumes each of one, two, three, and four servings per day. Among these adults, those consuming none or only one serving per day would be required to make truly dramatic dietary changes from eating no fruit and vegetables to consuming five servings per day - perhaps an unattainable change.

When interpreting results of intervention studies, we must also consider the reach of the program within the population. This has an impact on the overall population benefit that can be achieved with widespread dissemination of the intervention.

The apparent limited effectiveness of previous efforts also may be due, at least in part, to their inattention to the social contexts of the populations they are designed to influence. Behavioral interventions are likely to be most effective when they are embedded in the social context of the environment in which people live. Community interventions are needed which incorporate into their design and delivery the influence of social networks on behavior change, cultural factors that may influence health behaviors and receptivity to change, and barriers posed by restricted access to social and material resources.

An example may be useful to illustrate how social context can be addressed in a cancer prevention intervention. There are substantial differences among neighborhoods in the availability and cost of healthy foods. Studies have shown that middle-class neighborhoods have proportionally more pharmacies, restaurants, banks, and specialty stores while low-income neighborhoods have more fast food restaurants, check cashing stores, liquor stores, and laundromats. There are four times as many people per food market in poor neighborhoods. Typical food purchases cost approximately 15 percent more in poor neighborhoods, and produce may cost as much as 22 percent more than in higher income areas. In addition, the quality of the food on average is poorer in low-income neighborhoods. Relatively higher food costs in low-income neighborhoods may be associated, in part, with limited access to supermarkets, and reliance on small and medium size stores in which the quality, quantity, and variety of both fresh fruits and vegetables are limited. As a result, people in low in come neighborhoods are much less likely to meet their grocery needs in their local area. Such realities must be addressed is interventions are to be effective in influencing the eating patterns of persons living in low-income neighborhoods.

Given such realties it is not surprising that cancer morbidity and mortality as well as behavioral risk factors are distributed unevenly within the population, with higher risk associated with lower income and lower education (see chapters 9 and 23). Shifting the distribution of risk in the population may require a departure from the one-size-fits-all intervention strategy n order to enhance the effectiveness of community interventions. It may be necessary instead to match or tailor the intervention with the distribution of risk factors in the population, which are concentrated in defined "pockets of prevalence".

3.   CONCLUSIONS

Studies are needed to assess comprehensive, systemic interventions that use multifaceted approaches to behavior change. To be effective, these studies must attend to the social context of the populations they are designed to influence. Ultimately, these community interventions must be judged according to their impact on disease risk within the population, rather than at the individual level. Long term benefits will be best achieved through population wide changes in risk factors.

Three key strategies contributing to successful population based interventions are:

1. Designing interventions that target multiple levels of influence
2. Involving communities in program planning and implementation

3. Incorporating approaches for tailoring interventions at the population level

3.1   Targeting multiple levels of influence

Health behaviors respond to multiple levels of influence, including intrapersonal factors, interpersonal processes, institutional factors, community factors, and public policy. The social ecological model offers a theoretical framework that integrates multiple perspectives and theories in identifying effective strategies for interventions across these levels. We might best illustrate such a comprehensive strategy using tobacco control as an example. Public policy initiatives might include increases in taxation, thereby making tobacco less accessible through increased price, or policies banning advertising. Community initiatives may focus on increasing "social capital" within communities or neighborhoods. Social capital includes overall level of trust or social cohesion within the community, the extent of reciprocity between neighbors, and the level of participation in civic affairs. Applying this community-level construct to tobacco control, community initiatives may include increasing citizen involvement in efforts to reduce youth access through the development of community coalitions and actions targeting tobacco control. At an institutional level, policies banning tobacco use in worksites or other public settings are important in shaping overall norms about smoking. Interventions to build social support for quitting smoking may be included as part of interpersonal influences on tobacco control. Smoking cessation initiatives targeting individuals are thus part of an overall, comprehensive tobacco control effort, and are supported by influences across other levels.

3.2   Involving communities in program planning and implementation

Community interventions have relied on community organizing principles as a means of involving communities in program planning and implementation. Varying models have been applied, attending to different goals. Interventions are likely to be most successful when communities have a voice in the process.

3.3   Approaches to "tailoring" interventions

The majority of community intervention trials have employed a one-size-fits all approach to intervention. "Tailoring" offers a strategy for increasing the intensity of interventions delivered to at-risk populations. Tailored interventions typically use print communication or telephone counseling to enhance the relevance of interventions to the daily lives of the target population, thereby increasing the likelihood of achieving short-term or sustained intervention effects. Although few studies have assessed the efficacy of tailored interventions delivered at the community level, a growing body of evidence supports the efficacy of these types of interventions at the individual or micro level. These principles may also be applied to communities. Tailoring at the macro-level is consistent with social marketing approaches, which recommend that a target audience should be "segmented" into subgroups with similar geographic, demographic, psychological and problem-relevant characteristics.

3.4   Addressing social inequalities in disease risk

Inverse relationships between social class and disease have been found consistently across diseases. In addition, such differentials are increasingly prominent in the prevalence of health behaviors. Increasing attention is being given to the role of income inequality, rather than absolute income levels, in determining health outcomes; in a study of income distribution in the U.S., income inequality was associated not only with mortality, but also with rates of smoking and sedentary behavior. Community interventions to date have been most effective with well-educated, upper-to-middle income populations, compared to low income, less educated populations. Community interventions are needed to address the "pockets of prevalence" of risk related behaviors in order to reduce social inequalities of risk. Interventions designed for low-income populations must also take into account the social context influencing health behaviors.

SUMMARY POINTS

- Population wide change is the most important way to reduce the burden of cancer.
- Small changes at the individual level can translate to substantial changes in the burden of cancer within the population if the changes are distributed across the entire population.

RECOMMENDATIONS

- For successful population-based interventions we need to design interventions that target multiple levels of influence.

- We need to involve communities in program planning and implementation
- We need to incorporate approaches for tailoring interventions at the population level.

SUGGESTED FURTHER READING

1. Willett W, Colditz G, Mueller N (1996) Strategies for minimizing cancer risk. *Scientific Am* **275:** 88-95.
2. Sorensen G, Emmons K, Hunt MK, Johnston D (1998) Implications of the results of community intervention trials. *Annu Rev Public Health* **19:** 379-416.

REFERENCES

1. Willett W, Colditz G, Mueller N (1996) Strategies for minimizing cancer risk. *Scientific Am* **275:** 88-95.
2. Rose G (1981) Strategy of prevention: lessons from cardiovascular disease. *Br Med J - Clin Res* **282:** 1847-51.
3. Law MR, Frost CD, Wald NJ (1991) By how much does dietary salt reduction lower blood pressure? III-Analysis of data from trials of salt reduction. *Br Med J* **302:** 819-24.
4. Cook N, Cohan J, Hebert P, Taylor J, Hennekens C (1995) Implications of small reduction in diastolic blood pressure for primary prevention. *Arch Intern Med* **155:** 701-9.
5. McGovern P, Pankow J, Sharar E, Doliszny K, Folsom A, Blackurn H, *et al.* (1996) Recent trends in acute coronary heart disease. Mortality, morbidity, medical care, and risk factors. *N Engl J Med* **334:** 884-90.
6. Armitage P, Doll R (1954) The age distribution of cancer and a multistage theory of carcinogenesis. *Br J Cancer* **8:** 1-12.
7. Armitage P, Doll R (1957) A two-stage theory of carcinogenesis in relation to the age distribution of human cancer. *Br J Cancer* **11:** 161-9.
8. Brown C, Chu K (1987) Use of multistage models to infer stage affected by carcinogenic exposure: example of lung cancer and cigarette smoking. *J Chron Dis* **40**(Suppl 2): 171s-179s.
9. Hegmann K, Fraser A, Keaney R, *et al.* (1993) The effect of age at smoking initiation on lung cancer risk. *Epidemiology* **4:** 444-448.
10. Kawachi I, Colditz GA, Stampfer MJ, *et al.* (1993) Smoking cessation in relation to total mortality rates in women: a prospective cohort study. *Ann Intern Med* **119:** 992-1000.
11. Devesa S, Blot W, Fraumeni J (1989) Declining lung cancer rates among young men and women in the United States: a cohort analysis. *J Natl Cancer Inst* **81:** 1568-71.
12. Giovannucci E, Stampfer M, Colditz G, Hunter D, Fuchs C, Rosner B, *et al.* (1998) Multivitamin use, folate, and colon cancer in women in the Nurses' Health Study. *Ann Intern Med* **129:** 517-24.
13. Giovannucci E, Egan KM, Hunter DJ, Stampfer MJ, Colditz GA, Willett WC, *et al.* (1995) Aspirin and the risk of colorectal cancer in women. *N Engl J Med* **333:** 609-614.

14. Wallack L, Wallerstein N (1986) Health education and prevention: designing community initiatives. *Int Q Commun Health Educ* **7**: 319-42.
15. Rose G (1992) *The Strategy of Preventive Medicine.* New York: Oxford University Press.
16. Manley M, Pierce J, Rosbrook B, *et al.* (1997) Impact of the American Stop Smoking Intervention Study (ASSIST) on cigarette consumption. *Tob Control* **6**(Suppl 2): S12-6.
17. The COMMIT Research Group (1995) Community Intervention Trial for Smoking Cessation (COMMIT): 1. Cohort results from a four-year community intervention. *Am J Public Health* **85**: 183-92.
18. Sorensen G, Thompson B, Glanz K, *et al.* (1996) Final results of the working well multicenter cooperative trial: the effectiveness of a worksite cancer prevention intervention. *Am J Public Health* **86**: 939-47.
19. US National Cancer Institute. *The Cancer Letter* 1997 March 28.
20. Glynn T, Manley M (1989) *How to Help Your Patients Stop Smoking. A National Cancer Institute Manual for Physicians.* Bethesda, MD (USA): US Department of Health and Human Services; Report No.: NIH Pub No 89-3064.
21. Oster G, Delea T, Huse D, Regan M, Colditz G (1996) The benefits and risks of over-the-counter availability of nicotine polacrilex ("nicotine gum"). *Med Care* **34**: 389-402.
22. Susser M (1995) The tribulations of trials - intervention in communities. *Am J Public Health* **85**: 156-60.
23. Fielding J (1996) Great expectations, or do we ask too much from community-level interventions? *Am J Public Health* **86**: 1075-6.
24. Pate R, Pratt M, Blair S, *et al.* (1995) Physical activity and public health. A recommendation from the Centers for Disease Control and Prevention and American College of Sports Medicine. *JAMA* **273**: 402-7.
25. Cook J, Owen P, Bender B, Senner J, Davis B, Left M, *et al.* (1997) Monthly estimates of leisure-time physical inactivity – United States 1994. *MMWR* **48**: 393-7.
26. Stephens T (1998) Physical activity and mental health in the United States and Canada: evidence from four population surveys. *Prev Med* **17**: 35-47.
27. Colditz GA, Cannuscio CC, Frazier AL (1997) Physical activity and colon cancer prevention. *Cancer Causes Control* **8**: 649-67.
28. Krebs-Smith S, Cook D, Subar A, Cleveland L, Friday J (1995) US adults' fruit and vegetable intakes, 1989 to 1991: a revised baseline for the Healthy People 2000 objective. *Am J Public Health* **85**: 1623-9.
29. Steinmetz KA, Potter JD, Folsom AR (1993) Vegetables, fruit, and lung cancer in the Iowa Women's Health Study. *Cancer Res* **53**: 536-543.
30. Zeigler R, Mayne S, Swanson C (1996) Nutrition and lung cancer. *Cancer Causes Control* **7**: 157-77.
31. U.S. Department of Health and Human Services (1991) *Healthy People 2000: National Health Promotion and Disease Prevention Objectives.* Washington DC: Department of Health and Human Services, Report No.: Vol. DHHS Pub No PHS-91-50212.

Summary – Prevention of Cancer

Graham A. Colditz, M.D., Dr.P.H.
Channing Laboratory, Department of Medicine, Brigham and Women's Hospital and Harvard Medical School, Boston, MA

PREVENTION OF CANCER

In this book we first documented the overall contribution of lifestyle factors to the occurrence of cancer in the United States and other countries with established market economies. The overall contribution of these modifiable factors is summarized at the end of the section on causes of cancer. We then set forth a social strategy for the prevention of cancer through reducing the major risk factors in the United States. Each chapter in the section on prevention reviews the recent literature on strategies for prevention through the major cancer risk factors. It then follows the plan for social strategy as set forth by Richmond and Kotelchuk [1] and offers a summary statement on what can be done through preventive services delivered by health care providers, through structural interventions implemented by government and industry, and through local activities to promote healthier environment and lifestyle.

1. POPULATION CHANGES IN RISK

A key conclusion of this book is that for prevention to be successful changes must be implemented through all components of the social strategy. Repeatedly, it has been seen that interventions that focus on only one component of the strategy fail or achieve only minimal shifts towards lower cancer risk. For major reductions in the burden of cancer to be achieved, we need broad scale interventions that will shift the behavior of the whole

G.A. Colditz et al. (eds.), Cancer Prevention: The Causes and Prevention of Cancer - Volume I, 325–335.

population. Rather than focus on individuals defined as being at "high risk", a shift in behavior by the whole population can achieve greater reductions in cancer. Take for example activity and colon cancer. Lack of activity is now a defined cause of colon cancer [2]. However, the linear relation between increasing activity and lower risk of colon cancer means that even men and women who currently meet a specific national goal for activity can achieve further reduction in their risk of colon cancer by increasing their level of activity. Thus, rather than focusing solely on getting all individuals to meet the national goal, having the total population increase their weekly activity by the equivalent of 30 minutes of brisk walking per day will result in a greater reduction in the burden of colon cancer.

As discussed in Chapter 18, we estimate that if the entire population increased their level of physical activity by 30 minutes of brisk walking per day (or the equivalent energy expenditure) we would observe a 15 percent reduction in the incidence of colon cancer. This reduction in colon cancer is predicted for both men and women as the magnitude of the relation between physical activity and colon cancer is comparable across gender [3]. For the entire US population this translates to approximately 15,000 cases per year. This assumes that even those who are already active increase their level. If, on the other hand, the 22 percent of the population who already meet the year 2000 goals do not undertake any additional increase in their activity, then the benefits for the total population are substantially truncated. In addition, even those who increase their activity from currently low levels but who fail to reach the national goals will gain substantial protection against colon cancer from the increase in activity that they adopt.

To achieve the goal of cancer prevention, strategies that fold the prevention efforts into our patterns of daily life and shift social norms will be better sustained. This emphasizes the importance of structural changes that support the prevention of cancer. Examples illustrated in this book include the regulation of indoor clean air which has contributed to the reduction in cigarette smoking through shifting social norms and increasing motivation for smoking cessation. But it is noteworthy that in parallel with such regulatory changes, messages from health care providers and behavioral interventions aimed at individuals have fostered the increase in smoking cessation among adults. Here and elsewhere in the book we emphasize the need for coordinated interventions through all components of the social strategy to achieve reduction in the cancer burden. With the implementation of the strategies outlined in this book, we believe that the United States can realistically reduce cancer rates by as much as one-third.

One means to support these changes is the Harvard Center for Cancer Prevention web site, www.yourcancerrisk.harvard.edu, which provides tabulated feedback on strategies to change risk and tips to get started.

2.   TOBACCO

An estimated 30 percent of all US cancer deaths can be attributed to smoking. Thus, stemming the epidemic of tobacco smoking is our most effective means of preventing cancer.

Tobacco smoking causes cancer both by initiating cellular changes that lead to cancer, and also through action late in the carcinogenic process, promoting the growth of tumors such as lung cancer. We therefore address smoking both in terms of adult cessation from smoking, and also prevention of youth uptake of the habit. We conclude that the shift to a public health perspective on smoking cessation has resulted in a successful increase in the rate of cessation from smoking. Behavioral programs and pharmacotherapies such as nicotine replacement therapies are the major individual level cessation strategies currently used. Health care provider advice and support along with community level regulations that support non-smoking norms can impact smoking cessation by enhancing motivation to quit and by preventing relapse among those who achieve initial cessation.

- At the individual level it is important to have both behavioral and pharmacological interventions available to smokers
- Health care providers have a responsibility to their patients to ask about tobacco use, giving strong advice to quit and provide support for their efforts
- Individual and health care provider efforts must be supported by organizational and community level investment of resources in providing training and supportive material to health care providers and in enforcement of regulations.

With regard to the initiation of smoking by America's youth, a comprehensive approach to youth smoking prevention is required [4]. We need to integrate youth smoking prevention into schools, community, media, and policy efforts to create an environment that consistently discourages tobacco use. A well-structured mass media campaign can be focused on youth and used to reinforce awareness and educational messages; to support school and community programs; encourage public debate on the cost, availability and promotion of tobacco, and to create a climate of support for policy changes that will discourage tobacco use.

- Public health advocates should look to increased tobacco excise taxes to fund comprehensive state anti-tobacco campaigns
- Prevention programs should go beyond awareness and education to bring about basic change at the institutional, community, and public policy level

- A well-funded mass media campaign should be central part of prevention efforts aimed at youth, both at the state and national level.

Tips for quitting smoking
- Keep trying! Quitting is tough but not impossible. Over 1,000 Americans quit for good every day.
- Talk to a health care professional for help.
- Talk to the human resources office where you work. Your employer may offer quit-smoking programs for employees.

---

3.   DIET AND OBESITY

An estimated 25 percent of all US cancer deaths can be attributed to diet in adult life, including its effect on obesity. Evidence indicates that a diet that reduces cancer risk should be high in fruit and vegetables, high in whole grains, low in red meat, and low in salt.

There is clear evidence that intensive educational and behavioral interventions are effective for teaching and persuading motivated individuals and small groups to change their diets. However, no single type of intervention has proven consistently successful. The most intensive strategies such as those implemented in clinical trials have produced the greatest effects on dietary change. The cost per person increases with greater intensity of the intervention. On the other hand, policy interventions and changes in food and nutrient supply have great potential to enhance the effect of individual focused interventions.

- Dietary change research should aim toward specifying the minimum necessary level of intervention to achieve a meaningful impact on dietary behavior
- There is need for continued advances in the areas of design, measurement, and analysis in dietary change research
- Innovative communication technologies should be adopted and tested for their impact on cancer preventive dietary change
- Health care providers should counsel patients regarding dietary change to reduce the risk of cancer

---

Tips for eating a healthy diet
- Make fruits and vegetables part of every meal. Put fruit on your cereal. Eat vegetables as a snack.
- Choose chicken, fish, or beans instead of red meat. The less red meat the better.
- Choose foods like pasta, brown rice, and whole wheat bread.

4.　　SEDENTARY LIFESTYLE

Higher levels of physical activity can reduce the incidence of colon cancer and may help reduce the risk of breast and prostate cancers. Intervention approaches within worksites, schools, and by health care providers, have shown modest effects in increasing the physical activity level of participants, but many sites lack such programs. Public and environmental polices can powerfully encourage physical activity. Examples include the construction of sidewalks, bikeways and safe recreational spaces. Interventions can profitably aim to increase the entire distribution of physical activity in the populations, including reducing sedentary time as well as increasing moderate and vigorous physical activity.

Tips for maintaining a healthy weight
- Be physically active
- Balance the amount of food you eat with the amount of energy you use

---

- Consistent messages to increase levels of moderate and vigorous physical activity need to be embedded within multiple institutional settings: worksites, schools, health care providers, mass media and public spaces
- Opportunities to be more active exist throughout our daily environments. Individuals and organizations need encouragement to creatively identify new opportunities for increasing physical activity levels.
- Interventions need to address differences in perceptions, needs and impact within in population subgroups including those defined by age, gender, socioeconomic status, race and ethnicity, and those with physical disabilities.

Tips for exercise
- Get at least 30 minutes of physical activity every day
- A lot of things count as physical activity, maybe even your job if you are active at work. Try walking, jogging, or dancing – whatever you enjoy!
- Any amount of physical activity is better than none. In general, the more you do the better.

5.　　ALCOHOL

Use of alcohol interacts with tobacco smoking in the causation of cancers of the upper respiratory and gastrointestinal tracts. Moreover, alcohol also causes cancer of the breast and large intestine. Because epidemiologic findings are complicated, advice to minimize risk is complex. The US dietary guidelines recommend no more than one drink per day for women and no more than two drinks per day for men [5]. In addition to causing cancer, youth drinking is responsible for a large burden of premature mortality through motor vehicle accidents and violence.

School based prevention education needs to be reinforced through a community-based coalition that seeks restrictions on irresponsible alcohol advertising and marketing, strict enforcement of laws to reduce youth access, and new polices to reduce alcohol availability, including higher excise taxes. In addition to providing prevention messages, mass media campaigns can be used to enhance school based and community programs, encouraging public debate on policy initiatives to reduce alcohol consumption, and publicize new laws and regulations or increased enforcement efforts. Community wide responsible beverage service programs, for example, can be effective in preventing alcohol service to minors, decreasing the number of patrons who become intoxicated, and preventing those who are impaired from driving.

- Alcohol control programs should go beyond awareness and education to bring about basic change at the institutional, community and public policy level to create an environment that discourages youth drinking and excessive alcohol consumption
- Public health advocates should work for a wide range of policy initiatives that reduce the availability of alcohol, strongly enforce minimum age laws, eliminate irresponsible advertising and marketing practices, and require responsible beverage service programs
- Public health advocates should look to increased alcohol excise taxes to find comprehensive community-based campaigns for effective alcohol control

---

Tips for drinking less alcohol
- Choose non-alcoholic beverages, like juices and sodas, at meals and parties.
- Avoid occasions centered around alcohol
- Talk to a health care professional if you feel you have trouble limiting alcohol consumption.

6. VIRUSES AND INFECTIOUS AGENTS

Overlooked as a cause of cancer until the recent past, infectious agents are now considered as the cause of approximately five percent of cancers in the United States [5]. Among the more significant agents are human papilloma viruses (HPV), which cause cancer of the uterine cervix, and hepatitis B virus (HBV) which causes in liver cancer. Sexually transmitted viruses are a major preventable cause of cancer. Primary prevention can be achieved through delaying onset of sexual activity, abstaining from sex with individuals not known to be infection free, regularly using latex condoms, and being vaccinated against hepatitis B. Secondary prevention is possible through screening, early detection and treatment of cervical cancer.

- Health care providers should proactively inquire about risky sexual behaviors and provide client-centered counseling to reinforce safer sexual practices
- Community leaders should be recruited to help change sexual norms and promote healthier sexuality
- Policy makers must provide leadership and resources to make healthy sexual behaviors a standard part of cancer prevention strategies.

Tips for protecting yourself from sexually transmitted infections
- Consider not having sex. Abstinence is the best way to protect yourself.
- If you're sexually active, always use a condom and follow other safe sex practices.
- Never rely on your partner to have a condom. Be prepared.

---

7. OCCUPATIONAL FACTORS

The control of occupational exposure to carcinogens in the US represents an important triumph in the primary prevention of cancer. Collectively, occupational factors are thought to cause about five percent of cancer deaths, mostly of the lung, bladder, and bone marrow [6]. Application of a systematic hierarchy of controls is effective in reducing this risk of occupational exposure to carcinogens. Manufacturers, employers, workers, unions, health care providers, and occupational health professionals all play important roles in workplace cancer prevention. Regulatory standard setting and enforcement are an essential complement to voluntary efforts.

- Approaches that emphasize controlling workplace carcinogen exposures to the extent feasible should be broadly applied in individual, community, and regulatory interventions
- Expanded efforts in pre-market testing, occupational exposures and disease surveillance, and epidemiology are needed to characterize and control recognized carcinogens as well as to identify and prevent exposure to new ones
- Renewed political and budgetary support for ASHA and NIOSH are needed to protect workers from preventable work-related cancers.

8.   SOCIOECONOMIC STATUS

Cancers of the lung, stomach, uterine cervix, and possibly other sites are particularly common among poor and underprivileged population groups. Poverty may be though of as an important underlying cause for these cancers since it is associated with increased exposure to tobacco smoke, alcoholism, poor nutrition, and certain infectious agents. The primary prevention of cancer among the poor ultimately depends on altering the social environment that systematically stratifies cancer risk according to socioeconomic position.

- Reducing the increasing socioeconomic disparity in smoking prevalence will require stronger efforts aimed at influencing government action such as raising taxes and banning cigarette advertising
- Strategies to eliminate socioeconomic differentials in cancer must involve intersectoral collaboration -- government, business, and communities -- to modify the structural cancer risks encountered by disadvantaged populations.

9.   SUN EXPOSURE

Melanoma rates have risen rapidly in the US over the past 40 years. Childhood and adolescent sun exposure is the major cause of melanoma. Campaigns such as those implemented in Australia to reduce exposure to the sun between 11 AM and 3 PM to increase the use of broad brimmed hats, and to use sunscreen with SPF 15 or higher, have also emphasized community level support for apparently individual behavior changes. Town regulations have been modified to increase access to shade at town swimming pools, public awareness of sun exposure has been increased through collaboration with the weather service, and now architects compete annually for design awards that reward the use of sun protection in building design. A multi-pronged approach has dramatically shifted social norms, reduced high-risk behaviors, and the number of sunburns reported among children and adolescents has decreased.

Tips for protecting yourself from the sun
- Stay out of direct sunlight 10 AM to 4 PM
- Use hats, long-sleeve shirts, and SPF 15 sunscreens or higher.
- Avoid getting sunburned.
- Do not use sun lamps or tanning booths.

---

10.   SCREENING TESTS

While the focus of this book has been on prevention of the onset of cancer, it is important to remember that some cancers can be diagnosed at an early stage, when they are still highly responsive to treatment. Thus appropriate testing on a regular basis can save lives. In addition. Screening tests for cervical cancer and for colon cancer can detect preclinical or precursor lesions, lesions that if left without treatment might go on to become cancerous. For these cancers a test and subsequent treatment can prevent the cancer from developing in the first place.

Talk to your health care professional about tests for
- Colon and rectal cancer
- Breast cancer
- Cervical cancer

CONCLUSION

Although we cannot pretend that preventing cancer deaths in the United States will be easy, the broad individual and social changes that must occur are outlined in this report. Change is possible. Rates of smoking have halved among men since the first report of the Surgeon General on smoking in 1966. Rates in women have declined since peaking in 1960. Dietary change has also been substantial. Our challenge is to harness the knowledge that we have about cancer risk and use this to our collective advantage. We know that cancer risk is malleable. Rates of cancer have changed over time and within populations upon migration and change in lifestyle. Implementing the strategies outlined in this report we believe we can reduce the burden of cancer in the United States by as much as one-third. We have substantial knowledge about causes of human cancer. This report summarizes a broad range of social strategies to implement cancer prevention. We require the political will to make resources available to implement these strategies. Currently only 5 percent of the national health expenditure, which exceeds one trillion dollars annually, are allocated to disease prevention.

Our ability to prioritize strategies for cancer prevention would be enhanced by rigorous cost-effectiveness evaluations of both primary and secondary prevention. To date, insufficient resources have been allocated to this avenue of inquiry. Hence, we are left to informally weight the likely benefits of prevention efforts, the time frame from intervention to observed benefit, and the magnitude of the lifestyle or regulatory change that can be achieved. Because cigarette smoking remains the leading cause of cancer, efforts addressing the prevention of adolescent smoking and cessation from smoking among adults must be our highest priority in cancer prevention. Adding greater public awareness of other strategies for cancer prevention as outlined in this book should add hope, and speed widespread modification to lifestyles that will result in lower cancer risk and overall healthier lifestyles. Change in diet, increase in physical activity, reduction in alcohol intake, and improved contraceptive practices can each be implemented now. The benefits will be maximized when strategies are implemented concurrently through health care providers, through regulatory changes, and through individual on community level changes. The tips for behavior change set forth in this section are one aid to individual behavior change. Additional tips for prevention are presented in the Harvard Center for Cancer Prevention web site: www.hsph.harvard.edu/cancer.

REFERENCES

1. Richmond J, Kotelchuck M (1991) Coordination and development of strategies and policy for public health promotion in the United States. In: Holland W, Detel R, Know G, eds. *Oxford Textbook of Public Health*. Oxford: Oxford University Press.
2. U. S. Department of Health and Human Services, Centers for Disease Control and Prevention, National Center for Chronic Disease Prevention and Health Promotion, The President's Council on Physical Fitness and Sports (1996) *Physical Activity and Health: A Report of the Surgeon General*. Washington, DC: Office of the Surgeon General.
3. Colditz GA, Cannuscio CC, Frazier AL (1997) Physical activity and colon cancer prevention. *Cancer Causes Control* **8**: 649-667.
4. U.S. Department of Health and Human Services (1994) Preventing Tobacco Use among Young People: A Report of the Surgeon General. Atlanta, GA: U.S. Department of Health and Human Services, Centers for Disease Control and Prevention, National Center for Chronic Disease Prevention and Health Promotion, Office on Smoking and Health.

5. U. S. Department of Agriculture, U. S. Department of Health and Human Services (1995) *Nutrition and Your Health: Dietary Guidelines for Americans.* Washington, DC: U.S. Government Printing Office; Report No.: Home and Garden Bulletin No. 232.

6. Colditz GA, DeJong D, Hunter DJ, *et al.* (1996) Harvard Report on Cancer Prevention. Volume 1. Causes of Human Cancer. *Cancer Causes Control* 7(Suppl 1): 1-59.

Index